DYNAMICS OF SPEECH PRODUCTION AND PERCEPTION

NATO Science Series

A series presenting the results of scientific meetings supported under the NATO Science Programme.

The series is published by IOS Press and Springer Science and Business Media in conjunction with the NATO Public Diplomacy Division.

Sub-Series

I. Life and Behavioural Sciences	IOS Press
II. Mathematics, Physics and Chemistry	Springer Science and Business Media
III. Computer and Systems Sciences	IOS Press
IV. Earth and Environmental Sciences	Springer Science and Business Media
V. Science and Technology Policy	IOS Press

The NATO Science Series continues the series of books published formerly as the NATO ASI Series.

The NATO Science Programme offers support for collaboration in civil science between scientists of countries of the Euro-Atlantic Partnership Council. The types of scientific meeting generally supported are "Advanced Study Institutes" and "Advanced Research Workshops", although other types of meeting are supported from time to time. The NATO Science Series collects together the results of these meetings. The meetings are co-organized by scientists from NATO countries and scientists from NATO's Partner countries – countries of the CIS and Central and Eastern Europe.

Advanced Study Institutes are high-level tutorial courses offering in-depth study of latest advances in a field.
Advanced Research Workshops are expert meetings aimed at critical assessment of a field, and identification of directions for future action.

As a consequence of the restructuring of the NATO Science Programme in 1999, the NATO Science Series has been re-organized and there are currently five sub-series as noted above. Please consult the following web sites for information on previous volumes published in the series, as well as details of earlier sub-series:

http://www.nato.int/science
http://www.springeronline.nl
http://www.iospress.nl
http://www.wtv-books.de/nato_pco.htm

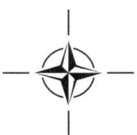

Dynamics of Speech Production and Perception

Edited by

Pierre Divenyi
Veterans Affairs Medical Center and East Bay Institute for Research and Education, Martinez, California, USA

Steven Greenberg
Silicon Speech, Santa Venetia, California, USA

and

Georg Meyer
Liverpool University, UK

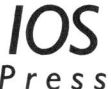

Press

Amsterdam • Berlin • Oxford • Tokyo • Washington, DC

Published in cooperation with NATO Public Diplomacy Division

Proceedings of the NATO Advanced Study Institute on
Dynamics of Speech Production and Perception
Il Ciocco (Lucca), Italy
23 June – 6 July 2006

ISBN 1-58603-666-1
Library of Congress Control Number: 2006932184

Publisher
IOS Press
Nieuwe Hemweg 6B
1013 BG Amsterdam
Netherlands
fax: +31 20 687 0019
e-mail: order@iospress.nl

Distributor in the UK and Ireland
Gazelle Books Services Ltd.
White Cross Mills
Hightown
Lancaster LA1 4XS
United Kingdom
fax: +44 1524 63232
e-mail: sales@gazellebooks.co.uk

Distributor in the USA and Canada
IOS Press, Inc.
4502 Rachael Manor Drive
Fairfax, VA 22032
USA
fax: +1 703 323 3668
e-mail: iosbooks@iospress.com

To Ludmilla's memory

In Memoriam
Ludmilla Andreevna Chistovich
1924 - 2006

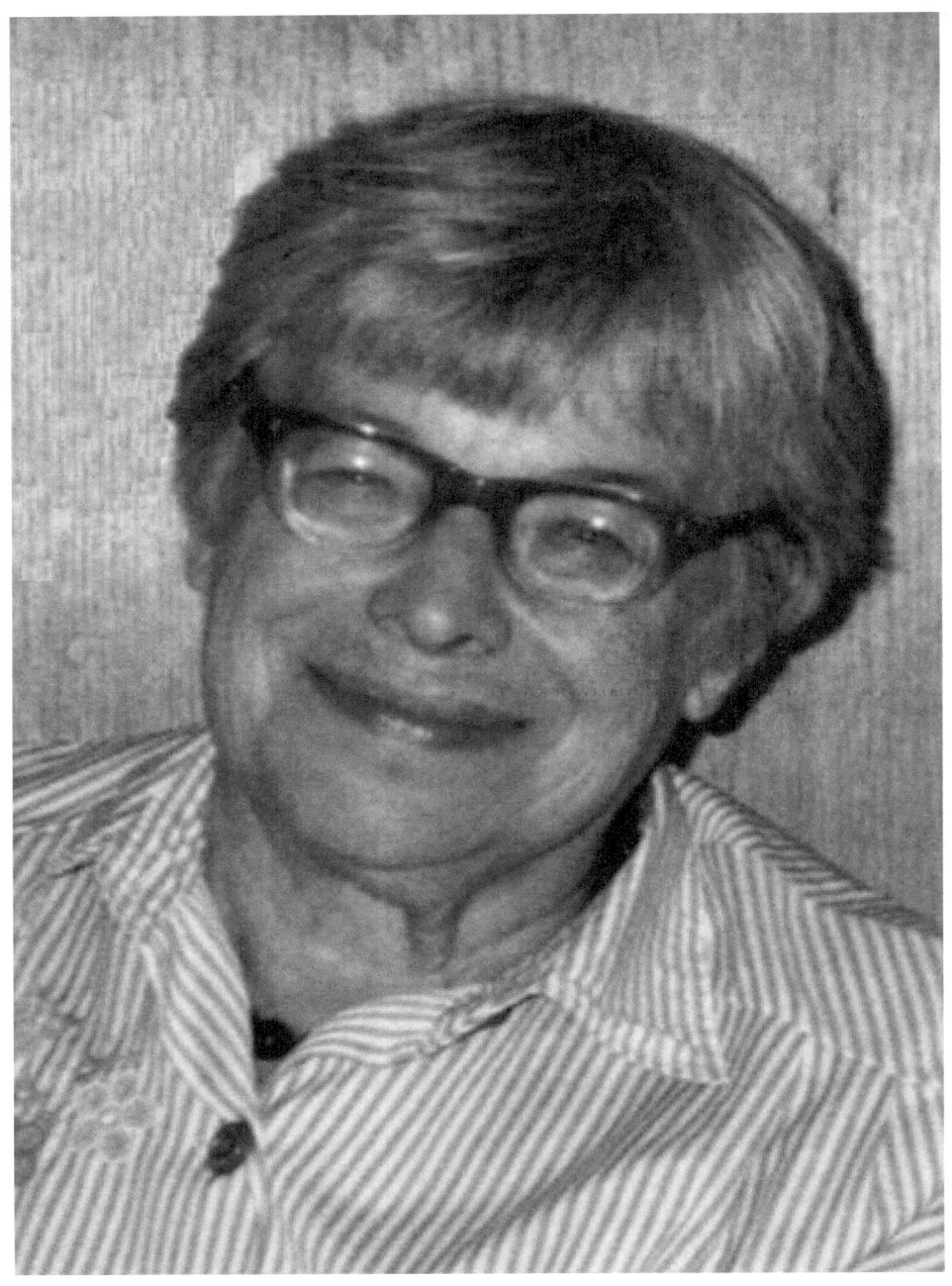

This book is dedicated to the memory of Ludmilla A. Chistovich. Her pioneering research blazed an important path for the scientific investigation of speech that many others have followed in recent years. As the founder of the "Leningrad School" (along with her husband, Valeriy A. Kozhevnikov) she headed one of the most dynamic and creative groups investigating the production and perception of speech. The influence of Chistovich and her colleagues has been profound, as many of the chapters in this volume attest. Her work was among the first to integrate nonlinear dynamics into models of speech production and perception. She was also among the first to appreciate the importance of auditory nonlinearities for the neural representation of speech.

Ludmilla Chistovich was born in Leningrad in 1924. She trained as a medical doctor prior to her research career at the Pavlov Institute of Physiology in Leningrad. In 1960, she founded the Laboratory of Speech Physiology at the Pavlov Institute. At the same time, Valeriy Kozhevnikov established the Laboratory of Speech Biophysics. The two worked in close collaboration until Kozhevnikov's untimely death 20 years later.

The group's early research was summarized in a monograph entitled *Speech: Articulation and Perception*, a translation from the Russian of *Rech: Artikulyatsiya i Vospriyatiye* (Moscow-Leningrad, 1965). This book introduced what were radical concepts for the time: nonlinear dynamics, the syllable as a basic unit of production and perception, and the importance of studying production and perception as reflections of a single, integral process. In 1976, a second monograph was published: *Speech Physiology and Speech Perception by Man* (in Russian). This book was one of the first attempts to apply a comprehensive approach to speech research, integrating phonetics, psychoacoustics, physiology signal processing and modeling. Although this interdisciplinary approach is common today, it represented a radical departure from the way in which speech was studied in the 1970s.

Given all that she and her group accomplished, Ludmilla Chistovich was entitled to retire to a life of ease and relaxation. Instead, after her official retirement in 1986, she began a second career, this one focused on developing social charities and public interest organizations. It was the era of "perestroika," and many things were changing in the Soviet Union. Chistovich was among the founders of the Mercy Society, the first charitable organization established in the former USSR. She also founded the Leningrad Consumers Society, where she oversaw the department concerned with the rights of ill and disabled individuals. As part of her efforts, she organized an important conference on the topic of the sick and disabled, which was the beginning of Leningrad's publicly funded programs for the elderly and young.

In 1991, Chistovich, together with her daughters Elena Kozhevnikova and Inna Chistovich, established the St. Petersburg Early Intervention Institute (EII, http://www.eii.ru). The EII was set up as a means of fostering the language development of young children through providing auditory screening in infants and early intervention programs for hearing-impaired children. During the last years of her life, Ludmilla Chistovich worked with EII to establish early intervention programs in other locations, first in St. Petersburg and eventually throughout Russia and other parts of the former Soviet Union. She passed away on April 11, 2006, shortly before this book went to press.

Additional information about Ludmilla Chistovich's scientific accomplishments can be found in *Speech Communication*, Volume 4 (1985) as well as http://www.mindspring.com/~rjporter/SeattlePavlovRev.htm.

Dynamics of Speech Production and Perception
P. Divenyi et al. (Eds.)
IOS Press, 2006

Preface

"Natural speech is not a simple sequence of steady-state segments. To represent the speech signal, as perceived by the listener, as if it were a succession of discrete segments
(analogous to alphabetic characters) or even as a sequence of
phonetically meaningful elements is simplistic at best. It is
only possible to portray speech as a succession of elements
when the ensemble of complex information transformations
that comprise speech perception are fully taken into account."

Ludmilla Chistovich [1, p.10]

That speech is a dynamic process strikes as a tautology: whether from the standpoint of
the talker, the listener, or the engineer, speech is an action, a sound, or a signal continuously changing in time. Yet, because phonetics and speech science are offspring of classical phonology, speech has been viewed as a sequence of discrete events-positions of
the articulatory apparatus, waveform segments, and phonemes. Although this perspective has been mockingly referred to as "beads on a string" [3], from the time of Henry
Sweet's 19th century treatise [5] almost up to our days specialists of speech science and
speech technology have continued to conceptualize the speech signal as a sequence of
static states interleaved with transitional elements reflecting the quasi-continuous nature
of vocal production. After all, there must be static, stable elements internally if listeners
can perceive and label individual phonemes in the speech stream. While this discrete
representation-static targets reached during production and recovered during percep-
tion-may describe, at best, clearly pronounced "hyper" speech in which departures from
the canonical are rare, it badly fails to characterize spoken language where such departures constitute the norm. A good example for the inadequacy of phonemic representation is a recent analysis of 45 minutes of spontaneous conversational speech in which 73
different forms of the word "and" were seen, and yet all of them were unambiguously
identified by listeners [2]. Obviously, we need to part with the phoneme as the basic unit
of speech if we want to study verbal communication.

Fortunately, an alternative approach was developed in the latter half of the twentieth
century by a team of scientists at the Pavlov Institute of Physiology in St. Petersburg,
the then-Leningrad. Headed by Ludmilla Chistovich and her husband Valeriy
Kozhevnikov, two great pioneers of speech research, this remarkable team recognized
that even in clear speech the phoneme could not be considered without the context in
which it appeared. In their view, the phoneme was an epiphenomenon, derived from the
more basic unit of the syllable [1]. In this, as in so many aspects of speech models, the
so-called "Leningrad group" was far ahead of its time. In the groundbreaking volume
"Speech: Articulation and Perception," [4] this group introduced the concept of dynamic
systems to speech research-as early as in the mid-1960s. For decades, their research was
considered more of an exotic curiosity than serious work because of its unusual and dis-

x

tinctive nature. Most speech scientists outside of the Soviet bloc did not know what to make of physical concepts such as dynamics because they lay outside the traditional realm of research. But Chistovich and Kozhevnikov understood that dynamics and the phoneme did not mesh. Looking back from the year 2006, it's easy to forget how radical the Leningrad group's perspective was at the time of its inception in the 1960s. Nowadays, dynamics-linear and nonlinear-is all the rage in many scientific fields, and the syllable is no longer controversial.

This book, a collection of papers each of which looks at speech as a dynamic process and highlights one of its particularities, is dedicated to the memory of Ludmilla Andreevna Chistovich. At the outset, it was planned to be a Chistovich festschrift but, sadly, she passed away a few months before the book went to press. The 24 chapters of this volume testify to the enormous influence that she and her colleagues have had over the four decades since the publication of their 1965 monograph. The book is divided into five sections, each examining the dynamics of speech from one particular perspective.

The first section treats the dynamics of speech production. Lindblom *et al.* look at the role of gestures in speech and sign language; Saltzman et al. show the multiple components of articulatory movements; Tremblay and Ostry show how speech targets are mediated by somatosensory targets; Slifka talks about the role of breath; Carré demonstrates the power of a simple dynamic production model; Pols and van Son trace the dynamic signal from its acoustic signature to its perception.

The second section's topic is the dynamics of speech perception. In it, Lublinskaja *et al.* show the capacity of amplitude modulation to generate speech from simple nonspeech signals; Feth *et al.* present experimental proof of the power of the Leningrad school's frequency center-of-gravity principle; Meyer *et al.* demonstrate the coexistence of different auditory and speech perception mechanisms; Divenyi addresses the question of segregation of speech-like streams consisting of different amplitude- and frequency-modulation patterns; Stern *et al.* show the importance of frequency transitions in spatial localization of speech; Turner *et al.* present a model that accounts for vowel normalization and perception of the physical size of the talker; Greenberg *et al.* demonstrate how temporal dynamics, in particular the amplitude modulation spectrum, is responsible for robust speech intelligibility.

The third section is focused on the role of speech dynamics in speech processing and other applications. Lee focuses on a human model-oriented approach to automatic speech recognition (ASR); Atlas introduces the reader to his method of obtaining amplitude modulation spectra and discusses its utility in speech technology; Hermansky discusses novel methods for the extraction of dynamic temporal patterns in speech; Mihajlik et al. present a rule-based automatic phonetic transcription system and discuss its application in ASR; Sorokin shows solutions to the seemingly intractable problem of mapping the acoustic wave of speech back to articulatory gestures; Vicsi presents a computer-assisted language learning system explicitly based on dynamic changes in the speech waveform.

The fourth section treats the dynamics of the singing voice. Riquimaroux shows how the amplitude envelope of lyrics alone is able to convey melody in noise-vocoded Japanese songs; Ross and Lehiste discuss how the conflict between duration-based prosodic stress and musical rhythm is solved in Estonian folk songs.

The final section focuses on how speech dynamics is looked at by the central nervous system. Shamma argues that spectrotemporal receptive fields obtained in the primary auditory cortex in response to simultaneously amplitude- and frequency-modulated complex sounds can explain the robustness of speech intelligibility; Nelken and Ahissar discuss how the auditory cortex uses auditory information processed at lower levels for higher-level processing necessary to decode the speech signal; Gaschler-Markefsky *et al.* present functional magnetic resonance imaging (fMRI) results that show functional differentiation of activity over cortical areas evoked by simple and complex sounds and requiring simple or complex responses, and discuss the interaction of these processes during listening to speech.

Our book is based on a NATO Advanced Study Institute, held at Il Ciocco, in the mountains of Tuscany, between June 24 and July 6, 2002. Over 100 established and young scientists, representing 30 countries in Europe, North America, Asia and Australia, participated in this meeting (for further details, see http://www.ebire.org/speechand-hearing/asi2002.html). The ASI's intent was to provide a rigorous, multidisciplinary scientific overview of speech regarded as a dynamic process. Diverse aspects of speech dynamics were presented in lectures interspersed with sessions devoted to discussion. In addition, over 50 young scientists presented posters of their work related to the general topic. Although Ludmilla Chistovich was invited to join the faculty of the ASI, she was unable to accept due to ill health. Fortunately, both her daughter Elena Kozhevnikova and her long-time colleague Valentina Lublinskaja came to the ASI and gave interesting presentations on the history of the Leningrad school. Frequent references during the ASI to work by Chistovich and her colleagues revealed the significant influence the Leningrad school had on the lecturers and other participants.

We would like to express our appreciation and gratitude to the ASI Faculty (René Carré, András Illényi, Hynek Hermansky, Björn Lindblom, Valentina Lublinskaja, Georg Meyer, Israel Nelken, Roy Patterson, Louis Pols, Jaan Ross, Elliot Saltzman, Shihab Shamma, Victor Sorokin, and Klára Vicsi) for their excellent lectures and the intriguing ideas they expressed during the discussions. We also want to thank all other participants and attendees who contributed to the ASI's success, in particular the over 50 ASI students and postdoctoral participants who presented their work in the poster sessions.

We would also like to express our appreciation to the North Atlantic Treaty Organization Science Programme, Life Science and Technology Division, which provided the lion's share of funding required to support the meeting through its Office of Scientific and Environmental Affairs. In particular, we thank the help offered by Dr. Walter Kaffenberger, Director of the Division, and his secretary Ms. Janet Lace throughout the process of organizing the ASI. We also want to thank the U.S. Office of Naval Research International Field Office and U.S. Air Force Office of Scientific Research for the additional funding they provided. For this, we want to personally thank Michael Pestorius and Keith Bromley from ONRIFO and Willard Larkin from the AFOSR Directorate of Chemistry and Life Sciences. We wish to express our appreciation to the U.S. National Science Foundation, the International Speech Communication Association, and the scientific student exchange programs between NATO and the governments of Greece, Portugal, and Turkey for offering support for the travel of student and postdoctoral participants to the meeting. In particular, we want to thank Sheryl Balke from the NSF's Directorate for Education and Human Resources for her help. We also want to thank the

Oticon Foundation and Phonak AG for their generous support of the ASI, and wish to express our gratitude to Claus Elberling, Oticon Foundation, and Stefan Launer, Phonak AG.

We are grateful to Bruno Gianassi and his staff at Il Ciocco, who continuously went beyond the call of duty to ensure that everything ran smoothly during the course of the meeting. We also want to express our gratitude to Brian Gygi and Ariani Richards for their intelligent and devoted work leading up to and during the ASI, to Joanne Hanrahan for the initial layout of the book chapters, as well as to Theresa Azevedo and Jill Anderson at the East Bay Institute for Research and Education for their support and their efficient handling of financial matters.

Finally, we would like to express our deepest appreciation to the authors for taking the time to prepare their chapters for this volume, as well to thank them for their patience and understanding during the lengthy preparation of the book.

Pierre Divenyi and Steven Greenberg
June, 2006

References

[1] Chistovich, L.A. and V.A. Kozhevnikov. *Theory and methods on the perception of speech signals [Voprosy teorii i metodov issledenovaniya vospriyatiya rechevykh signalov]*, Washington, D.C.: National Technical Information Service, U.S. Department of Commerce, 1970.

[2] Greenberg, S., H.M. Carvey, L. Hitchcock, and S. Chang. "Beyond the phoneme A juncture-accent model for spoken language", in *Proceedings of the Second International Conference on Human Language Technology Research*, 36-43, 2002.

[3] Hockett, C. "The origin of speech", in Scientific American, (pp. 89-96), 1960.

[4] Kozhevnikov, V.A. and L.A. Chistovich. Speech, articulation, and perception. NTIS, US Dept. of Commerce JPRS-30543, 1965.

[5] Sweet, H. *A Handbook of Phonetics.* (Reprint of the 1877 original edition), College Park, MD: McGrath, 1970.

Contents

Speech Processing and the Auditory Cortex

Production Dynamics of Speech

Dynamics of Speech Production and Perception
P. Divenyi et al. (Eds.)
IOS Press, 2006

Production Dynamics of Speech

Steven Greenberg
Silicon Speech
Santa Venetia, California, USA

Ludmilla Chistovich and Valery Kozhevnikov were perhaps the first to model the production and perception of speech as inherently nonlinear dynamic systems. As early as 1965, they characterized the speech signal as reflecting dynamic processes [2]. At that time, most speech scientists still portrayed the speech signal as a sequence of static states interleaved with transitional elements reflecting the quasi-continuous nature of vocal production. After all, there *must* be static, stable elements internally if listeners can perceive and label individual phonemes in the speech stream. Chistovich and Kozhevnikov understood that nonlinear dynamics and the phoneme did not mesh. In their view, the phoneme was an epiphenomenon, derived from the more basic unit of the syllable. In this, as in so many aspects of speech modeling, their "Leningrad School" was far ahead of its time (see this volume's Preface and Dedication to Ludmilla Chistovich for more detail). From the perspective of 2006, it's easy to forget how radical was their perspective at the time of its inception in the 1960s. Nowadays, nonlinear dynamics is all the rage in many scientific fields, and the syllable is no longer controversial. The chapters in this section testify to the enormous influence that Ludmilla Chistovich and her colleagues have had over the intervening decades.

In the first chapter, Lindblom and colleagues examine the concept of "target" in both speech and American Sign Language (ASL). The concept of "undershoot" in speech has been well known since the pioneering studies of Lindblom [5] and Öhman [7]. For many years, it was unclear whether this failure to reach specific acoustic (and articulatory) targets (associated with individual segments) was fundamental to perception and production. Beginning in the 1980s, many researchers in the West began to adopt the Leningrad perspective that most of the speech signal's information lay in the dynamics. Undershoot came to be understood as an intrinsic component of speech, not an ideal curiosity. In an elegant series of experiments, Lindblom and colleagues discuss some striking parallels between gestures in ASL and speech production. In their view, the essence of the message contained in each lies in the patterns of movement, rather than in the specific targets to which the motions point. Consonants and vowels cannot be readily distinguished in terms of their articulatory motion; they appear to influence each other. This is very much in the spirit of the Leningrad School and lends implicit support for the syllable.

Consistent with this dynamic perspective is the work described by Saltzman and colleagues in Chapter 2. Their work focuses on the principles governing the movement of the speech articulators – and other parts of the body. In their view, there is nothing special about the motion of the lips, tongue and jaw during speech production to distinguish them from the movement of the arms, legs and other parts of the body. This is, indeed, an interesting perspective, for it provides some potential insight as to how language may have evolved from non-linguistic, motor activity. It can also account for why the dynamics of spoken language are so similar to those of signed gestures (as described by Lindblom and colleagues in Chapter 1). The essential problem that Saltzman and colleagues address is how does the tongue and other articulators "know" where to go, and how fast to move in the course of producing speech? This is a non-trivial issue, one that has bedeviled scientists over the years (in many areas of motor behavior, not just in speech). In the authors' view, the underlying representation for speech is in the form of task dynamics, which are highly skilled movements learned over many years. There is no detailed coordinate system guiding the movement of the articulators. This view is consistent with what is known about cortical control of movement in general. The cortex sends very general commands to the spinal column in the form of general goals, not detailed actions. The latter are worked out in the spinal column and cerebellum, which translate the task goals into specific patterns sensitive to context (e.g., [1][9]).

Tremblay and Ostry discuss the all-important issue of context in their chapter. They focus on what happens when speech production is perturbed in controlled ways. A mechanical robot applies a certain amount of force to a talker's jaw that constrains articulation in measurable ways. One can then quantify the effect of this externally applied force on jaw movement to ascertain the extent to which talkers compensate for this perturbation and how quickly. Adaptation of the jaw depends on a variety of factors, including the nature of the vowel and whether it occurs at the beginning or end of a word. Talkers also vary in how they adapt to the perturbations. Tremblay and Ostry conclude "…the pattern of adaptation observed …is not due to mechanical aspects of the experiment." Rather, the results are consistent with "a somatosensory goal, independent of the acoustics, [which] is pursued in speech production." In other words, their results are consistent with the task-dynamic perspective of Saltzman and colleagues; the patterns of motor movement in speech production are difficult to reconcile with specific target or coordinate systems.

Respiration is the Rodney Dangerfield of speech production – it rarely receives the respect it deserves. Janet Slifka, in her chapter, examines lung pressure during the course of spoken material. Many decades ago, Stetson described the importance of breath groups in speech [8], work that was followed by a number of investigations in the 1950s (e.g.,[3]) and 1960s (e.g.,[4]) but which has received relatively little attention in recent years. Slifka raises the intriguing possibility that respiratory activity could reflect the prosodic organization of utterances, and therefore could be used to infer how a talker transforms an abstract, linguistic representation into concrete form.

The final chapters in this section examine the relationship between production and perception of speech – very much in the framework that Chistovich and her colleagues developed in the 1960s. Rene Carré, the author of the chapter on speech gestures, collaborated with the Leningrad group in the 1970s. In his view, the internal organization of perception and production must be closely related. Rather than focus on superficial properties of the signal, such as formant patterns *per se*, Carré seeks an underlying representation common to both production and perception, one that is relatively simple and of low-dimensional order. Like Chistovich, Carré believes that the syllable is the most basic unit of representation in speech. He focuses on vowel and glide transitions as emblematic of dynamic gestures in general. His "Distinctive Region Model" (DRM) divides the vocal tract into eight compartments. From this simple vocal tract model he is able to deduce many properties of production and perception through elegant synthesis and listening experiments. The percept of a vowel-consonant-vowel sequence can change dramatically through relatively subtle alteration of certain temporal properties. In his view "…the direction of gestures … is more important than the static targets to be reached." In other words, the perception and production of speech is dynamic, not static – consistent with other chapters in this section as well as with the general approach of the Leningrad School.

The authors of the final chapter, Louis Pols and Robert van Son, examine the issue of speech dynamics from the perspective of acoustic primitives (e.g., frequency sweeps) and information theory. They are also concerned with the "efficiency" of communication in terms of how the production (as reflected in the acoustics) adjusts to specific environmental conditions and communicative tasks. Pols and van Son observe that "…any vowel reduction seems to be mirrored by a comparable change in the consonant, thus suggesting that vowel onsets and targets change in concert." This is another way of stating that speech is organized in units larger than the segment, and is consistent with Chistovich's championing of the syllable. One of the most interesting aspects of their data concerns the importance of context on identification of vowels and consonants. Vowels are generally more accurately identified in full syllabic form. Prosodic factors are also important. In other words, segmental processing is facilitated by syllabic context. The linguistic nature of the material is also important. At any given signal-to-noise ratio, highly redundant material (such as spoken digits or predictable sentences) is more accurately identified than relatively unpredictable words or syllables. This observation (which dates to the 1940s, see [6]) can be interpreted in a variety of ways. One interpretation is that speech is not decoded phoneme by phoneme. If it were, there would be relatively little difference in intelligibility of nonsense syllables, infrequent words and common words (both in isolation and in sentence context). These data suggest that the process of speech decoding must operate at a much higher level, perhaps at the phrasal or sentential (or even higher) level, and is consistent with the work of Chistovich and her colleagues.

Although the chapters in this section cover a broad range of topics, the underlying theme is remarkably consistent. The organization of speech production (and perception) must occur at a level considerably longer than the phonetic segment. Whether the relevant unit of organization is the gesture, the syllable, the prosodic phrase or some other quanta is not so important. What is crucial is that the brain operates in terms of dynamic, not static representations, and this is reflected in how speech is produced and (as will be discussed in the following section) how it is perceived.

Several chapters in the "Perceptual Dynamics" section discuss the concept of the "complex modulation spectrum." This is a quantitative method for measuring the frequency, magnitude and phase of dynamics in the acoustic speech signal (see Les Atlas' chapter in particular). Much of the mathematics describing articulatory dynamics can be rendered into an equivalent form, raising the prospect that a uniform representation underlies the production and perception of speech. Although the Leningrad School used different terminology to describe the intimate connection between production and perception, contemporary models are very much in the spirit of their pioneering work.

References

[1] Himmelbach, M. & Karnath, H.O. "Goal-directed hand movements are not affected by the biased space representation in spatial neglect." *J. Cogn. Neurosci.* 15: 972-980.

[2] Kozhevnikov, V.A. and Chistovich, L.A. *Speech: Articulation and Perception*. Washington, D.C.: U.S. Department of Commerce, 1965. (Translated from the Russian).

[3] Ladefoged, P. (1967) *Three Areas of Experimental Phonetics*. Oxford: Oxford University Press, 1967.

[4] Lieberman, P. *Intonation, Perception and Language*. Cambridge: MIT Press, 1967.

[5] Lindblom, B. "Spectrographic study of vowel reduction." *J. Acoust. Soc. Am.* 35:1773-1781, 1963.

[6] Miller, G.A. *Language and Communication*. New York: McGraw-Hill, 1951.

[7] Öhman, S. "Coarticulation in VCV utterances: Spectrographic measurements." *J. Acoust. Soc. Am.* 39: 151-168, 1966.

[8] Stetson, R.H. *Motor Phonetics*. Amsterdam: North-Holland, 1951.

[9] Winstein, C.J., Grafton, S.T. and Pohl, P.S. "Motor task difficulty and brain activity: Investigation of goal-directed reciprocal aiming using positron emission tomography." *J. Neurophysiol.* 77: 1581-1594, 1997.

Dynamics of Speech Production and Perception
P. Divenyi et al. (Eds.)
IOS Press, 2006

Dynamic Specification in the Production of Speech and Sign

Björn LINDBLOM[1], Claude MAUK[2] and Seung-Jae MOON[3]
[1]Stockholm University, Sweden
[2]University of Pittsburgh, Pittsburgh, Pennsylvania, USA
[3]AJOU University, Suwon, Korea

Abstract. Sensory systems prefer time-varying over static stimuli. An example of this fact is provided by the dynamic spectro-temporal changes of speech signals which are known to play a key role in speech perception. To some investigators such observations provide support for adopting the gesture as the basic entity of speech. An alleged advantage of such a dynamically defined unit - over the more traditional, static and abstract, phoneme or segment - is that it can readily be observed in phonetic records. However, as has been thoroughly documented throughout the last fifty years, articulatory and acoustic measurements are ubiquitously context-dependent. That makes the gesture, defined as an observable, problematic as a primitive of phonetic theory. The goal of the present paper is to propose a resolution of the static-dynamic paradox. An analysis of articulatory and sign movement dynamics is presented in terms of a traditional model based on timeless spatial specifications (targets, via points) plus smoothing (as determined by the dynamics of speech effectors). We justify this analysis as follows: A first motivation is empirical: As illustrated in this chapter both articulatory and sign data lend themselves readily to a target-based analysis. The second part of the argument appeals to the principle of parsimony which says: Do not unnecessarily invoke movement to explain movement. Until a deeper understanding is available of how the neuro-mechanical systems of speech contribute to its articulatory and acoustic dynamics, it would seem prudent to put dynamic (gestural) motor commands on hold. Thirdly, if the schema of static-targets plus dynamic-smoothing is an intuitive way of conceptually parsing movements, it is only natural that phoneticians should have given many speech sounds static labels in traditional descriptive frameworks. Static-target control in speech production should in no way be incompatible with dynamic input patterns for perception. Once that fact is acknowledged, there is no paradox.

Keywords. Speech dynamics, speech production, American Sign Language

Introduction

A paradox

Experimental findings show that perception is more sensitive to changing stimulus patterns than to purely static ones. In speech articulatory movement and spectral changes are pervasive whereas steady-state intervals are rare. In view of those observations, it may seem curious that the traditional frameworks for describing speech should tend to emphasize static attributes. For instance, the IPA framework specifies consonants and vowels using terms the majority of which refer to speech production steady-states, e.g., *labial, high, voiced, stop, nasal* etc.

If perception likes change, why is phonetic specification built mainly around steady-state attributes?

The dynamic specification approach

A development that responds to this paradox is the "dynamic specification" approach proposed by Winifred Strange. It is based on a series of experiments [24][25] demonstrating that listeners are able to identify vowels with high accuracy although the center portions of CVC stimuli have been removed leaving only the first three and the last four periods of the vowel segment. In other words, vowel perception is possible also in 'silent-center' syllables - that is, syllables that lack information on the alleged 'target' but include an initial stop plosion and surrounding formant transitions. Strange takes her findings to imply that vowel identification in CVC sequences is based on more than just the information contained within a single spectral slice sampled near the midpoint "target" region of the acoustic vowel segment. Rather the relevant information is distributed across the entire vowel and it includes formant frequency time variations. According to the "dynamic specification" approach,

> ... vowels are conceived of as characteristic gestures having intrinsic timing parameters (Fowler, 1980). These dynamic articulatory events give rise to an acoustic pattern in which the changing spectrotemporal configuration provides sufficient information for the unambiguous identification of the intended vowels. (from [24], p. 2135-36).

It should be noted that the term 'target' has been used with several different meanings. Strange's definition refers to an *observable*, the spectral cross-section sampled at a vowel's quasi-steady-state midpoint. An alternative meaning is target as a *virtual* (underlying, asymptote) phenomenon - a point in multi-dimensional articulatory control space that may, or may not, be realized articulatorily and acoustically. This sense of target is the one found in the literature on "undershoot" (more anon).

Phonetic gestures

The term gesture is widely used informally in phonetics but also in the more technical sense of the quote from Strange. The history of the term gesture (as a theoretical primitive) goes back to the days when researchers at Haskins Laboratories were attempting to build reading machines for the blind. Using an alphabet of static acoustic patterns did not work. As a result of this failure a notion began to take shape, *viz.* the idea of the ultimate building blocks of speech as dynamic units [26]. From there the phonetic gesture can be traced through the writings on the motor theory, direct realism and articulatory phonology. Its current status is reviewed by [26].

A gesture is a "unit of action", "a change in position by an articulator", a movement "selected for linguistic use" and "made with communicative intent". Studdert-Kennedy agrees with Strange on the perceptual importance of spectral time variations:

> Motorically, a gesture is the act of forming and releasing a constriction of variable degree and location, at some point in the vocal tract, thus effecting a dynamic sequence of vocal tract configurations. (The reason for including both formation and release of a constriction within a single gesture is the fact, established by many per-

ceptual studies, that acoustic information specifying any given gesture is distributed over the spectral structure both before and after the peak or center of the gesture itself). (from [28])

Chapter outline

The last two sections raise a question that sets the stage for the remainder of this chapter. If, as suggested above, the perceptually relevant information is temporally distributed across the entire vowel segment, how is the motor control of this behavior organized? To what extent is the specification of the input task itself dynamic? We will return to those issues in two steps. First we exemplify the target-based approach with data on hand movements in American Sign Language and tongue shape variations in VCV sequences. Second, we shall review some current work on the physiological modeling of non-speech movements.

1. Experimental Observations

1.1 Vowel dynamics: Effect of consonantal context

In a classic study of American English vowels [23] observed that the formant pattern of a given vowel tended to be systematically displaced in the direction of the frequency values of the consonant context. Those shifts were interpreted to indicate that articulatory movements tended to fall short of hypothetical vowel targets. Similar effects were reported for Swedish by [11]. The measurements were numerically summarized with the aid of a 'target undershoot' model which successfully predicted formant frequency displacement as exponential functions of vowel duration, vowel-invariant 'targets' and consonant context information (extent of CV formant transitions).

Subsequent research has confirmed the existence of formant undershoot but has sometimes also failed to demonstrate the duration-dependence postulated by the target undershoot model [4][27]. The key to resolving such discrepancies lies in recognizing the fact that vowel formant values depend not only on duration and consonant context but also on a previously neglected parameter: the rate of formant frequency change. The motivation for this addition comes from biomechanics [17] which suggests that, everything else being equal, a more forceful movement is associated with greater peak velocity (greater "articulatory effort"), in other words a more rapid approach to target, and should therefore give rise to less undershoot.

This interplay between duration, extent and velocity of movement is documented in the kinematic data in [9], [3] and [18]. The findings of [16] also lend credence to this three-way interaction. They found duration- and context-dependent formant undershoot in [w_l] sequences produced with identical main stress but with varying vowel durations elicited by means of the word-length effect (*e.g., will, willing, willingly*). The duration- and context-dependence was less severe in clear overarticulated speech than in normal casually spoken syllables (Figure 1). This finding was consistently linked with more rapid formant transitions as expected from the biomechanical perspective.

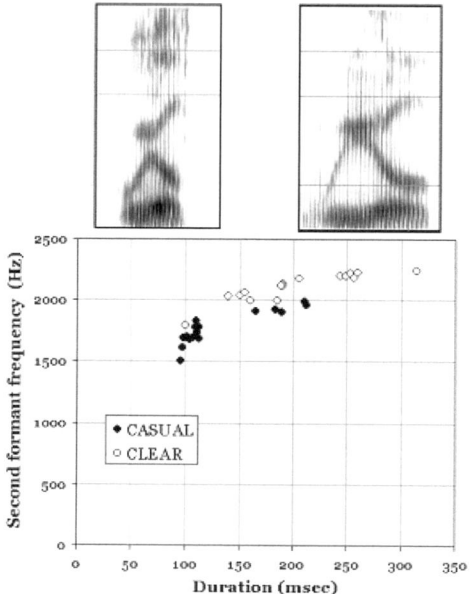

Figure 1. The phenomenon of 'undershoot'. *Upper panels*: Spectrograms of long and short variants of the word 'wheel'. *Lower diagram*: Second formant measured at vowel midpoint in [i] and plotted as a function of vowel duration for two speaking styles.

1.2 From vowels to ASL

Some recent experimental work on the movements of sign language [14] allows us to examine the undershoot phenomenon more closely in terms of its kinematics. The data include measurements of hand shape and hand location from two male and two female signers all born deaf with American Sign Language (ASL) as their primary mode of communication. For the present discussion we limit the presentation to the location data and to phrases in which sequences of three signs were used. Subjects were asked to sign these phrases in four different ways: a) normal signing, b) signing faster than normal but not so fast as to jeopardize intelligibility, c) signing even faster than in b) but without concern for possible loss of clarity, d) signing "as fast as possible". Movements were recorded at 60 frames per second with a Vicon 250 system with five infrared cameras tracking the x, y and z positions of reflective markers placed on the subject.

Figure 2 shows a representative example of the vertical location of the hand as defined by a wrist marker (placed at the protrusion of ulna at the back of the wrist). The data are from one of the subjects signing at the normal rate condition. Ten repetitions of SMART-CHILDREN-SMART are plotted as clusters at their relative time locations. Intermediate data points are omitted and replaced by straight lines.

The sign SMART starts with contact between the forehead and the side of the index closer to the thumb. It involves moving the hand away from the forehead (top left insert). The sign for CHILDREN begins with the two hands palm down relatively close to the signer's midline. The hands make two or three up-and-down movements as they move apart away from the midline (top right insert). Movement along the vertical

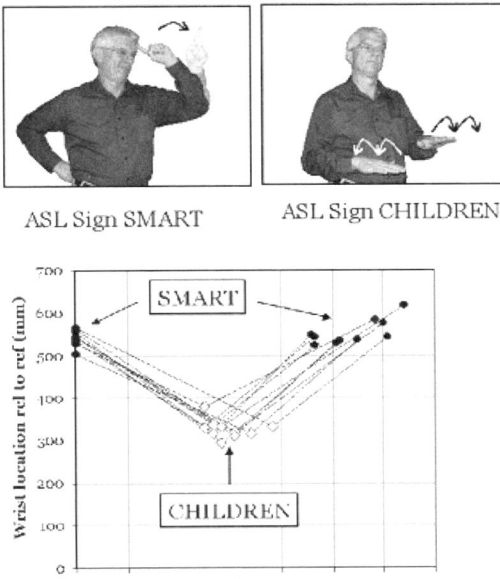

ASL Sign SMART   ASL Sign CHILDREN

Figure 2. Representative from an investigation of hand movement in ASL. The diagram shows data from one of the subjects signing at the normal rate condition. Ten repetitions of SMART-CHILDREN-SMART are plotted as clusters at their relative time locations. Intermediate data points are omitted and replaced by straight lines.

dimension was sampled where the signs for SMART showed a maximum value (near contact between index finger and the forehead). The location of the sign for CHILDREN was taken at the minimum of the record. Figure 2 shows that hand movement in this sequence resembles the point-to-point movements found in a symmetrical phonetic CVC sequence.

Figure 3 plots the measurements of the minima in CHILDREN for all the rate conditions. The ordinate shows the extent of the movement relative to its starting value in the first SMART sign. The x-axis shows the duration of the movement defined as the interval between the samples in CHILDREN and the first SMART. As duration decreases the extent of the downward movement is reduced. The smooth curve depicts the duration-dependence of the displacement. Arrows indicate average wrist locations in the normal condition. If we interpret the arrows as target values maintained constant throughout the four tempo conditions, it is clear that, for decreasing values of duration, these movements exhibit an increasing degree of undershoot.

The smooth curve of Figure 3 does a crude job of describing the somewhat noisy data points. However, 'noisy' is not necessarily appropriate here, since Figure 3 examines the duration dependence but says nothing about the role of peak velocity. To further refine the description, we performed a multiple regression analysis aimed at predicting wrist displacement from duration and peak movement velocity. The dependent variable was wrist displacement. The two independent variables were each point's deviation from the smooth curve of Figure 3 and the corresponding point's peak velocity. The data were taken from movement in the segment between SMART 1 and CHILDREN.

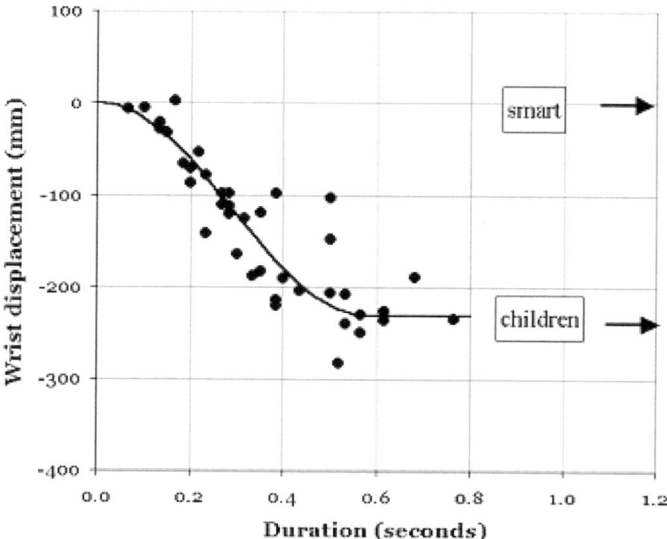

Figure 3. Undershoot in sign language. Extent of wrist marker displacement in transition from SMART to CHILDREN plotted as a function of the duration of the movement. Arrows indicate average wrist locations in slow reference productions.

Figure 4 indicates that the variations in hand location can be accounted for with high accuracy with the aid of these two variables. An r^2 score of 0.98 is obtained.[1] We conclude that the three-parameter undershoot model is supported also by kinematic ASL data.

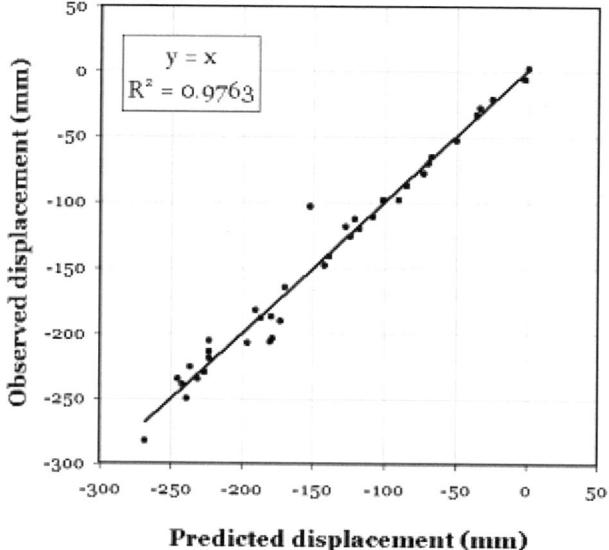

Figure 4. Prediction of degree of undershoot in hand movement based on movement duration and peak velocity of movement.

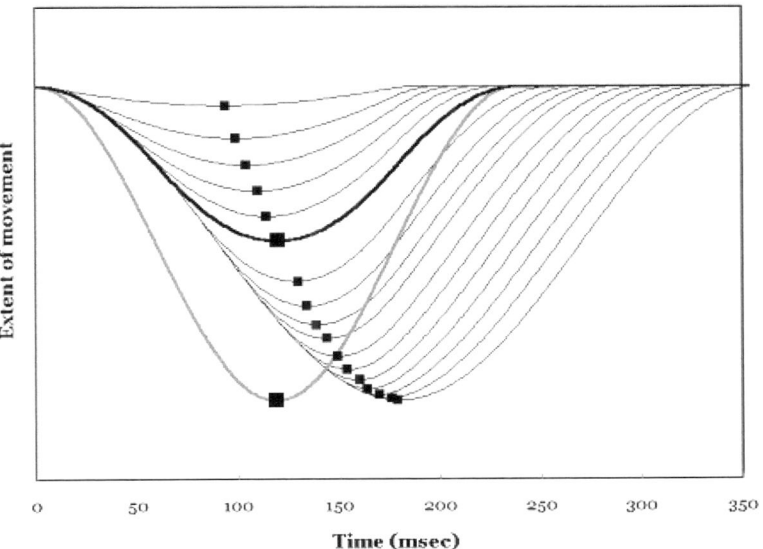

Time (msec)

Figure 5. Geometric model of movement undershoot. Thin contours were generated by adding together two constant-amplitude cosines of opposite sign and varying the delay of the second cosine. As the interval between the two movements is decreased the extent of the downward excursion is reduced (filled squares at minima). Larger solid squares are associated with two movements of equal duration but with different frequencies (peak velocities). The curve with higher velocity avoids the undershoot seen in the other curve.

1.3 A "gestural" account of target undershoot

In Figure 5 an attempt is made to summarize the discussion so far by means of a geometric blending exercise. The diagram was generated using two fixed curve shapes: a downward time function (a half cosine) and an upward movement (the same half cosine with opposite sign). By varying the delay of the upward movement and then summing the two components we obtained the family of curves shown in the diagram. The minimum values (solid squares) highlight the fact that smaller delays are associated with more reduced downward excursions. The curve in gray breaks away from the general pattern because the frequency of its two cosine components was set to higher value. Its durational characteristics is comparable to one of the time functions in the curve family but, because of its more rapid movement, it does have time to complete the downward movement whereas the corresponding curve with slower transitions does not (larger squares).

The point of the exercise is to illustrate how the depth of the minimum (read: undershoot) co-varies with the relative timing of the components and the speed of their excursions. In other words, the variability arising from failure to complete the full extent of the downward movement can be explained as the result of a superposition of two fixed curve shapes, their temporal overlap and their velocity characteristics. Restated in kinematic terms: Movement undershoot need not arise from a change in the intended extent of movement (read: target) but can occur simply as a result of movement duration getting shorter, and/or speed of movement becoming slower.

Let us view the curves of Figure 5 as stylizations of real articulatory transitions from high to low and then from low to high positions, as in the movement of the upper lip during the production of a labial closure. The diagram gives a partial description of the 'gesture' of labial closure. In citation form speech, a voiced bilabial stop must be made with a contact between the lips that is sufficiently deep and is maintained for a certain time period so as give rise to significant acoustic characteristics including a stop gap with a low F1, a release burst and formant transitions. For normal running speech, laboratory records would typically show that the degree of closure can vary and that the lips are capable of moving into the closure (and away from it) from (to) arbitrary positions. In other words, kinematically defined, labial closures and other gestures are not invariants.

1.4 Consonant dynamics: effect of vowel context

Is undershoot confined to vowel dynamics? A brief summary of a Principal Components analysis (PCA) of tongue shapes will demonstrate that it is not.

A 20-second X-ray film of a Swedish male speaker provided the data presented in this section [15]. The speech materials included [ɛCV] sequences in which C = [b p d g] and V = [i e a ɑ ɔ u]. The film taken at 50 frames/second displays the subject's vocal tract in lateral profile. The acoustically relevant articulatory structures were traced using the Osiris software package.[2] Tongue contours were defined in a mandible-based coordinate system and resampled at 25 equidistant 'fleshpoints'. The data consisted of about 200 tongue contours each specified by the x and y coordinates of its 25 fleshpoints. Accordingly the input to the PCA was a 25-by-400 matrix. For the present results this matrix was split into two tables, one for the tongue body (first 16 fleshpoints) and one for the tongue tip (9 fleshpoints). A separate analysis was run for each set. For both sets a single PC was found to give better than 85% accuracy while two PC's achieved more than 95%.

PC analysis produces a small number of PC functions, a set of basic tongue shapes, and a table of weights in which rows refer to a given articulatory profile and the columns represent a PC. Every profile gets two sets of weights since the input matrix contained two values per point, x and y. To recreate an observed shape the following expression was used:

$$s(i, x, v) \;=\; w_1(i, v) \cdot PC_1(x) + w_2(i, v) \cdot PC_2(x) + \ldots \qquad (1)$$

where $PC_n(x)$ refers to a principal component, $w_n(i,v)$ is the weight, x is fleshpoint number, i identifies the contour/image, and v selects the x or y coordinate. The formula expresses the idea that any observed contour is a linear combination of a set of basic tongue shapes.

Figure 6 presents a summary limited to the tongue body results for [d] as portrayed in terms of the most important component, the first PC. The diagram shows the weight values for tongue shapes observed at the moments of release (triangles) in [di], [de], [da], [dɑ], [dɔ], and [du] and the weights for the contours sampled at the vowel quasi-steady-states of those syllables (circles). The horizontal component of PC1 is plotted along the x-axis from back to front. The vertical component is on the y-axis its values spanning low to high positions.

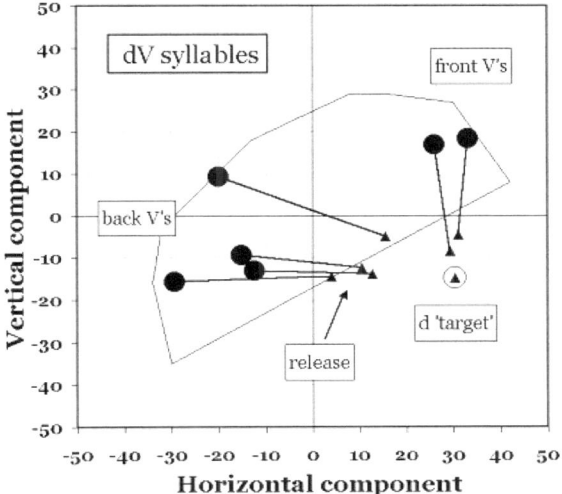

Figure 6 **[dV]** tongue shapes pictured in a Principal Components space. Axes show the vertical and horizontal components of the first PC. Tongue shapes sampled at release of [d] (triangles) and the following vowel [i e a ɑ ɔ u] (large circles). The transitions are approximated by straight lines. The average intersection of the lines was used to define a hypothetical 'target' state for an ideal [d] tongue shape.

The front vowels are located to the right in the semi-circle. The central and back vowels fall in the left, and hence more posterior, region of the space. The semi-circular figure shows the subject's vowel space. It encloses all vowel points.

The straight lines are simplified representations of the CV transitions between the releases and the vowels. This stylization brings out a systematic pattern in the data creating the impression of the [dV] tongue movements as originating from a common 'locus' and then diverging towards their respective vowel destinations. This effect is enhanced by adding a point (encircled triangle) corresponding to the average point of intersection of the line pairs.

A possible interpretation of this intersection is to think of it as a virtual target. The subject's [d] is likely to be aimed at producing the acoustic attributes significant for this segment such as a voice bar and spectrally appropriate release burst and formant transitions. Conceivably, from experience, he has discovered that the method of achieving this is to move toward the virtual [d] target until a dental blade/palate contact of sufficient depth has been established. If that goal is set with a certain margin of tolerance, it would leave room for contextual vowel-dependent perturbations. It seems plausible that it is the combination of virtual target plus the tolerance margins that give rise to phenomenon of VCV coarticulation.

Given the data on releases (R), vowel (V) and virtual target (T), we computed the following ratio as a measure of 'degree of coarticulation' based on the Euclidean distances between R and T (RT), V and T (VT), in the PC space:

$$(degree\ of\ articulation = RT/VT) \qquad (2)$$

The numerical pattern pictured in Figure 6 lends strong support to the idea of a [d] target. This suggestion is paralleled by the work of [21] who successfully used a single

di	0.31
de	0.20
da	0.44
dɑ	0.44
dɔ	0.41
du	0.32

Table 1. Degree of coarticulation at release of [dV] syllables.

tongue shape, c(x), for [d] in his account of vowel-dependent coarticulation in VCV sequences.

The variable degrees of coarticulation of Table 1 tell us two things: First, the proposed measure indicates that coarticulation is not uniform across vowel contexts. Second, the values indicate the answer to the question raised at the beginning of the section: In no case is the vowel influence absent. The [d] target is never reached. In this sense, vowel-dependent coarticulation in stops is analogous to consonant-dependent undershoot in vowels.

2. Clues From Physiological Modeling

2.1 Spring-mass Models

Many speech production models include a level at which articulators are represented as spring-mass systems, that is, devices with mass, damping and elasticity. In such mechanisms movement is produced by applying a force of appropriate magnitude to an articulator so as to push it towards an intended goal. Because the articulator is strongly damped, the response to the force unfolds slowly along a roughly s-shaped path.

An example is the model of lip and jaw movement in [14] in which movement was controlled with the aid of positional targets each corresponding to a given input force. Despite its lack of physiological realism, the model offered an explanation for why open vowels tend to be longer than closed vowels. However, the coding of articulatory goals in terms of force values turns out not to be a viable approach [22]. This is so because the force needed to move an articulator towards a certain goal, by necessity depends on the distance between where the movement starts from and where that goal is. Hence, like kinematically defined gestures (but unlike positional targets), input force is not context-free.

2.2 Targets and the Equilibrium-point Hypothesis

The preceding remarks suggest that the level of control is located further upstream than the generation of muscle forces. Consequently, we need to probe more deeply into the physiology of movement. So doing we encounter the Equilibrium-Point (EP) hypothesis also known as the λ model. It was originally proposed by [3][4] in studies of arm and eye movement and has been applied extensively also to speech notably by David Ostry and his colleagues [12][7][23]. A paper by [22] provides a helpful overview for phoneticians particularly if read in conjunction with the commentaries by other leading speech physiologists [1].

The EP hypothesis was developed from the observation that muscles tend to behave like springs. An activated muscle that is stretched produces a restoring force that varies with the degree of stretch. If a limb is moved by some external action, it will return to its original position when the perturbation is removed. Its return path and speed of response are determined by its stiffness. The EP hypothesis assumes that voluntary movements result from shifting the equilibrium-point of the motor system. The mechanism is formalized in the λ model [4][23]. The input to the model is λ, the threshold length of a given muscle at which motorneuron recruitment begins. The neural signal driving muscle activation is determined by the difference between λ and reflex information on the muscle's current length and its rate of change. When the muscle length reaches the value of λ, muscle activation, and thus force generation, cease. The point in space at which force is zero defines an equilibrium-point [2].

The EP hypothesis provides a parsimonious account of how the central nervous system plans and executes movements. EP control bypasses the problem of "inverse dynamics" [2]. It suggests that the brain finds a unique and smooth trajectory by letting that path be automatically determined by the dynamics of the physiological system. The parsimony lies in the fact that neural control levels do not need an explicit representation of limb dynamics. Nor is any preplanning (predictive simulation of motor commands) required in the case of compensatory tasks since viscoelastic forces provide immediate corrective action in response to an external perturbation.

2.3 Movement paths as a result of optimization

Theoretically there is an infinite number of paths that a limb or articulator could take between two points. Studies of hand movement during reaching show that, for any given task, observed trajectories are highly consistent both from one trial to another and between subjects. This fact is handled by the EP hypothesis, but there are also competing answers to why movements take one specific path rather than others that are in principle possible [24]. A central idea in these accounts is that uniqueness and kinematic characteristics are products of optimization.

An often-mentioned fact about of natural motions is that the brain seems to have a preference for the 'smoothest' option. It has been suggested that motions are smooth because control processes are guided by criteria related to minimal energy consumption [19]. An empirically successful and widely embraced variant of this thinking is the 'minimum jerk' model [9] which finds the least 'jerky' pathway by optimizing the acceleration pattern. A third criterion, also in this category, is 'minimum muscle force change' [24].

A recent proposal takes a different route [8]. It argues that the dimension optimized is 'precision', not 'efficiency' as in the three studies just mentioned. This work starts from the observation that neural signals are inherently noisy. Because of the noise the same command does not guarantee reaching the same destination. The noise is activity-dependent: the stronger the command the larger the variability. The 'minimum variance' model of Harris and Wolpert optimizes the precision of endpoint control and in so doing generates motions exhibiting both smoothness and the kinematic properties closely matching those found in natural movements.

2.4 Emerging picture

We shall limit our observations to point-to-point movement tasks because they appear most analogous to phoneme-to-phoneme movements in speech. The evidence reviewed converges on the following picture.

1. *Target control.* First, all accounts appear to assume that the nervous system has information on the current location of the limb and a specification of where it has to go. Both EP and non-EP models postulate positional targets.
2. *Determinants of trajectory shape: stiffness tuning and optimization.* Another shared theme is that, once information on 'here' and 'there' is available, physiological constraints determine the shape of the path between those points. According to the EP hypothesis, movement paths are determined by the stiffness of the activated muscles. Since stiffness can be controlled separately from muscle lengths there exists a possibility of varying the time course of the trajectory. In non-EP approaches trajectories are derived by means of various forms of optimization. While the choice of optimality criterion may be a matter of lively debate [10], that debate seems to be, not about optimization per se, but about the parameter(s) to be optimized.

The literature review does not resolve the issue of static targets *vs.* dynamic gestures in phonetics, but it does provide some preliminary clues: It shows that the notion of 'target' as an object of control is pervasively paralleled in recent neuro-computational models of movement. It also suggests that, if the production of 'phonetic gestures' is assumed to be analogous to trajectory formation in point-to-point arm movements, they are better seen as interpolation phenomena arising as by-products of efficiency- and/or precision-optimized execution rather than as explicitly specified at the input level of speech production control.

3. Final Remarks - Making the Paradox Disappear

In the speech production mechanism the downstream responses to higher-level control signals distribute the acoustic consequences of those commands in complex patterns of spatial and temporal overlap along the time scale. It seems highly plausible that listeners make good use of this rich and redundant information in processing the signal. Therefore Strange's point about the perceptual insufficiency of single spectral target slices at vowel midpoints makes good sense and is supported by perceptual experiments. But does it logically necessitate abandoning target control in speech production and replacing it by dynamic gestures? In our judgment it does not.

The reason for this judgment is partly empirical, partly methodological. Invoking parsimony as our guiding principle, we can formulate the strategy as follows: Do not postulate dynamic control until a deeper understanding is available of how physiological and biomechanical system characteristics contribute to speech dynamics! Since there are solid, a priori reasons to believe that those 'filtering' characteristics cannot be ignored with impunity, the parsimony principle makes us put dynamic motor commands on hold until the downstream mechanisms have been more fully investigated and put to use for explanatory purposes.

> *To substitute an ill-understood model of the world for the ill-understood world is not progress. (from [17])*

The message becomes: do not explain dynamics with dynamics as long as much remains unknown about the response characteristics of the speech system.

If the schema of *static-targets plus dynamics-from-execution* is an intuitive way of conceptually parsing movements, it is only natural that phoneticians should have given many speech sounds static labels in traditional descriptive frameworks. Static-target control in speech production is in no way incompatible with dynamic input patterns for perception. Once that fact is acknowledged, there is no paradox.

Endnotes

1. It should be observed that, although there are three determinants of undershoot in the model, *viz.* 'inter-target distance', 'duration of movement' and 'peak movement velocity', only the latter two were used in the regression analysis. The reason for this omission is the assumption that 'inter-target distance' remained constant across all tokens of the SMART CHILDREN SMART phrase.

2. http://www.expasy.org/www/UIN/html1/projects/osiris/osiris.html

References

[1]   Abry, C., Badin, P., *et al. Les Cahiers de l'ICP.* Numéro 4 (Special issue), 1998.
[2]   Bizzi, E., Mussa-Ivaldi, F.A., *et al.* "computations underlying the execution of movement: A biological perspective." *Science* 253: 287-291, 1991.
[3]   Feldman, A.G. "Functional tuning of the nervous system with control of movement or maintenance of a steady posture - II. Controllable parameters of the muscle." *Biofizika* 11(3): 498-508, 1996.
[4]   Feldman, A.G. "Once more on the equilibrium-point hypothesis (model) for motor control." *J. Motor Behav.* 18: 17-54, 1986.
[5]   Flege, J.E. "Effects of speaking rate on tongue position and velocity of movement in vowel production." *J. Acoust. Soc. Am.* 84: 901-916, 1988.
[6]   Gay, T. "Effect of speaking rate on vowel formant movements." *J. Acoust. Soc. Am.* 63: 223-230, 1978.
[7]   Gribble, P.L., Ostry, D.J., *et al.* "Are complex control signals required for human arm movement?" *J. Neurophysiol.* 79: 1409-1424, 1998.
[8]   Harris, C.M. and Wolpert, D.M. "Signal-dependent noise determines motor planning." *Nature* 394: 780-784, 1998.
[9]   Hogan, N. and Flash, T. "Moving gracefully: Quantitative theories of motor coordination." *Trends Neurosci.* 10: 170-174, 1987.
[10] Kawato, M. "Internal models for motor control and trajectory planning." *Curr. Opin. Neurobiol.* 9: 718-727, 1999.
[11] Kuehn, D.P. and Moll, K.L. "A cineradiographic study of VC and CV articulatory velocities." *J. Phonetics* 4: 303-320, 1976.
[12] Laboissière, R., Ostry, D.J., *et al.* "A model of human jaw and hyoid motion and its implications for speech production." *Proc. 13th Int. Cong. Phon. Sci.*, 1995.
[13] Lindblom, B. "Spectrographic study of vowel reduction." *J. Acoust. Soc. Am.* 35: 1773-1781, 1963.
[14] Lindblom, B. "Vowel duration and a model of lip and mandible coordination." *STL/QPRS, Speech Transmission Laboratory*, KTH, Stockholm 4: 1-29, 1967.

[15] Lindblom, B. "A numerical model of coarticulation based on a principal components analysis of tongue shapes." *Proc. 15th Int. Cong. Phon. Sci*, 2003.

[16] Mauk, C. *Undershoot in Two Modalities: Evidence from Fast Speech and Fast Signing.* Ph.D. Thesis, Department of Linguistics, Austin, University of Texas, 2003.

[17] Maynard Smith, J. "Natural selection of culture?" *New York Review of Books*: Nov 6, pp. 11-12, 1986.

[18] Moon, S.-J. and Lindblom, B. "Interaction between duration, context and speaking style in English stressed vowels." *J. Acoust. Soc. Am.* 96: 40-55, 1994.

[19] Nelson, W.L. "Physical principles for economies of skilled movements." *Biol. Cybern.* 46: 135-147, 1983.

[20] Nelson, W.L., Perkell, J.S., *et al.* "Mandible movements during increasingly rapid articulations of single syllables: Preliminary observations." *J. Acoust. Soc. Am.* 75: 945-951, 1984.

[21] Öhman, S. "Numerical model of coarticulation." *J. Acoust. Soc. Am.* 41: 310-320, 1967.

[22] Perrier, P., Ostry, D.J., *et al.* "The equilibrium point hypothesis and its application to speech motor control." *J. Speech Hear. Res.* 39: 365-378, 1996.

[23] Sanguineti, V., Laboissière, R., *et al.* "A dynamic biomechanical model for neural control of speech production." *J. Acoust. Soc. Am.* 103: 1615-1627, 1998.

[24] Soechting, J.F. and Flanders, M. "Movement planning: kinematics, dynamics, both or neither?" *In Vision and Action.* L.R. Harris and M. Jenkin (eds.), Cambridge: Cambridge University Press, 1998.

[25] Stevens, K.N. and House, A.S. "Perturbation of vowel articulations by consonantal context: An acoustic study." *J. Speech Hear. Res.* 6: 111-128, 1963.

[26] Strange, W. "Dynamic specification of coarticulated vowels spoken in sentence context." *J. Acoust. Soc. Am.* 85: 2135-2153, 1989.

[27] Strange, W. "Evolving theories of vowel perception." *J. Acoust. Soc. Am.* 85: 2081-2087, 1989.

[28] Studdert-Kennedy, M. "How did language go discrete?" In *Evolutionary Prerequisites of Language,*. M. Tallerman (ed.) Oxford: Oxford University Press, 2003.

[29] van Son, R.J.J.H. *Spectro-temporal Features of Vowel Segments.* Doctoral thesis, University of Amsterdam, 1993.

Dynamics of Speech Production and Perception
P. Divenyi et al. (Eds.)
IOS Press, 2006

Controlled Variables, the Uncontrolled Manifold Method, and the Task-Dynamic Model of Speech Production

Elliot SALTZMAN[1,2], Masayoshi KUBO[3], and Cheng-Chi TSAO[4]

[1]*Dept. of Physical Therapy & Athletic Training, Boston University, Boston, MA, USA*
[2]*Haskins Laboratories, New Haven, Connecticutt, USA*
[3]*Department of Physical Therapy University of Delaware, Newark, Delaware, USA*
[4]*Rehabilitation Institute of Chicago, Chicago, Illinois, USA*

Abstract. The task-dynamic model of sensorimotor coordination [20][21][22][23] is reviewed, highlighting the issues of the coordinate systems involved (e.g., articulator vs. task coordinates), the mappings between these coordinate systems, and the dynamics defined within these coordinate systems. The empirical question of which sets of coordinates are the most appropriate candidates for the control of speech and other tasks is addressed through the introduction of the uncontrolled manifold method [24][25]. This method is introduced using the non-speech example of planar reaching using a 3-joint arm, and is generalized to speech production. In particular, it is shown how the method can be applied to skilled behaviors, such as speech production, in which there is no analytic formula that can be (easily) derived between the hypothesized coordinate systems underlying the skill, e.g., the forward kinematic mapping from articulator positions to acoustic/auditory coordinates.

Keywords. Speech production, task dynamics, kinematics

Introduction

When investigating any skilled behavior, one of the key issues that must be addressed is the nature of the variables that are essential to the task's definition and that, hence, must be controlled by the actor during the performance of the skill. For example, reaching toward a target might involve defining the task's goals at the level of musculoskeletal coordinates (e.g., joint angular distances between current posture and a set of target joint angles) or, alternatively, the spatial relationships between the end-effector and the target (e.g., distances and relative orientations between hand and target). Similarly, in speech production, the articulators might be controlled with reference to musculoskeletal coordinates (e.g., distances between current and target positions for the component articulators – jaw, lips, tongue, etc.) or, alternatively, to more abstract, functional coordinates (e.g., differences between the current and target states of a bilabial constriction). There are, however, several lines of argument that support the hypothesis that the controlled variables are task coordinates rather than musculoskeletal ones.

One line of support comes from studies in which ongoing performance is perturbed mechanically at the articulatory level, and the articulatory motions automatically and swiftly readjust themselves to achieve the task goal, albeit with different final articulatory postures than in the unperturbed situation. For example, in an elegant experiment by [14], subjects were asked to produce the syllables /bæb/ or /bæz/ in the carrier phrase "It's a ___ again", while recording (among other observables) the kinematics of upper lip, lower lip, and jaw motion, as well as the electromyographic activity of the tongue-raising genioglossus muscle. During the experiment, the subjects' jaws were unpredictably perturbed downward as they were moving into the final /b/ closure for /bæb/ or the final /z/ constriction for /bæz/. When the target was /b/, for which lip but not tongue activity is crucial, compensation occurred remotely in the upper lip relative to unperturbed control trials, but there was normal tongue activity; when the target was /z/, for which tongue but not lip activity is crucial, compensation occurred remotely in the tongue but not the upper lip. The remote compensation was relatively immediate, i.e., 20-30 ms from the onset of the downward jaw perturbation to the onset of the compensatory activity. The swiftness of this response implies that there is some sort of automatic "reflexive" organization established among the articulators with a relatively fast loop time. However, the gestural specificity implies that the mappings from perturbing inputs to compensatory outputs are not hard-wired, and that such flexibility was not produced by a system in which task goals were defined as target positions for each of the articulators. Although such a system would be able to achieve the target posture in unperturbed situations, it would fail when perturbing forces prevented one of the articulators from attaining its target position. The compensatory articulation that is observed experimentally can, however, be captured by a model which specifies the task's goals in constriction (e.g., [20]) or acoustic (e.g., [1][8]) coordinates.

A second line of support for the hypothesis that the controlled variables in skilled behaviors are abstractly and functionally specified, rather than specified at the relatively concrete level of musculoskeletal states, comes from investigations that seek to characterize the invariant kinematic signatures of the behaviors in question. For example, it is a common observation that the shape of one's written signature is uniquely identifiable as one's own whether it is written with the dominant or non-dominant hand, or even with the pen held between one's toes or one's teeth. Less anecdotal, however, are data from a remarkable experiment by [17] that examined the kinematic organization displayed in an altered reciprocal aiming Fitts task. In the standard version of this task, a subject unimanually moves a pointer rhythmically between two stationary targets. [17] added conditions where the subject unimanually moved the *targets* (both targets were fixed on a moveable substrate) rhythmically relative to the stationary pointer, or bimanually moved *both* the targets and the pointer. They even added a condition where two subjects participated, with one subject moving the pointer and the other moving the targets. The authors showed that, when the pointer and target motions were projected into a task-space coordinate defined by the distance between pointer and target, the kinematics of all conditions were effectively identical despite the use of different effectors within and between subjects to produce these movement patterns.

It is thus relatively accepted that the controlled variables in skilled behaviors are abstractly and functionally specified at the level of task-space coordinates, rather than at the relatively concrete level of musculoskeletal coordinates. However, there still remains the issue of *which* task-spaces are the most appropriate for the control of a given skilled activity. For example, in a sit-to-stand transition, the controlled variable might be the position of the head or of the body's center of mass (e.g., [24]).

In what follows, we will first review briefly the *task-dynamic* model of sensorimotor activity that has been used to simulate skilled actions of the limbs (e.g., [22]) and speech articulators (e.g., [23][21]), with an emphasis on how it has been applied to modeling the gestural patterning observed during speech production. We then address the issue of which task spaces are the most appropriate candidates for the controlled variables of speaking, and describe the *uncontrolled manifold* method (e.g., [24][25]) that may be used to distinguish between these candidates. Finally, we describe a computational neural network procedure for implementing this method.

1. The Task-Dynamic Model

The major hypothesis underlying the task-dynamic model is that the principles governing the control and coordination of the speech articulators – e.g. tongue, lips, jaw, etc. – during speaking are the *same* as those involved in skilled actions of the limbs and torso. In applying the task-dynamic framework to understanding a particular skilled behavior, four questions must be addressed. The first is what "objects" are being controlled? For example in many skills, what is being controlled is the gap between two surfaces or objects – hand-to-target distance in reaching, the distance between a wielded hammer and its targeted nail, the horizontal orientation of a full-to-the-brim beer glass *en route* from table to lips, the aperture between the lips in speaking or between the hands in clapping. The second question is what are the *sets* of variables (reference frames) that are entailed in controlling the intended action, and what are the dimensionalities of these spaces? Answering this question typically entails defining or hypothesizing an *articulator/musculoskeletal* space that is relatively high-dimensional and a *task/goal* space that is relatively low-dimensional. As discussed in the previous section, examples of articulator spaces are joint angle positions for reaching or hammering, and speech articulator positions for speaking. Examples of task space coordinates are the three spatial translation axes along which distance of hand to target is defined for reaching, and the vocal tract constriction location and degree values or acoustic formant values for speaking. The third question is what kind of dynamics is defined along each of the task axes? For example, point attractor dynamics would be defined for discrete motion tasks such as reaching, while limit cycle dynamics would be defined for rhythmic task such as polishing a car or erasing a blackboard. Finally, the fourth question is what are the kinematic/geometric *relationships* between the articulator and task reference frames? Understanding these relationships is crucial, since they are the means by which task-space dynamics can harness the articulators in order to produce task-specific patterns of coordinated motion. These relationships are bidirectional, and include both afferentation (i.e., perceptual input is transformed into task relevant form) and efferentation (i.e., motoric output is shaped into task-relevant form). For reaching, afferentation refers to the means by

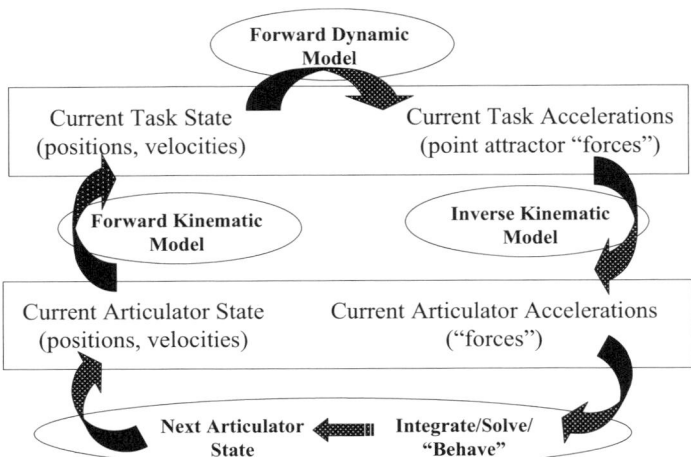

Figure 1. Schematic of task-articulator space relationships (forward and inverse kinematics) and task-dynamics specification (forward dynamics).

which joint angles and target information are transformed into distance-of-hand-from-target information, and efferentation refers to the way that synergistic muscle activation patterns are produced to shape task-specific patterns of hand motion toward the target.

In the task-dynamic model of speech production, the spatiotemporal patterns of speech emerge as behaviors implicit in a dynamical system with two functionally distinct but interacting levels. The *interarticulator* level is defined according to both *model articulator* (e.g. lips and jaw) coordinates and task-space coordinates called *tract-variables* (e.g. lip aperture and protrusion); the *intergestural* level is defined according to a set of *activation* coordinates. Invariant gestural units are posited in the form of context-independent sets of dynamical parameters (e.g. target, stiffness, and damping coefficients) that define the *point attractor* dynamics of damped mass-spring systems in the task-space and that serve, for example to close the lips, raise the tongue tip, etc. Further, each gestural unit is associated with a corresponding subset of model articulator, tract-variable, and activation coordinates. During the simulated production of a given utterance, each unit's activation coordinate reflects the strength with which the associated gesture's point attractor (e.g., for bilabial closing) "attempts" to shape vocal tract movements at any given point in time. The tract-variable and model articulator coordinates of each unit specify, respectively, the particular vocal-tract constriction (e.g. bilabial) and articulatory synergy (e.g. lips and jaw) whose behaviors are affected directly by the associated unit's activation. The interarticulator level accounts for the coordination among articulators at a given point in time due to the currently active gesture set. The intergestural level governs the patterns of relative timing among the gestural units participating in an utterance and the temporal evolution of the activation trajectories of individual gestures in the utterance.

For the purpose of addressing the issue of how to identify the controlled variables for speech production, we will focus on the interarticulator level of the task-dynamic model and on the geometric relationships between the articulator and tract-variable coordinates. As illustrated in Figure 1, the processes involved in simulating a particular gestural sequence begin with the "afferent" *forward kinematic* map from articulator state (i.e., positions, velocities) to tract-variable state. This map is defined explicitly by a set of closed form equations. Once specified, the tract-variable state, in conjunction with the current set of activated gestural point attractors, is used to define a set of tract-variable "forces" according to a *forward dynamic* model. Next, the "efferent" *inverse kinematic* map from tract-variable to articulator "forces" is defined by the Jacobian pseudoinverse of the forward mapping (see [23] for details on the computation of this pseudoinverse). Finally, these articulatory forces cause a change in articulatory state, which is then transformed into a new tract-variable state, and so on.

Although the task-dynamic model posits task-space coordinates defined according to the set of vocal tract constrictions used in a particular language (e.g., [5][2][3][4][23]; see also [13][15]), there are other possible candidates. In particular, several researchers [1][9][10][11][18] have proposed that speech targets should instead be specified in auditory or acoustic coordinates (e.g., formant frequencies). However, the distinction between auditory/acoustic and tract-variable coordinate spaces is not always a clear one, since tract-variables define the locations and degrees of the constrictions produced by the gestures comprising a given speech sequence, and these constriction variables are primarily responsible for shaping the formant patterns of the vocal tract. Thus, for a given articulator configuration, and hence vocal tract area function and formant pattern, the formant changes that result from changes in the configuration are small if those changes do not alter the area function in the region of the main constriction. For example, it is known that the region of maximum constriction is approximately preserved during bite-block productions of steady-state vowels, and that the resulting formant patterns are thereby minimally, although systematically, altered relative to the non-bite-block versions of the same utterances [7][16]. How might one distinguish between these constriction-based and acoustics-based hypotheses?

2. The Uncontrolled Manifold Method

In many skilled speech and non-speech behaviors it is unclear or controversial which set of task coordinates is the most appropriate candidate to define the primary controlled variables for that behavior. The *uncontrolled manifold* method (e.g., [24][25]) allows this issue to be addressed empirically. Briefly, this method allows one to partition the overall kinematic variability observed during a movement or sustained posture into two parts – a task-specific component and a task-irrelevant component. These variability components are defined at the level of articulator coordinates, and are computed using the forward kinematic relationship between the (observed) articulator positions and the corresponding positions of each set of hypothesized task-space coordinates. In particular, the variability is partitioned into motion patterns within both a controlled manifold (CM), defined by motion patterns in articulator space that correspond to motions in the hypothesized task space, and an uncontrolled manifold (UCM), defined by motion patterns in articulator space that correspond to no motion ("do no harm") in task space. It is assumed that the system controls motions "tightly" along the CM and relatively "loosely" if at all along the UCM. The "best" of several hypothesized task spaces will show the smallest ratio of CM-variability to UCM-variability, i.e., σ_{CM}/σ_{UCM}.

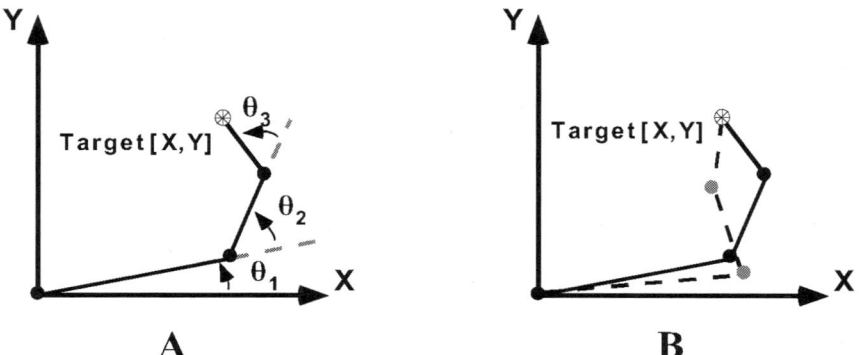

Figure 2. (a) Planar 3-joint arm showing joint angles and endpoint's target position. (b) Two possible postures for a given endpoint position.

2.1 Example: Planar Reaching

We will illustrate these concepts using the relatively simple example of planar reaching using the three-joint arm illustrated in Figure 2(a), where the task coordinates are defined by the x and y positions of the end-effector (i.e., the "fingertip"), and the articulator coordinates are defined by the joint angles θ_1, θ_2, and θ_3. In this figure, the end-effector is positioned at the target and the task can be thought of as one of maintaining the fingertip at the target. Since there are more articulator coordinates than there are task coordinates, there are (infinitely) many postures for each hand position (two are shown in Figure 2(b)). This type of geometric relationship between articulator space and task space is called *redundancy*, and confers postural flexibility to the system in tasks such as reaching to a target in an obstacle-filled environment. Given the system is redundant and given, for example, the task of maintaining the fingertip at the target position, one can define an uncontrolled manifold (UCM) for every task space position using the forward

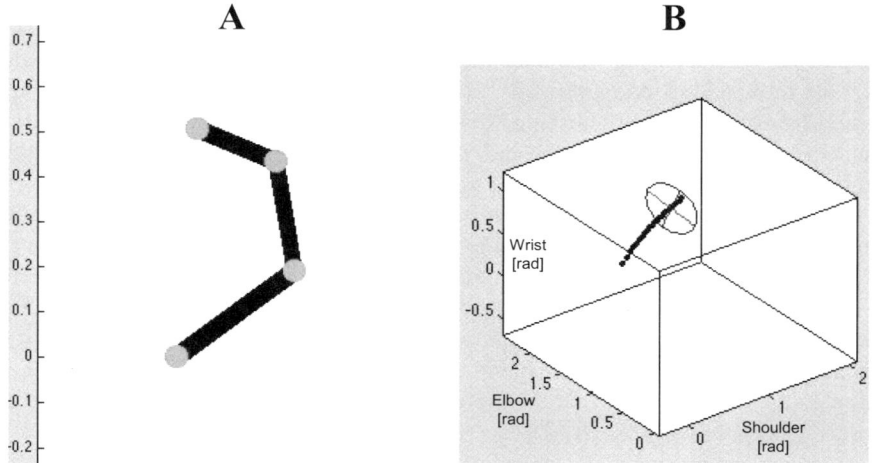

Figure 3. (a) Planar 3-joint arm showing joint angles and endpoint's target position. (b) Three-dimensional joint space containing the arm's 1-dimensional UCM for the endpoint position shown in 3(a), and the CM centered at the arm posture shown in 3(a).

kinematic mapping from articulator space to task space. Intuitively, the UCM is the *set* of postures defined in articulator space that correspond to a given task-space position. For the end-effector position of the three-joint arm shown in Figure 3(a), the postures corresponding to the UCM can be represented as the one dimensional path in joint space shown in Figure 3(b) (the current posture shown in Figure 3(a) corresponds to the location on the UCM defined by the intersecting ellipse). The controlled manifold (CM) is defined relative to the current posture in articulator space as the "leftover" set of postures that do not lie along the UCM. Since the joint space is three dimensional, and the UCM is one dimensional, the CM is two dimensional. In Figure 3(b) the basis vectors that define the dimensions of the CM are represented as the major and minor axes of the ellipse intersecting the UCM at the current posture. When the endpoint moves, for example, from the position in Figure 3(a) to the position in Figure 4(a), the UCM changes accordingly from that shown in Figure 3(b) to that shown in Figure 4(b) (Note that the current posture and its corresponding CM are not highlighted in Figure 4(b)).

The key to computing both the UCM and the CM is the forward kinematic mapping from articulator- to task-space coordinates. For the *xy* task space shown in Figures 2-4, the forward kinematic model is defined as:

$$x = f_1(\theta) = L_1\cos(\theta_1) + L_2\cos(\theta_1 + \theta_2) + L_3\cos(\theta_1 + \theta_2 + \theta_3) \quad \text{(1a)}$$

$$y = f_2(\theta) = L_1\sin(\theta_1) + L_2\sin(\theta_1 + \theta_2) + L_3\sin(\theta_1 + \theta_2 + \theta_3) \quad \text{(1b)}$$

where θ is the column vector of joint angles $(\theta_1, \theta_2, \theta_3)^T$ (the superscript T denotes the matrix or vector transpose operation). This forward kinematic map can be rewritten in vector notation as:

$$x = f(\theta) \quad \text{(2)}$$

where x is the column vector of task coordinates $(x, y)^T$, and f is the column vector function $(f_1(\theta), f_2(\theta))^T$. Equation (2) can be differentiated to give a forward differential ("small") displacement map:

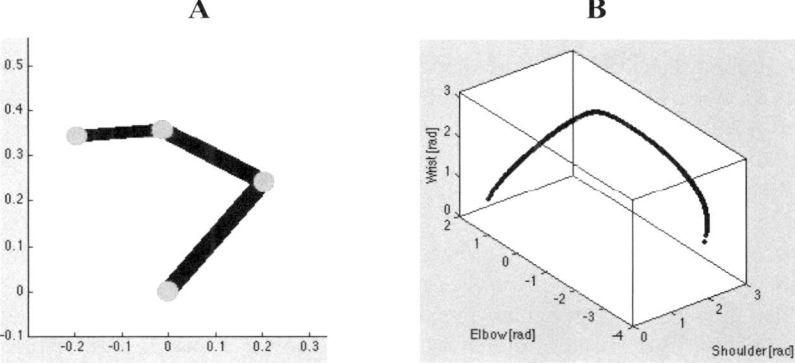

Figure 4. (a) Planar 3-joint arm showing joint angles and endpoint's target position different from those shown in Figure 3(a). (b) Three-dimensional joint space containing the arm's 1-dimensional UCM for the endpoint position shown in 3(a), which differs from the UCM in Figure 3(b).

$$dx = J(\theta)d\theta, \text{ where} \tag{3}$$

dx and $d\theta$ = small displacements in the task- and joint-spaces; and

$J(\theta)$ = the *Jacobian* of the position mapping, *defined at the current posture* (joint angle configuration). Thus, the Jacobian elements are functions of the current posture and, as arm posture changes, the values of the Jacobian elements change correspondingly;

= matrix of partial derivatives, $[\partial x_i / \partial \theta_j]$, that transform small joint-space deviations from the current posture into corresponding small task-space displacements.

The Jacobian matrix in Equation (3) is the crucial element in computing both the UCM and the CM. In linear algebra terms (e.g., [6]), the UCM is the *null space* of the Jacobian matrix, and is computed by finding the set of displacement *directions* in joint space that cause no motion in the task space. These directions are defined (spanned) in joint space by the eigenvectors of $J^T J$ having eigenvalues of zero, where $J^T J$ is the *major product moment* of J. The CM is the *orthogonal complement* of the null space, and is defined by the remaining set of displacement directions in the joint space. These directions are defined (spanned) in joint space by the eigenvectors of $J^T J$ having *non*-zero eigenvalues.

We now illustrate the UCM method using a planar three-joint arm in a task whose goal is to maintain the arm's endpoint (the fingertip) at a given target position. We hypothesized that the arm was controlled according to task-space control that minimizes the xy distance between fingertip and target, i.e., we hypothesized a point attractor for the arm's endpoint at the target xy position. According to this hypothesis, the forward kinematic map and its Jacobian would be defined using Equations 1-3. We then tested this endpoint control hypothesis across two simulations: 1) Task-space control, using task-dynamics to define point-attractors along the x and y task-space axes to stabilize the endpoint position; and 2) Joint-space control, using point attractors directly defined at each joint to stabilize a particular "target" posture that was associated with the endpoint's desired target position. We started both simulations "on target" with the same posture, and added random perturbing "forces" (identically distributed gaussians) at the joints for both the joint- and endpoint- control cases. Finally, we computed the UCMs and CMs in both cases, and compared variability ratios (σ_{CM}/σ_{UCM}) for the endpoint control hypothesis across the two (known) control schemes. For the joint control simulations, we found that the postural dispersion about the mean joint configuration was isotropic, i.e., it showed no predominant directionality, with the result being that $\sigma_{CM}/\sigma_{UCM} = .0017/.0018 = .94$. On the other hand, for the endpoint control simulations we found that the postural dispersion about the mean joint configuration was directed predominantly along the UCM, i.e., the system took a random walk along the UCM, with the result that $\sigma_{CM}/\sigma_{UCM} = .0015/.0124 = .12$. Thus, the endpoint control hypothesis was supported (small ratio) when there was an underlying endpoint control regime, but *not* when there was an underlying *joint space* control regime (large ratio). This is a comforting albeit obvious result given how we defined the two simulations, but it provides a simple and useful illustration of the UCM method's power in probing the nature of a system's controlled variables.

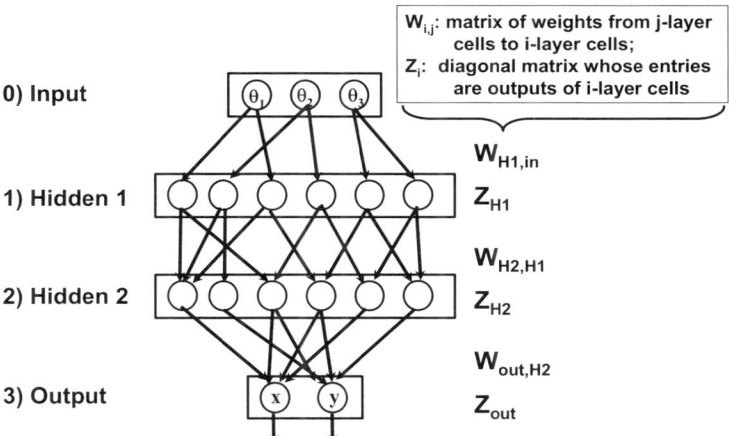

Figure 5. Feedforward neural network for the forward kinematic model in the case of a 3-joint planar arm with task-space endpoint control.

2.2 The Problem with Speech Production

Recall that for speech production, two types of task space coordinates have been hypothesized: constriction coordinates and acoustic/auditory coordinates. It is relatively easy to apply the UCM method using vocal tract constriction coordinates such as lip aperture, tongue tip constriction location and degree, etc. Given experimental data consisting of articulator measurements in the sagittal plane, it is possible to write relatively simple forward kinematic equations that map articulator positions to constriction coordinates. This means that one can differentiate these forward equations and derive the equation for the constriction hypothesis' Jacobian. In turn, therefore, one can computationally derive the UCM/CM variability ratio for this hypothesis. However, for the hypothesis of control by acoustic/auditory coordinates, there is a problem – it is not possible to write a set of forward kinematic equations from articulator positions to formants (or nonlinear auditory transforms of formants). Without these equations, there is no way to analytically derive the corresponding Jacobian that lies at the heart of the UCM method.

However, there is a way out of this dilemma. One can generate the Jacobian elements using the computations inherent in relatively standard connectionist neural network training algorithms. Specifically, one can train a feedforward neural network using backpropagation training methods [19] to instantiate the forward kinematic mapping, and then recover the Jacobian elements from the trained neural network [12]. For simplicity's sake, we will illustrate this technique using our earlier example of a 3-joint planar arm controlled according to endpoint dynamics defined in *xy* task coordinates. The feedforward neural net in this case is shown in Figure 5. The network consists of an input layer with three units corresponding to the arm's joint angles, an output layer with two units corresponding to the endpoint's *x* and *y* position, and two hidden layers that allow the network to acquire the nonlinear mapping from joint to task coordinates. This mapping is represented in the pattern of interlayer weights learned during network backpropagation training. Once the network training is complete and the forward kinematic mapping is learned, the Jacobian elements for a given posture can be recovered in a relatively straightforward manner [12].

Specifically, the joint angles for a particular posture are applied as inputs to the trained network and, for each cell in the hidden and output layers, the derivative (δ) of the cell's output (z) with respect to its input is computed. For typical cells with "logistic" activation functions,

$$\delta = z(1-z) \tag{4}$$

When all δ's for the ith layer are arranged into the elements of a diagonal matrix, Δi, the Jacobian matrix, $J(\theta)$, for the input posture is given as:

$$J = \Delta_{out} W_{out, H2} \Delta_{H2} W_{H2, H1} \Delta_{H1} W_{H1, in} \tag{5}$$

where W_{ij} denotes the matrix of weights connecting layer-j to layer-i. Note that the elements of J change as the input posture changes, due to the corresponding changes in the network cells' output values in the Δ_i matrices, thus capturing the posture-dependence of the ideal, analytic Jacobian, $J(\theta)$, described by Equation (3).

This same method can be used for computing the "acoustic" Jacobian using articulator positions as inputs and, for example, formants as outputs. Once the corresponding "acoustic" Jacobian is derived, the UCM method can be used to test the hypotheses of constriction and acoustic controlled variables against one another.

3.   Summary And Conclusions

The issues faced in general when investigating the controlled variables in skilled movement were described. Evidence was reviewed supporting the position that these variables are abstractly and functionally defined at the level of *task space* coordinates rather than at the more concretely defined level of musculoskeletal coordinates. The issue of deciding which task-space coordinates comprise the controlled variables for a given skill was discussed, with an emphasis on the alternate hypotheses for speech production of constriction vs. acoustic/auditory task spaces. A promising method for distinguishing among hypothesized task spaces, the *uncontrolled manifold method*, was reviewed in detail using a relatively simple example of a planar three joint arm. Central to this method is the specification of the forward kinematic mapping from articulator position to task space position, and the Jacobian of this mapping. It was shown how neural network methods could be used to define both this mapping and its Jacobian even in cases, such as the mapping from articulator position to acoustic coordinates in speech production, where the mapping can not be written analytically in equation form. We conclude that this method is a promising one and are currently attempting to implement it to distinguish between constriction and acoustic task spaces for vowel production (at Haskins Laboratories), as well as between center of mass position and head position task spaces for the control of locomotion (at Boston University).

Acknowledgements

This work was supported by NIH grant DC-03663

References

[1] Bailly, G., Laboissière, R., and Schwartz, J.L. "Formant trajectories as audible gestures: An alternative for speech synthesis." *J Phonetics*, 19, 9-23, 1991.

[2] Browman, C.P. and Goldstein, L. "Articulatory gestures as phonological units." *Phonology*, 6, 151-206, 1989.

[3] Browman, C.P. and Goldstein, L. "Tiers in articulatory phonology, with some implications for casual speech." In J. Kingston and M.E. Beckman, eds., *Papers in laboratory phonology: I. Between the grammar and the physics of speech.* (pp. 341-338) Cambridge, England: Cambridge University Press, 1990.

[4] Browman, C.P. and Goldstein, L. "Articulatory phonology: An overview." *Phonetica, 49,* 155-180, 1992.

[5] Browman, C. and Goldstein, L. "Towards an articulatory phonology." In C. Ewan and J. Anderson eds., *Phonology yearbook 3* (pp. 219-252). Cambridge: Cambridge University Press, 1986.

[6] Carroll, J.D., Green, P.E., and Chaturvedi, A. *Mathematical tools for applied multivariate analysis.* New York: Academic Press, 1997.

[7] Gay, T.J., Lindblom, B., and Lubker, J. "Production of bite-block vowels: Acoustic equivalence by selective compensation." *J Acoust Soc Am, 69,* 802-810, 1981.

[8] Guenther, F.H. "A neural network model of speech acquisition and motor equivalent speech production." *Biological Cybernetics*, 72, 43-53, 1994.

[9] Guenther, F.H. "Speech sound acquisition, coarticulation, and rate effects in a neural network model of speech production." *Psychological Review*, 102, 594-621, 1995.

[10] Guenther, F.H., Hampson, M., and Johnson, D. "A theoretical investigation of reference frames for the planning of speech movements." *Psychological Review*, 105, 611-633, 1998.

[11] Johnson, K., Ladefoged, P., and Lindau, M. "Individual differences in vowel production." *J Acoust Soc Am*, 94, 701-714, 1994.

[12] Jordan, M.I. "Constrained supervised learning." *Journal of Mathematical Psychology*, 36, 396-425, 1992.

[13] Kaburagi, T, and Honda, M. "A trajectory formation model of articulatory movements based on the motor tasks of phoneme-specific vocal tract shapes." *Proc. Internat. Conf. on Spoken Lang. Processing (ICSLP 94), Yokahama, Japan.*, vol. II (pp. 579-582). Acoustical Society of Japan, 1994.

[14] Kelso, J.A.S., Tuller, B., Vatikiotis-Bateson, E., and Fowler, C.A. "Functionally specific articulatory cooperation following jaw perturbations during speech: Evidence for coordinative structures." *J Exp Psych: Human Percep and Perform*, 10, 812-832, 1984.

[15] Kröger, B.J., Schröder, G., and Opgen-Rhein, C. "A gesture-based dynamic model describing articulatory movement data." *J Acoust Soc Am*, 98, 1878-1889, 1995.

[16] Lindblom, B., Lubker, J., and Gay, T. "Formant frequencies of some fixed-mandible vowels and a model of speech motor programming by predictive simulation." *J Phonetics*, 7, 147-161, 1979.

[17] Mottet, D., Guiard, Y., Ferrand, T., and Bootsma, R.J. "Two-handed performance of a rhythmical Fitts task by individuals and dyads." *J Exp Psych: Human Percep and Perform*, 27, 1275-1286, 2001.

[18] Perkell, J.S., Matthies, M.L., Svirsky, M.A., and Jordan, M.I. "Trading relations between tongue-body raising and lip rounding in production of the vowel /u/: A pilot motor equivalence study." *J Acoust Soc Am*, 93, 2948-2961, 1993.

[19] Rumelhart, D.E., Hinton, G.E., and Williams, R.J. "Learning internal representations by error propagation." In D.E. Rumelhart and J.L. McLelland, eds., *Parallel distributed processing: Explorations in the microstructure of cognition, Vol 1. Foundations.* Cambridge, MA: MIT Press, 1986.

[20] Saltzman, E. "Task dynamic coordination of the speech articulators: A preliminary model." *Exp Brain Research,* Series 15, 129-144, 1986.

[21] Saltzman, E. and Byrd, D. "Task-dynamics of gestural timing: Phase windows and multifrequency rhythms." *Human Movement Science,* 19(4), 499-526, 2000.

[22] Saltzman, E.L., and Kelso, J.A.S. "Skilled actions: A task dynamic approach." *Psychological Review,* 94, 84-106, 1987.

[23] Saltzman, E.L., and Munhall, K.G. "A dynamical approach to gestural patterning in speech production." *Ecological Psychology*, 1, 333-382, 1989.

[24] Scholz, J.P., and Schöner, G. "The uncontrolled manifold concept: Identifying control variables for a functional task." *Exp Brain Research*, 126, 289-306, 1999.

[25] Scholz, J.P., Schöner, G., and Latash, M.L. "Identifying the control structure of multijoint coordination during pistol shooting." *Exp Brain Research*, 135, 382-404, 2000.

Dynamics of Speech Production and Perception
P. Divenyi et al. (Eds.)
IOS Press, 2006

The Achievement of Somatosensory Targets as an Independent Goal of Speech Production – Special Status of Vowel-to-Vowel Transitions

Stéphanie TREMBLAY[1] and David OSTRY[1,2]
[1]*McGill University, Montreal, Quebec, Canada*
[2]*Haskins Laboratories, New Haven, Connecticut, USA*

Abstract. A number of studies have explored the contribution of auditory information in speech production. On the other hand, little attention has been devoted to the possible role of somatosensory feedback in the achievement of speech goals. Nevertheless, the ability of individuals who become deaf as adults to produce intelligible speech could indeed be maintained by somatosensory information. This paper presents the use of a method which manipulates somatosensory feedback independent of speech acoustics, allowing direct assessment of the importance of somatosensation in speech. A robotic device applied mechanical loads to the jaw during speech production. The device significantly altered somatosensory feedback without perturbing the speech acoustics. In a previous study (Tremblay, Shiller & Ostry, 2003), we showed that sensorimotor adaptation to mechanical loads is observed during both vocalized and silent speech. That is, even in the absence of acoustic perturbation, subjects modified their motor commands in order to reach desired somatosensory targets. Thus, the Tremblay et al. study provided direct evidence that somatosensory input is central to the achievement of speech targets. However, in that experiment, the observed patterns of adaptation were specific to movements involving a vowel-to-vowel transition. To investigate this somewhat surprising outcome, the present study explores patterns of adaptation by manipulating the location of the vowel-to-vowel transition within the speech utterance. The goal was to identify the linguistic units for which the achievement of specific somatosensory targets might be important. The present results are consistent with the findings of the previous study: adaptation to a mechanical load is only achieved in portions of speech movements that are associated with a vowel-to-vowel transition. The results are discussed in terms of mechanical and acoustic properties of vowel production.

Keywords. Somatosensory feedback, speech production, motor learning

Introduction

A common view in speech research is that the motor system controlling speech is organized with the aim of achieving acoustic goals. One finding that has been used to support this idea is the demonstration that subjects compensate for perturbations in which acoustic feedback is altered, while somatosensory feedback remains unchanged. For example, Jones and Munhall [7] have altered fundamental frequency ($F0$) feedback during vowel production. Subjects were asked to repeat vowels while hearing the acoustic feedback of their own speech production through earphones. The feedback was transformed such that the pitch was slowly and progressively shifted to a lower or a higher level (depending on the condition). The authors showed that subjects gradually compensated for an increase in $F0$ by lowering their pitch, and vice versa. Therefore, pitch seems to be sensitive to altered acoustic feedback. In another study, Houde and Jordan [6] used a different approach to alter acoustic information. They used an apparatus that provided feedback of shifted formant frequencies. They asked subjects to produce consonant-vowel-consonant (CVC) utterances that contained the sound /ɛ/. The first and the second formant frequencies were increasingly shifted until the actual production of the sound /ɛ/ provided acoustic feedback corresponding to /i/ or /æ/, depending on the treatment condition. They found that subjects gradually altered their production of speech utterances to a point where they actually articulated the vowel /a/ in order to hear /ɛ/. These two studies show situations in which acoustic feedback plays a fundamental role in the production of speech targets.

The capacity of intelligible speech by deaf speakers suggests that somatosensory information may similarly play a role in the achievement of speech goals [5]. A number of techniques have resulted in the alteration of somatosensory feedback during speech production. In a series of experiments, Baum and McFarland report that speakers can compensate for the presence of an artificial palate that modifies the internal shape of the vocal tract [1][2][8]. Other investigators have used perturbations that impede jaw or lip movements — such as bite blocks and lip tubes — that have modified somatosensory feedback [3][9][10]. Similarly, they found that subjects can adapt to such perturbations. These results indicate the importance of somatosensory information in the production of speech: speakers adapt to the perturbations in order to achieve specific vocal tract shapes, that this, somatosensory targets. However, in these experiments, perturbations which alter somatosensory feedback simultaneously produce an effect on the acoustic output. Therefore, one cannot rule out the possibility that the adaptation has been achieved in order to maintain desired acoustic feedback.

In a previous study [11], we reported the first demonstration of an alteration of somatosensory feedback in the absence of acoustic perturbation. We have borrowed a technique used in studies of arm movements to apply mechanical loads to the jaw. The perturbation was sufficiently strong to create a deviation in the movement path of the jaw, and hence somatosensory feedback, without affecting the associated acoustic output. It consisted of forces which pulled the jaw in the protrusion direction. The strength of the forces was correlated with the jaw instantaneous vertical velocity. We have altered somatosensory feedback in three different conditions: (1) normal vocalized speech, in which the subjects had to repeatedly produce the utterance *siat* (pronounced see-at) at a subject chosen rate and volume, (2) "silent speech" (speech without vocalization), in which subjects were required to articulate the utterance *siat* without producing any sound, and (3) non-speech jaw movements, in which the subjects had to produce movements that are matched in amplitude and duration to those observed in the speech conditions. There was no reference whatsoever to speech production in the description of the third task. The first two conditions were tested to assess the extent to which adaptation to a somatosensory perturbation might occur in the presence of unaltered acoustic feedback (condition 1) and when acoustic feedback was absent altogether (condition 2).

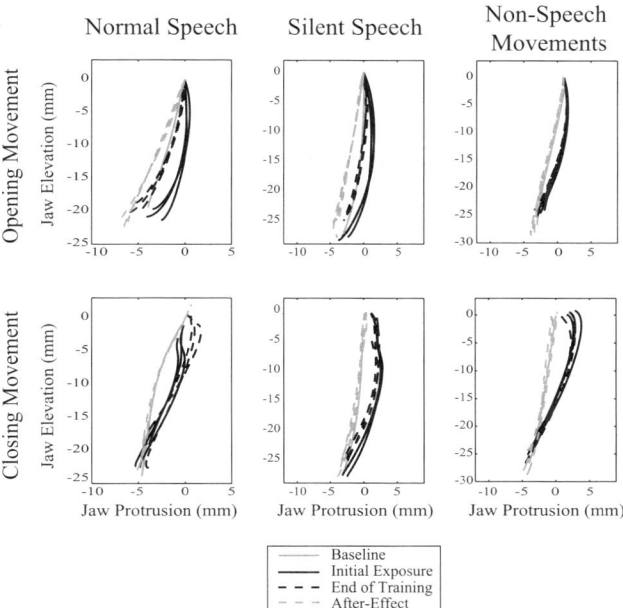

Figure 1. Sagittal plane jaw motion paths during the baseline condition (shown in gray), initial exposure to the force-field (black), at the end of training (black dotted lines), and following unexpected removal of the field (gray dotted lines). The figure shows individual trials for single subjects. Top panels show the opening phase of the movements, whereas the bottom panels show the closing phase. Adaptation to the force-field is represented by both a restoration of the jaw path from initial exposure to the force field to baseline movements, and a subsequent motion dependent after-effect in a direction opposite to the force field. A. During vocalized speech, adaptation to the force-field is observed in the opening phase of the movement, but not in the closing phase. B. During silent speech, the pattern of adaptation observed in vocalized speech is unaltered by removal of acoustic feedback: adaptation is observed in the opening phase only. C. Matched non-speech movements show no adaptation in any phase of the movement.

The third condition examined whether adaptation would occur in matched jaw movement tasks in which the speech component has been removed.

Our results showed that adaptation to a velocity dependent force field can be observed on the basis of somatosensory feedback alone (Figure 1). Subsequent acoustic analyses confirmed that the perturbations had no effect on the speech acoustics. For example, no difference was found in F1 and F2 frequencies during the transition between vowels when the subjects repeated utterances in the force field as compared to when the movements were produced in the baseline condition. Moreover, a perceptual discrimination task revealed that listeners were unable to identify the utterances that were produced during the initial exposure to the force field [11]. These results showed that, even when the acoustic goal is achieved, subjects modify their motor commands in order to reach somatosensory targets. The adaptation was not observed in the third condition, in which the speech component had been removed. This indicates that matching jaw movements on amplitude and duration is not sufficient to achieve the adaptation observed in the normal vocalized and the silent speech groups. Moreover, this is an indication that in speech, subjects work to maintain an entire articulatory trajectory, and not, for example, just movement start and end.

Another outcome of that study was that subjects compensated for the perturbation only in portions of the movement that held the vowel-to-vowel transition, that is, in the opening portion of the movement (s-i- æ). This pattern of adaptation was observed in both normal vocalized speech and silent speech (Figure 1(a) and 1(b)). The present study was performed with two purposes. Firstly, we wanted to replicate the findings that in speech, subjects work to maintain somatosensory targets independent of the acoustic output. Secondly, we were interested in exploring to what extent the sensorimotor adaptation to the mechanical load is specific to portions of the speech movement that held a vowel-to-vowel transition. More precisely, we wanted to know whether the lack of adaptation in the closing movement was due to the mechanical or geometrical components of the task or whether it was a consequence of the absence of a vowel-to-vowel transition. For that purpose, we varied the location of the vowel-to-vowel transition in the speech utterance in order to examine whether the subjects would restrict their adaptation to the opening phase of the movement or if they would adapt in the portion of the movement that held the vowel-to-vowel transition.

1. Methods

Eight subjects were randomly assigned to one of the two experimental conditions. The subjects had no known speech, hearing or other motor problems. Also, none of them had dental implants, prostheses, crowns or temporomandibular joint dysfunctions.

1.1 Materials

The force was delivered by a servo-controlled robotic manipulator; the Sensable Technologies Phantom 1.0 (www.sensable.com) (Figure 2(a)). The Phantom consists of a cable-drive mechanism with encoders for position measurement (0.03 mm nominal position resolution) and a six axis ATI Nano-17 force/torque sensor (www.ati-ia.com). The latter was mounted on the tip of the robot for measurement of subject's applied forces and torques. The subject's jaw was connected to the Phantom through a custom built 3D magnesium and titanium connector that links the ATI force/torque sensor to the subject's lower appliance and to the jaw (see below). A metal structure was built in order to eliminate head movements. The restraint was necessary since even small perturbations produce significant head motion. Movements were eliminated by fixing the position of the upper teeth and, consequently, the skull. Two metal sleeves situated at each side of the subject's mouth fit around the metal rods coming out of the upper appliance. These sleeves were connected to metal bars that were themselves fixed to a non-movable structure. All pieces were attached together by rotary joints that were locked in place such that every part of the head restraint was independently adjustable to the subject's comfort. When a subject was initially positioned *in* the head restraint, the rotary joints were unlocked, and the subject would move freely in every degree of freedom. However, once the subject was locked in position, the head stayed completely still. Two acrylic and metal appliances -one for the lower teeth and one for the upper teeth- were custom built for each subject and served to attach the subject to the robot (the lower appliance) and to the head restraint apparatus (the upper appliance). The appliances were glued to the subject's teeth with a dental adhesive (*Isodent*).

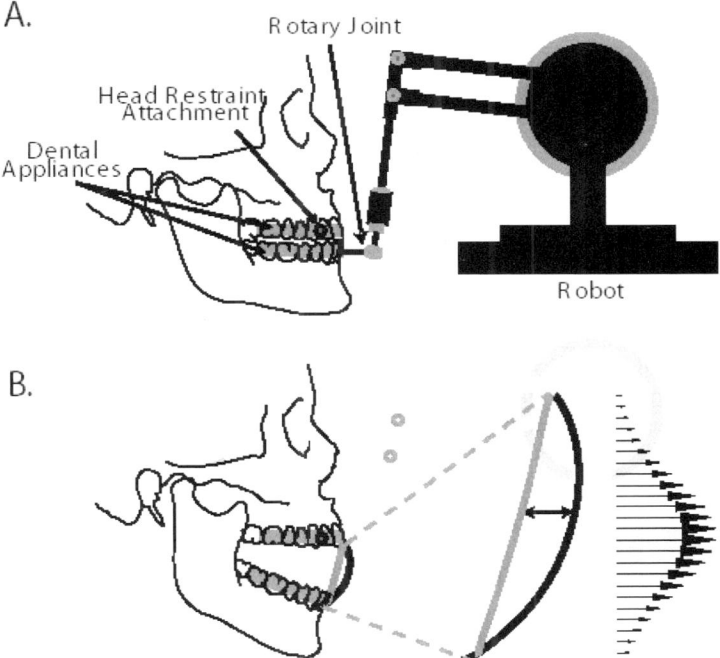

Figure 2. A. Schematic showing subject attached to the robotic device. B. Jaw opening movement with the force-field off (grey) and upon initial exposure to the field (black). Vectors depict the magnitude and direction of force applied by the robot over the course of the movement. The double headed-arrow shows the maximum horizontal deviation between null-field and force-field movements which served as a performance index.

1.2 Force Field

Perturbations produced by the robot pulled the jaw in the protrusion direction (Figure 2(b)). Force amplitude varied in proportion of the instantaneous vertical velocity of the mandibular incisors. When velocity of jaw opening and closing movements increased, perturbing forces increased in the direction of jaw protrusion. Similarly, when jaw velocity decreased, forces decreased. Consequently, no force was applied when the jaw was at rest, which has the advantage of reducing potential subject fatigue. A force of 0.02 N was delivered for each millimeter per second of jaw velocity. The maximum force during a typical opening and closing cycle ranged from 3 to 4 N at peak velocity. As a safety feature, no more than 7 N were delivered. Thus, if the jaw reached a speed of 350 mm/sec or above, the Phantom was automatically deactivated.

1.3 Tasks

The eight subjects were equally divided into two groups. The subjects of the first group were asked to repeatedly produce an utterance in which the vowel-to-vowel transition took place in the opening movement, namely *sias* (pronounced "s-i-æ-s"). The second group was trained with an utterance in which the vowel-to-vowel transition was in the

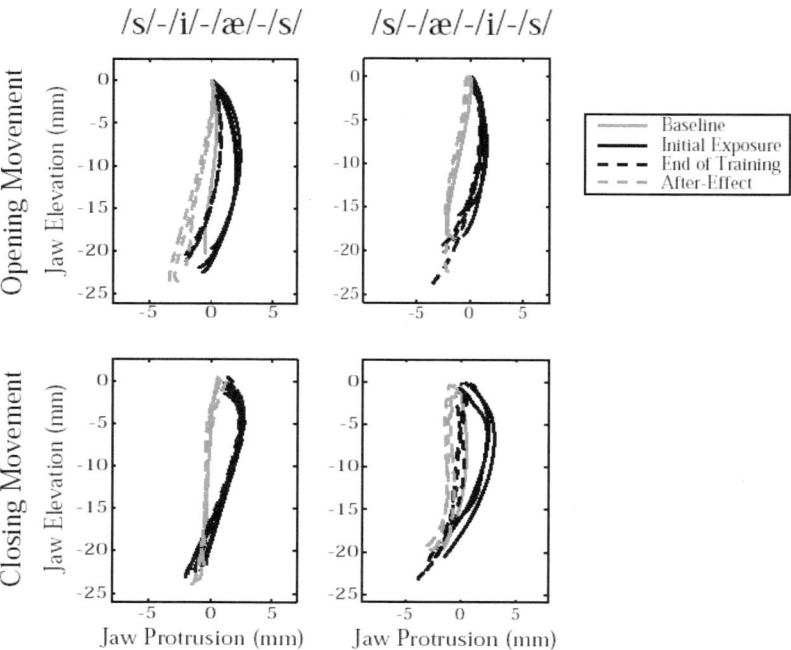

Figure 3. Sagittal plane jaw motion paths during the baseline condition (gray), initial exposure to the force-field (black), at the end of training (black dotted lines), and following unexpected removal of the field (gray dotted lines). The figure shows individual trials for single subjects. The top row shows the opening phase of the movements, whereas the bottom row shows the closing phase. During the production of siæs, adaptation to the force-field and a subsequent after-effect are observed in the opening phase, but not in the closing phase. During the production of sæis, the pattern of adaptation and after-effect are observed in the closing phase of the movement only.

closing portion of the speech movement (*sais*). Every subject was required to produce the assigned utterance at his preferred rate and volume. The experimenter monitored a real-time display of movement parameters and provided verbal feedback when amplitude, duration or volume deviated from their initial values by more than ~20%.

1.4 Experimental Design

The experiment began with three blocks of trials, each of which contained 10 repetitions of the test utterance. Note that during these three blocks, no force was applied to the jaw. This practice phase allowed the subject to familiarize himself with the head restraint and the robot. This practice phase was followed by the collection of a baseline dataset, which comprised one block of twenty utterances produced in the null field condition. This block served as a reference to which we compared the movements produced in the force field condition. A training phase consisted of 35 blocks of 15 trials each produced in the force field condition. In the final phase, the force field was suddenly turned off. This phase consisted of two blocks of 15 trials performed in the null field condition and measured a possible after-effect following the completion of the adaptation.

1.5 Data Analyses

The three dimensional position of the jaw at the incisors was sampled at 1KHz and digitally low-pass filtered at 10 Hz off-line. One complete jaw movement in the current experiment corresponded to an opening and a closing movement. The start and the end of each movement were individually scored based on 10% of the peak tangential velocity of the opening and closing movements respectively. Once scored, the representation of jaw motion was transformed into a 3D head-centered coordinate frame. The origin of this new coordinate frame was the tip of the maxillary incisors at occlusion and the horizontal axis was aligned with the occlusal plane. Motor adaptation was quantified by the decrease in the maximum horizontal distance (mm) between each movement and the baseline path over the course of the training phase. The baseline was derived from the average of movements produced in the initial null field phase. Maximum horizontal distances of the first 20% trials exposed to the force field were compared to the last 20% trials of the training phase. Statistical analyses using ANOVA were conducted for each subject separately. The analyses compared the four phases of the experiment (baseline, first 20% of the training trial, last 20% of the training trials, and null field trial after training – after-effect). Pair-wise comparisons of means were carried out using Tukey's method, where appropriate.

2. Results

Analyses of kinematic data revealed a systematic pattern of force-field adaptation in the portion of the speech movement that held the vowel-to-vowel transition. Figure 3 illustrates opening movements (top panels) and closing movement (bottom panels) for individual subjects in the group that produced the utterance *sias* (left panels), and the group that was tested with the utterance *sais* (right panels). As depicted by the black lines, the jaw path deviated in the direction of protrusion with the introduction of the force-field. Following training   (shown in black dotted lines), it can be noted that the group which produced the utterance *sias* reduced their deviation in the opening portion of the movements (s-i-æ), but not in the closing portion (æ-s). The opposite pattern was observed in the group that produced the utterance *sais*: the subjects did not adapt in the opening portion of the movement (s- æ), but did reduce their deviation in the closing portion (æ-i-s). A motion dependant after-effect (shown in gray dotted lines) was found in portions of the speech movements where adaptation was observed — i.e. in the opening movements of the *sias* group and in the closing movements of the *sais* group. This after-effect was measured at the end of the training session when the field was unexpectedly removed. It is characterized by a jaw path which is retracted as compared to the baseline, that is, in a direction opposite to the perturbation.

Figure 4 gives mean values of maximum horizontal deviation in opening and closing movements for each subject separately. The black lines indicate that the force-field similarly altered the path of the jaw both in opening and closing movements of each condition: movements at the start of training (in black) deviated significantly in the protrusion direction compared to the baseline ($p < 0.001$ for all subjects). After training (shown in black dotted lines), a significant reduction in deviation from baseline indicates that adaptation was achieved in the opening movement for all subjects of the *sias*

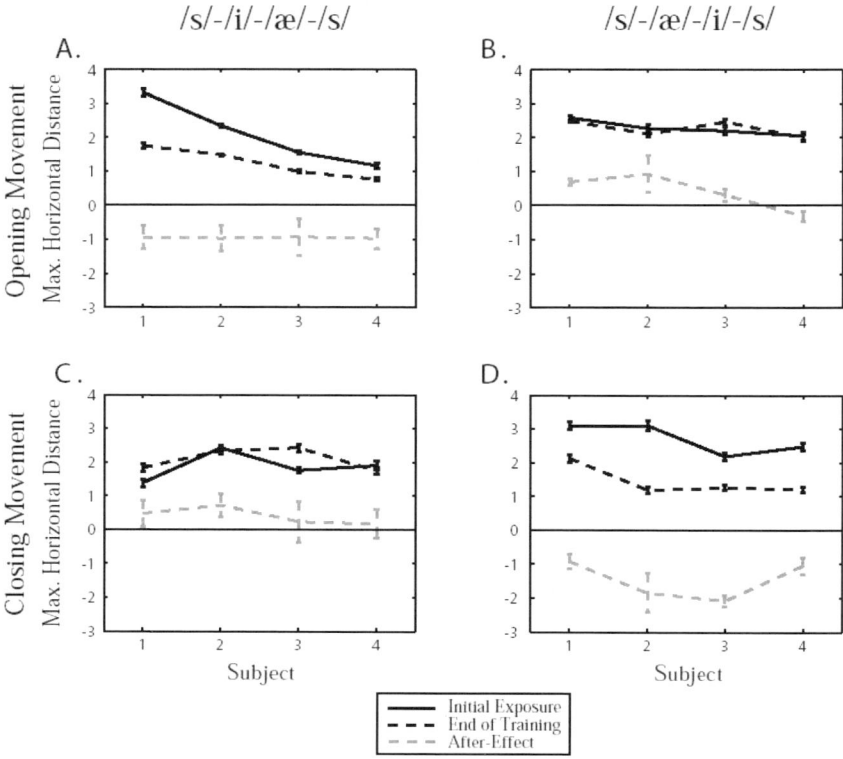

Figure 4. Average values of maximum horizontal deviation shown on a per subject basis for initial exposure to the force field (in black), end of the training session (in black dotted lines), and following the unexpected removal of the force field (in gray dotted lines). *A.* In the opening phase of the movement, all subjects of the *sias* group showed a decrease in the maximum horizontal deviation and a significant motion dependant after-effect, whereas in *B.* none of the subjects in the *sais* group adapted to the force field in this same phase of the movement. *C.* None of the subjects in the sias group showed adaptation in the closing movement, but *D.* all subjects of the sais group adapted to the force field in the closing phase of the movement.

group ($p < 0.001$) and in the closing movement for all subjects of the *sais* group ($p < 0.001$) (Figures 4(a) and 4(d)). In contrast, adaptation was not achieved in the closing movement of the *sias* group or in the opening movement of the *sais* condition. That is, movements at the end of training did not differ reliably from those at the beginning ($p > 0.05$), except for one subject (3rd subject of the *sias* group; closing movements), for which the deviation increased over time (Figure 4(c)). Finally, a motion dependent after-effect (depicted in gray dotted lines) was observed in the opening movement of the *sias* condition and in the closing movement of the *sais* condition ($p < 0.001$ in all cases). This suggests that the subjects adapted their jaw movements by modifying their motor commands in order to counteract the effect of the field. When the field was unexpectedly removed, resulting paths reflected the change in the motor commands the nervous system had to generate in order to cancel out the external perturbation and to produce adapted movements. An after-effect was not observed in portions of speech movements where adaptation was not achieved, i.e. in the closing portion of the *sias* movements and

	Peak Velocity; Null Field		Maximum Initial Deviation	
SIAS Condition	Opening	Closing	Opening	Closing
Subject 1	0.2221*	0.1739	3.3499	2.0056
Subject 2	0.2396	0.2249	2.5831	2.4630
Subject 3	0.1691	0.1919*	1.7729	2.1173
Subject 4	0.2188	0.2453	0.8509	2.3567*

* $p < 0.01$

Table 1. Peak velocity and maximum initial deviation for the *sias* group on a per subject basis. The first two columns display the mean peak velocity of the trials in the null field consdition for the opening and the closing movement separately. The third and the fourth columns show the average of the maximum horizontal distance between the average baseline and the trials of the initial block under force field conditions.

in the opening portion of the *sais* movements (Figure 4(b) and 4(c)) ($p > 0.05$ in all cases).

These results indicate that the lack of adaptation in the closing movement of the previous study (described in the introduction section of this chapter) was not a consequence the geometry or dynamics of the orofacial apparatus. It is possible to adapt to this force field in the closing phase of a speech movement, as long as it involves a vowel-to-vowel transition. So, why is this the case? One possibility is that vowel-to-vowel transitions involve a higher velocity movement, and consequently are associated with greater perturbations. It is reasonable to believe that subjects would tend to first restore the movement paths in which the perturbation is greatest. To investigate this possibility, we compared the peak velocity of the opening movements to the peak velocity of the closing movements in the null field trials preceding training. Statistical analyses using Paired-sample T-tests were carried out on a per subject basis. Results are given in Table 1 (*sias* condition) and Table 2 (*sais* condition). The peak velocity of the opening movement was significantly higher for one subject of the *sias* group and one subject of the *sais* group ($p < 0.01$). Moreover, one subject of the *sias* group and one subject of the *sais* group showed a significantly higher peak velocity in the closing movement portion of the movement ($p < 0.01$). Overall, no systematic pattern suggests that the peak velocity was higher in portions of the movement that held the vowel-to-vowel transition. We also explored the possibility that initial exposure to the force field

	Peak Velocity; Null Field		Maximum Initial Deviation	
SAIS Condition	Opening	Closing	Opening	Closing
Subject 1	0.2286*	0.2036	2.8013	3.6640*
Subject 2	0.1669	0.1543	2.0460	3.3760*
Subject 3	0.1801	0.2583*	1.7307	2.3113
Subject 4	0.2335	0.2603	2.2080	3.0767*

* $p < 0.01$

Table 2. Peak velocity and maximum initial deviation for the *sais* group on a per subject basis. The information provided in this table is comparable to the previous table, but concerns the subjects of the second condition (*sais* group).

had a greater effect in the portion of the movement that held the vowel-to-vowel transition than in the other half of the movement. Paired-sample T-tests were used to compare the maximum horizontal deviation of the opening movement and the closing movement during the very first block of the training session (15 repetitions). Results found in Table 1 and 2 show that one subject of the *sias* group and three subjects of the *sais* group were significantly more perturbed in the closing movement than in the opening movement during first exposure to the force field ($p < 0.01$). However, there was no systematic pattern to the initial perturbation effects. Overall, this suggests that the achievement of adaptation in the vowel-to-vowel transition is not due to higher velocity or greater perturbation in the vowel-to-vowel transition.

3. Discussion

The results of the present study can be summarized as follows: (1) as observed in the previous study, subjects adapted to a velocity dependent force field that altered somatosensory feedback during speech production and (2) adaptation was obtained in portions of the speech movement that held a vowel-to-vowel transition.

The reduction in maximum deviation is a demonstration that individuals adjust their speech movements when exposed to a velocity dependent force field, which indicates that the nervous system takes account of dynamics while planning speech movements. The presence of a motion dependent after-effect shows that subjects adjusted their motor commands to cancel out the effect of the field by applying a force which is equal but opposite to the one delivered by the robot. This *after-effect* is indicative of the adjustments that the nervous system makes in order to produce movements characterized by relatively normal kinematic output under the influence of the field. This shows that the subjects learned the relationship between the field strength and the jaw velocity and, based on this information, compensate for the force field by applying the appropriate amount of force in the opposite direction. Overall, the results are consistent with previous work [11], which shows that a somatosensory goal, independent of the acoustics, is pursued in speech production.

A second finding is that subjects adapt to the force field only in the portion of the speech movement that involved the vowel-to-vowel transition. We explore the possibility that the finding arose because of mechanical reasons. For example, the effect of the perturbation and/or the peak velocity could have been greater in the vowel-to-vowel transition than in the consonant-vowel or vowel-consonant transitions. Under such conditions, it would have been understandable for subjects to correct first for the more salient error. However, statistical analyses did not support this explanation: neither the peak velocity in null field nor the effect of the perturbation at initial exposure to the field was greater in the vowel-to-vowel transition than in the consonant-vowel or vowel-consonant transitions. It seems that the pattern of adaptation observed in this study is not due to mechanical aspects of the experiment.

A second possible explanation involves the acoustic properties of a vowel-to-vowel transition. It could be hypothesized that the required precision of speech movements is higher during vowel-to-vowel transitions than during consonant-vowel or vowel-consonant transitions. More specifically, it may be the case that the transition between two vocal tract shapes associated with vowels follows a precise kinematic pattern. This is consistent with a study carried out by Carré et al. [4], in which the experimenters manipulated the shape of the transition between the vowels *i* and *a* in F1 and F2 frequency space. In that study, two methods of deformation of the frequency transition between vowels were tested. A longitudinal deformation consisted of a displacement of the constriction location parallel to the main axis of the vocal tract, whereas the transversal deformation refers to a displacement perpendicular to the same axis. The authors presented to listeners pairs of vowel-to-vowel transitions that have been produced with either the same or two different methods of deformation. Then, they asked subjects if the transitions sounded similar or different, and if different which of the two sounded more natural. They found that subjects could easily detect when two different methods were used to produce the transitions. Moreover, unanimously, subjects preferred the transversal way of deforming F1 and F2 paths between the two vowel targets. These results suggest that during speech production, speakers might follow a precise pattern of kinematics while producing a vowel-to-vowel transition. Consequently, speakers would be more inclined to correct for a perturbation that disrupted this precise transition pattern. This could explain why the subjects of the present study showed adaptation in the portion of the movement that held the vowel-to-vowel transition. Extensions to this procedure may offer a means to explore the relative precision requirements of somatosensory feedback during speech.

References

[1] Baum, S.R. and McFarland, D.H. "Individual differences in speech adaptation to an artificial palate." *J. Acous. Soc. Am.* 107: 3572-3575, 2000.

[2] Baum, S.R. and McFarland, D.H. "The development of speech adaptation to an artificial palate." *J. Acous. Soc. Am.* 102: 2353-2359, 1997.

[3] Baum, S.R., McFarland, D.H. and Diab, M. "Compensation to articulatory perturbation: perceptual data." *J. Acous. Soc. Am.* 99: 3791-3794, 1996.

[4] Carré, R., Ainsworth, W.A., Jospa, P., Maeda, S. and Pasdeloup, V. "Perception of vowel-to-vowel transitions with different formant trajectories. *Phonetica* 58(3): 163-178, 2001.

[5] Cowie, R. and Douglas-Cowie, E. "Postlingually acquired deafness." In *Trends in Linguistics, Studies and Monographs* (Vol. 2), New York: Mouton de Gruyter, 1992.

[6] Houde, J.F. and Jordan, M.I. "Sensorimotor adaptation in speech production." *Science* 279: 1213-1216, 1998.

[7] Jones, J.A. and Munhall K.G. "Perceptual calibration of f_0 production: Evidence from feedback perturbation." *J. Acous. Soc. Am.* 108: 1246-1251, 2000.

[8] McFarland, D.H., Baum, S.R. and Chabot, C. "Speech compensation to structural modifications of the oral cavity." *J. Acous. Soc. Am.* 100: 1093-1104, 1996.

[9] McFarland, D.H. and Baum, S.R. "Incomplete compensation to articulatory perturbation." *J. Acous. Soc. Am.* 97: 1865-1873, 1995.

[10] Savariaux, C., Perrier, P. and Orliaguet, J.P. "Compensation strategies for the perturbation of the rounded vowel [u] using a lip tube: A study of the control of space in speech production." *J. Acous. Soc. Am.* 98: 2428-2442, 1995.

[11] Tremblay, S., Shiller, D.M. and Ostry, D.J. "Somatosensory basis of speech production." *Nature*, 423: 866-869, 2003.

Dynamics of Speech Production and Perception
P. Divenyi et al. (Eds.)
IOS Press, 2006

Respiratory System Pressures at the Start of an Utterance

Janet SLIFKA
Research Laboratory of Electronics
Massachusetts Institute of Technology
Cambridge, Massachusetts, USA

Abstract. When a person begins to speak, the motions of the respiratory system, vocal folds, and articulators are coordinated through relatively large excursions in a small window of time. As the pressure drive for creating a sound source is established and the articulators move appropriately for the initial sound segment, acoustic cues are generated that form the set of prosodic cues associated with the start of an utterance. The principles underlying variation in these acoustic cues could be better quantified given additional data on the coordination of the respiratory system actions. In this chapter, net muscular pressures from Campbell diagrams are analyzed for normal read speech in American English. As a speaker starts talking, the respiratory system executes a rapid and large change in net muscular pressure with very little volume change. Utterance onset generally begins during net inspiratory muscular pressure - prior to the point at which the respiratory system has generated a 'relatively constant working level' for alveolar pressure. A limited number of pauses within a breath group (silent and filled) are examined, and all show a distinct change in the momentum of the respiratory system. Respiratory system involvement is present for various types of sound segments at the pause as well as various locations of pauses within the utterance.

Keywords. Speech breathing, prosodic boundaries, respiratory physiology, utterance initiation, filled and unfilled pauses

Introduction

The speech production system involves a wide range of structures that includes the diaphragm and chest wall of the respiratory system, the vocal folds, and the articulators. One instance where the motions of these structures are coordinated through relatively large excursions is when a speaker starts talking. In a small window of time, the pressure drive for creating a sound source must be established, the constriction in the airway for generating sound must be created, and the articulators must move appropriately for the initial sound segment. These actions are also involved in creating the acoustic cues to the start of an utterance. Some of the physiological correlates to these cues are examined in this chapter, which looks more closely at the details of the motions and forces in the respiratory system when a speaker starts talking. The data include the acoustic signal as well as several physiologically-related signals for normal read speech as produced by four native speakers of American English. In an attempt to characterize the muscular

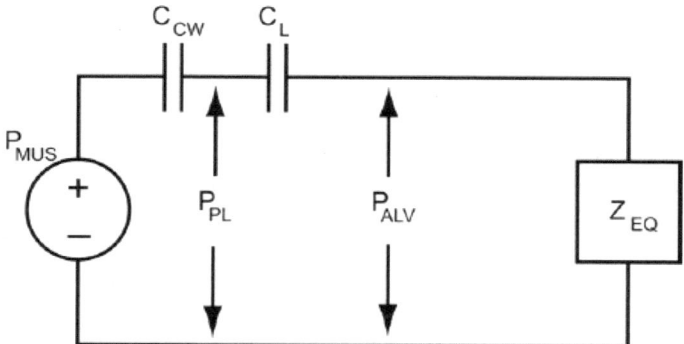

Figure 1. Simple model of the respiratory system using pressure as the across variable and volume velocity as the through variable. P_{PL} is the pleural pressure, and P_{ALV} is the alveolar pressure. C_{CW} is the compliance of the chest wall, and C_L is the compliance of the lungs. Z_{EQ} is the equivalent impedance facing air leaving the lungs. P_{MUS} is the net muscular force applied to the system.

habits of the subjects during speech, no special requests were made of the speakers regarding lung volume, syllable prominence, or loudness. The analysis concentrates on net muscular force and respiratory system dynamics. This methodology is extended, in some aspects, to speech boundaries that do not align with breath boundaries, such as pauses within a breath group.

1.   The Respiratory System

The respiratory system is dominated by two elastic elements: the lungs and the chest wall (as in Rahn et al. [10]). These can be thought of as two springs. One spring, the lungs, is relatively small at rest. The other spring, the chest wall, is relatively large at rest. When the two are coupled through the fluid-filled pleural space, the lungs/chest wall system reaches an equilibrium volume called the relaxation volume (V_{rel}) where the force of the lungs to collapse is countered by an equal and opposite force of the chest wall to expand. This is the rest position of the respiratory system. To breathe, a person applies muscular force to stretch the spring system. Passive recoil forces of the spring system are available to pull the lungs back down toward the rest position. Normal breathing requires work in just one direction - inhalation. The force applied to the lungs comes from the pressure in the fluid in the pleural space, called the pleural pressure (P_{PL}). Generally, in normal breathing, exhalation ends slightly above V_{rel}, (for example, Loring and Mead [9]), at the functional residual capacity (FRC). Vital capacity (VC) is the volume change between the maximally stretched and maximally compressed lungs/chest wall system. FRC is generally in the range of 30-40%VC.

These forces, the muscular force and the recoil force of the spring system, can be related in terms of a model, as shown in Figure 1, where the analogy is that of pressure as the across variable and volume velocity as the through variable. All pressures in the figure are referenced to atmospheric pressure. The active drive to the system is the net muscular force (P_{MUS}). P_{MUS} is zero when the lung volume is equal to the relaxation volume V_{rel}. The air pressure in the lungs is called the alveolar pressure (P_{ALV}). Subglottal pressure, the drive for sound sources in speech, can be considered to be equal to P_{ALV} when the airflow rate is not high enough to cause a significant drop across the airway resistance. High rates of flow generally occur during speech only for some aspirated consonants. There are two capacitors in the model, and these represent the elastic elements of the lungs (C_L) and chest wall (C_{CW}). The "springiness" of these elastic elements is described mathematically in terms of their compliances. Compliance is a measure of the volume change created for a given change in pressure and is normally measured in liters per cm H_2O.

These compliances are generally nonlinear and dependent upon the history of the system. For these reasons and others, the compliances are characterized through a graph of lung volume versus pleural pressure for static conditions with muscles relaxed rather than with a single number. (For example, see Knowles et al. [5]) Such graphs can be described mathematically from the model. From the pressure drops in the middle section of the model, the air pressure in the lungs, P_{ALV}, is the sum of the pleural pressure (P_{PL}) and the static recoil pressure of the lungs (P_L), i.e., the pressure across C_L in the model:

$$P_{ALV} = P_{PL} + P_L \tag{1}$$

The relaxation characteristic of the chest wall (P_{CW}) is the pressure exerted by the chest wall when the muscles of the chest wall are relaxed, and is the pressure across C_{CW} in the model. P_{PL} is the pressure between the two compliant elements (the lungs and the chest wall), and can be described using the pressure drops at the leftmost end of the model:

$$P_{PL} = P_{MUS} + P_{CW} \tag{2}$$

2. Acoustic and Physiological Data Acquisition

The data are from four subjects (two women, two men) who range in age from 21 to 28, report normal hearing, have no history of respiratory ailments, are non-smokers, and speak American English as their first language. In this document, the speakers are referred to as Subject #4 through Subject #7 for consistency with an existing publication [12]. All subjects signed a consent form and were compensated for their participation.

Simultaneous recordings of the acoustic signal, airflow, and physiological signals used to estimate lung volume and lung pressure were made at the Voice and Speech Laboratory of the Massachusetts Eye and Ear Infirmary. During signal acquisition, subjects read isolated utterances and short paragraphs. As a part of the calibration tasks, intraoral pressure was also recorded. Airflow estimates were made using a circumferentially vented pneumotachograph mask [11] from Glottal Enterprises, Inc. Lung volume is estimated from the cross-sectional areas of the ribcage and abdomen [6] as measured using respiratory inductive plethysmography (Respitrace, Ambulatory Monitoring, Ardsley, NY).

Alveolar pressure is estimated from measurements of esophageal pressure [14]. A thin latex balloon was passed through the nasal cavity and placed at a level below the trachea and above the diaphragm, and was inflated with at least 0.5 cm³ of air. Placement with respect to whether the tip of the balloon had crossed the diaphragm was checked by having the subject make inspiratory and expiratory efforts against an occlusion, as in Baydur et al. [1]. The balloon in the esophagus is separated from the lungs by the tissue of the esophagus and the pleural space. Pressure in the esophageal balloon will differ from that in the lungs because of these intervening structures. There is only a significant pressure drop across the esophageal tissue during a peristaltic wave. When muscular force is exerted, the lungs may deform non-uniformly; this non-uniformity will also contribute to the difference between pleural pressure and the esophageal pressure measurement. In general, however, the difference between esophageal pressure and pleural pressure is small and generally constant for the mid-range of lung volumes in an upright person [16]. All calibrated alveolar pressure data were derived from pleural pressure by compensating for the static recoil pressure of the lungs (P_L) for each speaker [7]. P_L is measured as pleural pressure across the range of lung volumes when P_{ALV} is zero. For details of the calibration process, see Slifka [13].

Calibration maneuvers were performed before and after the speech task segment of the experiment. All data recordings were digitized on-line at a sample rate of 10 kHz using the Axoscope (Axon Instruments, Inc.) recording software and Digidata digitizers. Signals were filtered to prevent aliasing, and were amplified using a Cyberamp 380 Programmable Signal Conditioner (Axon Instruments) prior to digitizing.

Utterances were excluded from analysis if there was evidence of a peristaltic wave during some portion of the utterance. Pressure and airflow for each utterance in the data set were checked at the point where flow crossed from negative to positive. At this point, the pressure in the lungs should be zero. Utterances where the magnitude of this difference was greater than 1.5 cm H_2O were excluded from analysis. Also evidence of any oddity in the reading such as disfluency or stumbling over the reading of an utterance caused the utterance to be excluded. Exclusions for all of these reasons across all four subjects amounted to 16%.

2.1 Utterances and acoustic landmarks

In the final utterance set, there are 241 utterances, where 80.2% were read as an isolated utterance, and 19.8% were read as part of a short paragraph. Onset speech segments

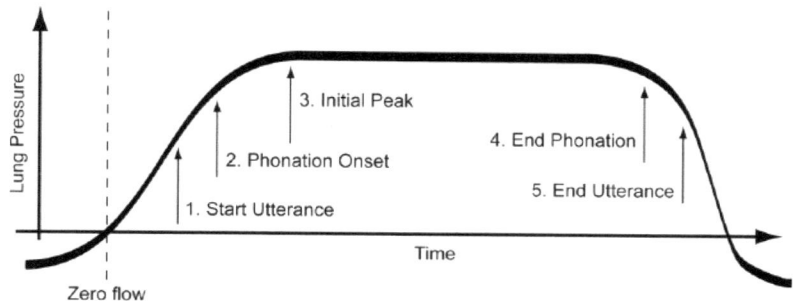

Figure 2. Various timing landmarks were determined from the audio, airflow, and pressure signals. These are: (1) the start of the utterance, (2) the start of phonation, (3) the initial peak in alveolar pressure for the utterance, (4) the end of phonation in the utterance, and (5) the end of the utterance.

contain primarily voiced sonorants (in this case, vowels and the segment /j/), stop consonants, fricatives, and the segment /h/. In the final utterance set, 33.6% contained a syntactic boundary denoted by a comma.

Based on the audio, airflow, and pressure signals, times were labeled for zero flow, start of the utterance, onset of phonation, initial alveolar pressure peak, end of phonation at the end of the utterance, and end of the utterance, as shown in Figure 2. Start pressure refers to the alveolar pressure at the start of the utterance. However, for voiced stop onsets such as /b/, the start of the utterance was set as the burst release if the segment was devoiced. Phonation onset pressure refers to the alveolar pressure at the onset of phonation. For utterances that began with a voiced phonetic segment, the start of the utterance was the same as the onset of phonation. The first peak in pressure was determined automatically from an algorithm which low-pass filtered the pressure and found the first occurrence of two consecutive points where the slope in the pressure curve was less than or equal to zero. The pressure peak time was set to the first of those two points.

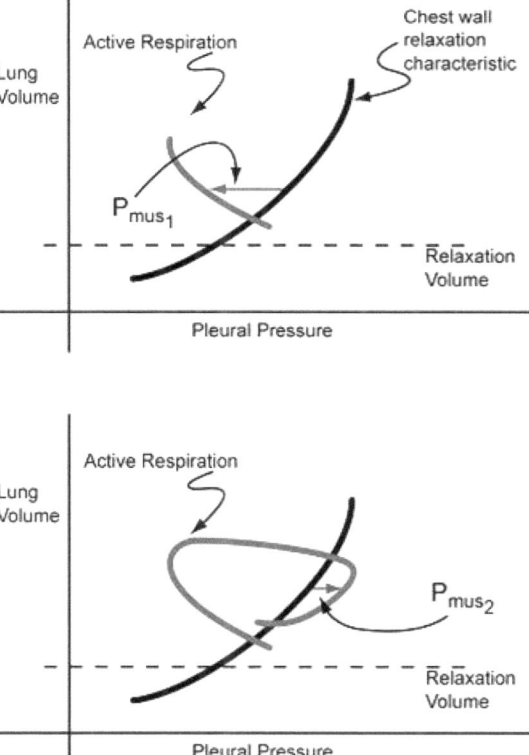

Figure 3. The Campbell diagram provides an estimate of net muscular force as given in the difference between the chest wall relaxation curve and the active respiration curve. (a) During a typical inhalation, lung volume increases and net muscular pressure (P_{mus1}) is to the left of the relaxation curve and is therefore inspiratory. (b) During a typical exhalation for speech, lung volume decreases and net muscular pressure (P_{mus2}) is to the right of the relaxation curve and is therefore expiratory.

3. Net Muscular Force

An estimate of regions of active muscular force and passive recoil can be derived from a graphical representation of equation 2. This plot is called a Campbell diagram [2] and is a graph of lung volume versus pleural pressure that includes, for reference, a curve representing the pressure-volume characteristic of the relaxed chest wall (P_{CW}). The relaxed chest wall curve was not directly measured for the subjects in this experiment because at the time of data acquisition it was not anticipated that it would be necessary. Estimates of the curves for each subject were made based on limited measured data and on landmarks from Knowles et al. [5]. (For details, see Slifka [12]) Discussions involving the relaxed chest wall characteristic will focus on broad trends rather than details.

Net muscular force can be estimated from the diagram as the distance between the curve representing the respiratory system gesture and the relaxation characteristic of the chest wall. Both inspiratory and expiratory muscles may be active simultaneously, but the pleural pressure is a result of net forces applied to the system. The schematic in Figure 3(a) shows a typical inhalation. Lung volume increases as the lungs/chest wall spring system is stretched further from the relaxation volume. The net muscular force at each point along the active inhalation curve is estimated as the difference in pressure between the chest wall relaxation characteristic and the active inhalation curve. This difference is demonstrated for a single point in the inhalation by the length of the line labeled P_{mus1}. A difference to the left of the chest wall relaxation characteristic is a net inspiratory pressure. Figure 3(b) completes the active respiration with an exhalation segment. When the respiration curve falls to the right of the chest wall relaxation characteristic, the net pressure is expiratory. An example is shown as P_{mus2}. If a person exhaled using net braking effort from a predominance of inspiratory muscle activity, that region of the exhalation would fall to the left of the relaxed chest wall curve. Any portions of the exhalation that trace the relaxed chest wall curve are times of zero net muscular force. During such portions, either there is no muscular force applied or else the inspiratory muscular force balances the expiratory muscular force. For a more detailed discussion see, for example, Rahn et al. [10] or Loring [8].

The Campbell diagrams used here are modified to include a time measure (Figure 4). Labeled vertical lines correspond to the previously defined timing landmarks in the utterance (see Figure 2). Figure 4(a) shows the time tracks for audio, P_{ALV}, airflow, and lung volume. In Figure 4(b), each circle along the pressure-volume curve is separated, in time, by 80 milliseconds. In this example, utterance onset occurs during a time of little volume change but rapid P_{PL} change. The pressure peak occurs to the right of the relaxed chest wall curve and the bulk of the utterance stays to the right of the curve. Regions that have large distances between the circles are times of rapid pressure changes, rapid volume changes, or rapid changes in both pressure and volume. If the circles are close together, the changes are much slower by comparison. Onset is a rapid action through the first pressure peak with little change in volume. After the initial pressure peak (point 3 in Figure 4(b)) the circles are more closely spaced through the offset of phonation (point 4). Between the offset of phonation and the end of the utterance, there is a quick drop in pleural pressure of about 4 cm H_2O.

Two typical examples are shown in Figure 5 for Subject #6. Figure 5(a) is an utterance read in isolation, and Figure 5(b) is an utterance read as part of a short paragraph. The time to move from the largest inspiratory P_{MUS} (leftmost point in the modified

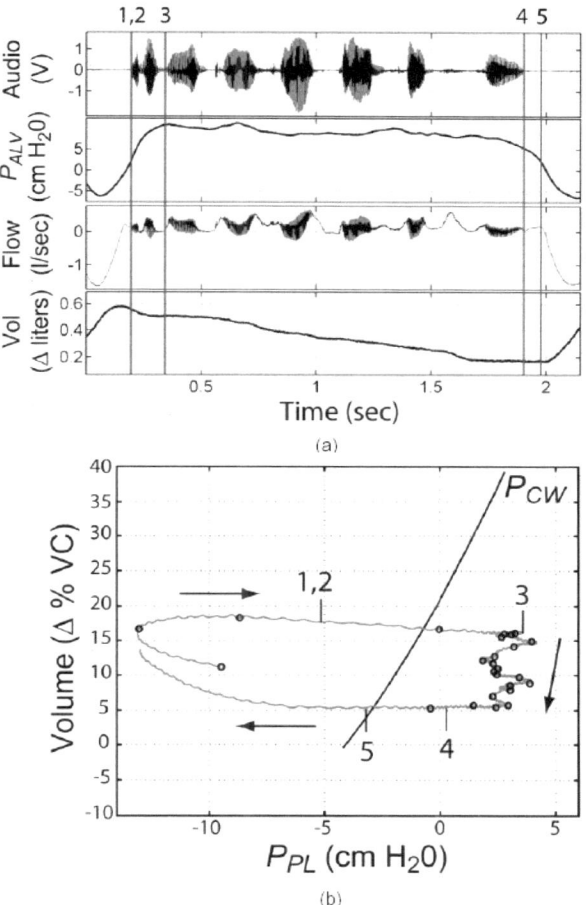

Figure 4. (a) Time tracks for audio, alveolar pressure, air flow, and lung volume (as measured in liters relative to FRC) from Subject #5. The utterance is "It'll be a brief walk down Fifth Street," and was read within a paragraph. Vertical bars denote timing landmarks (1=utterance onset, 2=phonation onset, 3=initial pressure peak, 4=phonation offset, 5=utterance offset) (b) Pressure-volume curve for the example in (a). P_{CW} is an estimate of the relaxed chest wall curve. The arrows indicate the direction of time progression. Open circles along the curve are separated by 80 milliseconds. Volume is measured in %VC relative to FRC.

Campbell diagram) to the peak in alveolar pressure at Point #3 is approximately 400 milliseconds for the utterance read in isolation and about 240 milliseconds for the utterance read as part of a paragraph. In the case of speech breathing, expiratory muscles are generally considered to become active as the inspiratory muscles reduce in activity. (For a review see Weismer [15]) In this view of speech breathing, both inspiratory and expiratory muscles may be continuously active throughout the utterance, to greater or lesser degrees, to meet the demands of the utterance without having to initiate from complete rest.

Two of the major initiation landmarks, utterance onset and the time of the initial alveolar pressure peak, are shown for all utterances in the data set and for all speakers in

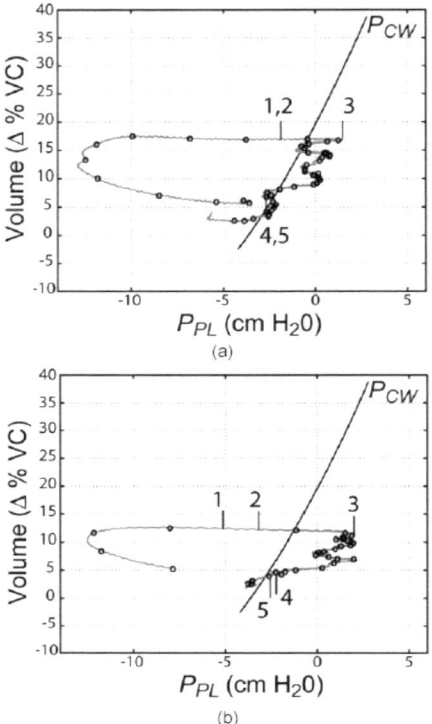

Figure 5. Pressure-volume examples from Subject #6. (a) The utterance, "Ali will have the best seat in the show," was read in isolation. (b) The utterance, "There is a large round rock in the path," was read as part of a short paragraph. (See legend for Figure 4.)

Figure 6. The 'x' symbols represent utterance onset, and the 'o' symbols represent the initial peak in alveolar pressure. Subject #4 and Subject #6 produced utterances that begin within a limited lung volume range. The pressure peak clusters close to, or slightly to the right of, the estimated relaxation curve. Subjects #5 and #7 use a wider range of lung volumes at utterance initiation. For the initial alveolar pressure peak data, values at higher lung volumes occur more to the left than values at lower lung volumes.

These four subjects predominantly begin utterances during net inspiratory muscular force; whether from a tapering of inspiratory activity prior to use of net expiratory force or from deliberate braking of the recoil force. The average time from utterance onset to the peak in alveolar pressure, across all speakers, was 162 milliseconds (63 milliseconds standard deviation, n=241). Hixon et al. [3] used pressure-volume curves to assess the muscular contributions of the ribcage and abdomen during speech production for sustained vowel tasks, reading, and conversational speech. During that study it was observed that, except for cases of high initial lung volume, speech was initiated to the right of the relaxation curve. In a recent study by Johnston et al. [4], a similar observation was made in a study using modified Campbell curves to compare the muscular effort of normal speakers with that of stutterers. The current study finds that sound is initiated as soon as the conditions permit; those conditions generally occur during the rapid transition from strong inspiratory effort toward a net muscular effort that is capa-

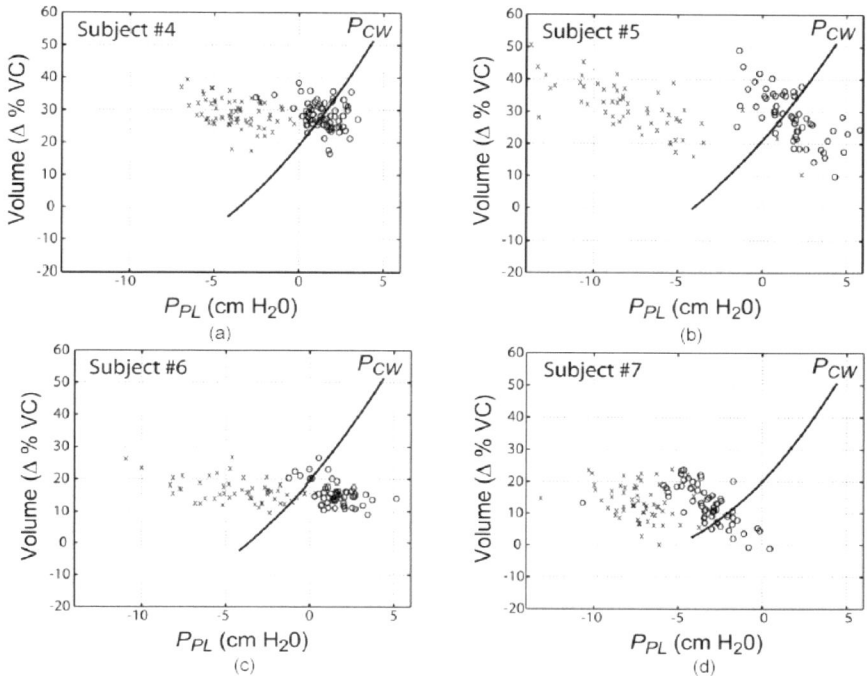

Figure 6. Pressure-volume onsets. The 'x' symbols correspond to utterance onset. The 'o' symbols correspond to the initial alveolar pressure peak. The relaxed chest wall curve is plotted for reference. (a) Subject #4, (b) Subject #5, (c) Subject #6, (d) Subject #7.

ble of generating the 'working level' of alveolar pressure A driving pressure is required to generate sound, yet in order to create that pressure, there must be an impedance or constriction in the vocal tract. Both the impedance and the pressure build-up as the articulators and/or vocal folds move into position to start an utterance. In general, this interdependence leads to low pressures generating low amplitude sounds in the initial milliseconds. (The exceptions are utterances that begin with a complete occlusion of the vocal tract.) Utterance onset occurs prior to the initial pressure peak and, in general, occurs as the articulators, vocal folds (if applicable), and the respiratory system structures are still in transition from their configuration for inhalation.

At utterance onset, the initial alveolar pressures are low and go through a substantial rise from the time of utterance onset until the initial pressure peak. This region of rapid change influences the acoustic realization of the initial segment(s). For the utterances in this study, mean start pressures range from 2.7 to 4.6 cm H_2O across the subjects and mean peak pressures range from 6.5 to 11.9 across the subjects. Signal amplitude changes are present at utterance onset and could be used by the listener as cues for the boundary. Additional cues could be present in the spectral content. For example, as the vocal folds move from a spread position to a more adducted position, there are changes in the coupling to the subglottal spaces as well as changes in the character of the contact between the folds.

4. Pauses

A pause, in terms of an acoustic definition, is a brief period of silence within the speech signal. Some pauses are associated with a phrase boundary within an utterance. The suspension of sound sources requires that vocal-fold vibration and/or noise-like sources be inhibited. This suspension may involve increasing the area of the constriction, by decreasing the pressure drive across the constriction, obstructing the airflow (as might be done by pressing the vocal folds together) or some combination of the above actions. However, a boundary may be perceived even when there is no suspension of sound. These cases are sometimes referred to as "filled pauses."

Each subject read 14 different utterances with a syntactic break indicated by a comma. Eight of those utterances were read twice at different points in the recording session, giving a total of 22 utterances. For all of these utterances, a boundary was perceived by a listening panel of five listeners at the syntactic break indicated by the comma. In some cases, additional pauses, not aligned with a comma, were also perceived by the panel. For details regarding the listening panel, see Slifka [12].

Figure 7 shows both airflow and alveolar pressure as functions of time for segments of speech around a perceived boundary within an utterance, as well as the corresponding Campbell diagram for the entire utterance. In the figure, three utterances are displayed as produced by Subject #5. Locations of perceived boundaries are marked with arrows. Three examples of sound segment pairs on either side of the boundary are given: a fricative to a stop consonant (Figure 7(a)), a vowel to a vowel (Figure 7(b)), and a stop consonant to a vowel (Figure 7(c)). In all cases, there is a distinct gesture by the respiratory system at the prosodic boundary. The action appears in the Campbell diagram as an almost horizontal inset in the pressure-volume curve. These curves are typical of those for all of the speakers. The gesture at the pause involves either a reduction in the net expiratory muscular force, a switch from net expiratory force to net inspiratory force, or an increase in the net inspiratory force. The exact details are subject to the accuracy of the estimate of the relaxed chest wall characteristic.

In some cases, there is a cessation of airflow at the boundary. An example is given in Figure 7(b) which shows a boundary between two vowel segments. The airflow is most likely stopped by pressing the vocal folds together. As seen in the Campbell diagram, P_{PL} falls quickly and then rises again during the period that the airflow is obstructed (the curve traces back on itself). Changes in the pressure during this time period do not influence the acoustics, as no sound is being produced. However, P_{ALV} and the momentum of the respiratory muscles are changing prior to and after the airflow obstruction.

In two series of utterances, an attempt was made to keep some variables constant in the utterance while moving the location of the syntactic break within the utterance. One series was as follows:

1. Ask Jeff, but speak with him well before the start of the show.
2. Ask to speak to Jeff, but call him well before the show.
3. Ask the operator if you can speak to Jeff, but call before the show.

These utterances were chosen to make a first assessment of whether the respiratory system would be involved to varying degrees depending on the recoil forces available from the lungs/chest wall spring system. An example of this series of utterances, in

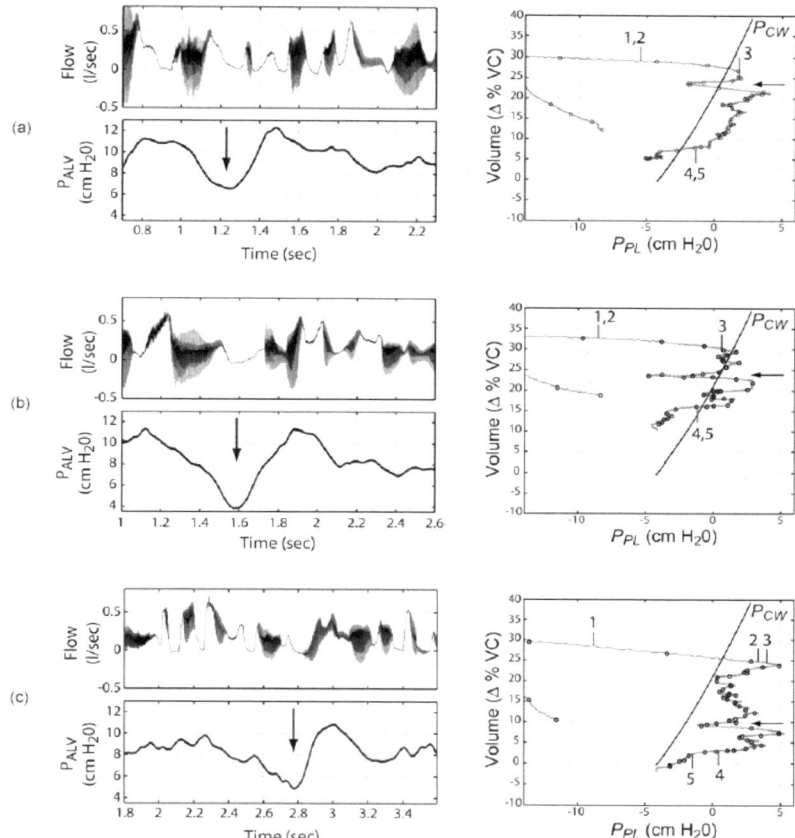

Figure 7. Utterances with pauses for Subject #5. On the left are the airflow and pressure traces for time segments around the boundary. On the right are the Campbell diagrams for the utterances. Arrows indicate the perceived boundary. Vertical bars denote timing landmarks (1=Utterance onset, 2=Phonation onset, 3=Initial pressure peak, 4=phonation offset, 5=utterance offset), and open circles are separated by 80 milliseconds. The text of each utterance is: (a) "Ask the operator if you can speak to Jeff, but call before the show." (b) "If you say the word show, Alissa will say the word sew." (c) "Six will be asked if they would be willing to participate, even though there could be eight."

terms of Campbell curves, is shown in Figure 8 for Subject #4. These three utterances were all initiated near 27% VC above FRC and all end near 10%VC above FRC. Recall that Subject #4 uses a narrow range of lung volumes to initiate utterances and shows little volume change while moving to the initial alveolar pressure peak. In all three utterances, a respiratory gesture is made that has an excursion of approximately 3 cm H_2O in pleural pressure and 3% VC in lung volume. The duration of the segment is about 0.56 seconds. Similar patterns were found for all four speakers for the utterance series used in Figure 8 as well as one other similar series of utterances.

In this data set, every perceived pause was accompanied by a gesture in the respiratory system. This gesture occurred as a rapid transition in muscular effort during a period of relatively little volume change. In the Campbell diagrams, the gesture appears as an almost horizontal line. This gesture occurred for (1) all speakers, (2) during both silent and filled pauses, (3) at various lung volumes (where various levels of recoil force

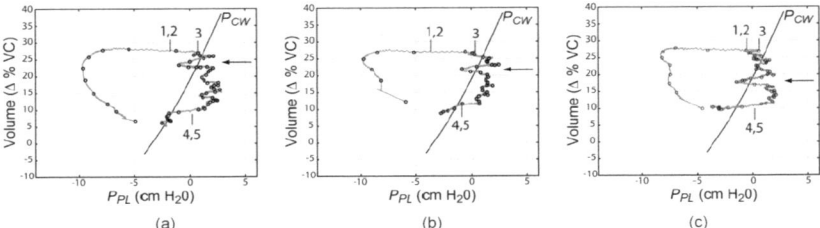

Figure 8. Three different locations for pauses within an utterance from Subject #4. Arrows indicate the perceived boundary. Vertical bars denote timing landmarks (1=Utterance onset, 2=Phonation onset, 3=Initial pressure peak, 4=phonation offset, 5=utterance offset), and open circles are separated by 80 milliseconds. (a) Text: "Ask Jeff, but speak with him well before the start of the show." (b) Text: "Ask to speak to Jeff, but call him well before the show." (c) Text: "Ask the operator if you can speak to Jeff, but call before the show."

are available), and (4) for various combinations of segments at the pause boundary.

A sound source could be suspended by increasing the area of the constriction, reducing the pressure drop across the constriction, obstructing the airflow or by combining these methods. This data set indicates that the pressure drive is reduced. If the speaker also spreads the vocal folds to suspend glottal vibration, the decrease in pressure controls the airflow from the widening glottis. If the speaker obstructs the airflow, the decrease in pressure may act to avoid an inappropriate build-up of pressure against the obstructed airway during the pause. In all cases, the gesture has implications on both sides of the pause: a reduction in drive going into the pause and a reversal of the momentum coming out of the pause. The changing momentum of the relatively large structures of the respiratory system (with correspondingly larger time constants) may be an important factor for the speaker in generating a pause. In these data, there is a similarity between the respiratory system dynamics, as shown on the Campbell diagram, at utterance boundaries aligned with a breath to the boundaries at perceived pauses which are not aligned with a breath. Both show the rapid and almost horizontal region.

5. Summary

As a speaker starts talking, there is a rapid action in the respiratory system showing a large change in the applied muscular pressure and very little volume change. Utterance onset generally begins during net inspiratory muscular force - prior to the point at which the respiratory system has generated a 'relatively constant working level' for alveolar pressure during speech. The modified Campbell diagrams in this study show that most utterances begin during a rapid transition in muscular force from a strong inspiratory force to the level of muscular force necessary to produce pressure in the speech range. In general, the alveolar pressure peaks close to or to the right of the estimated chest wall relaxation curve, except when utterances are produced at higher lung volumes.

Boundaries within an utterance, such as those at pauses within a breath group, are marked with a muscular gesture from the respiratory system. This gesture is present for perceived pauses in which there is a period of silence in the utterances as well as perceived pauses where phonation continues through the boundary. The respiratory system involvement is present for various types of sound segments at the boundary as well as various locations of pauses within the utterance. Evidence of this gesture is even seen when the airway is completely obstructed during the pause. There appears to be a distinct change in the momentum of the structures of the respiratory system at some prosodic boundaries that are not aligned with the initiation or termination of exhalation.

The coordinated set of acoustic cues that signal boundaries in speech includes changes in fundamental frequency, amplitude, voice source, and segmental duration. This array of cues could be considered to be a cognitively chosen set of cues. If that is the case, then the set of changes could have been chosen to be anything. However, it could be that the set of cues that are present at major prosodic boundaries are there because they are the consequences of the actions of the respiratory system as it ends, suspends, or initiates muscular action in controlling the driving pressure for speech.

Acknowledgements

This work greatly benefited from the advice and support of Prof. K. N. Stevens. It has also been influenced by the guidance of Stephen Loring, Bob Hillman, Martha Gray, and James Kobler. This work was supported in part by NIH grants #5T32DC0038, #5R01-DC00266-14, and #DC00075, the Clarence J. LeBel Chair at MIT, HST Fellowship, and a Dissertation Enhancement grant from the National Science Foundation INT 98-21048.

References

[1] Baydur, A., Behrakis, P.K., Zin, W.A., Jaeger, M. and Milic-Emili, J. "A simple method for assessing the validity of the esophageal balloon technique." *Am. Rev. Respir. Dis.* 126(5): 788-791, 1982.

[2] Campbell, E.J.M. *The Respiratory Muscles and the Mechanics of Breathing.* London: Lloyd-Luke, 1958.

[3] Hixon, T.J., Mead, J. and Goldman, M.D. "Dynamics of the chest wall during speech production: Function of the thorax, rib cage, diaphragm, and abdomen." *J. Speech Hear. Res.* 19: 297-356, 1976.

[4] Johnston, S., Yan, S., Sliwinski, P. and Macklem, P.T. "Modified Campbell diagram to assess respiratory muscle action in speech." *Respirology*, 4(3): 213-222, 1999.

[5] Knowles, J.H., Hong, S.K. and Rahn, H. "Possible errors using esophageal balloon in determination of pressure-volume characteristics of the lung and thoracic cage." *J. Applied Physiol.* 14(4): 525-530, 1959.

[6] Konno, K. and Mead, J. "Measurement of the separate volume changes of ribcage and abdomen during breathing." *J. Applied Physiol.* 22: 407-422, 1967.

[7] Kunze, L. "Evaluation of methods of estimating sub-glottal air pressure." *J. Speech Hear. Res.* 7: 151-164, 1964.

[8] Loring, S.H. "Mechanics of the lungs and chest wall." In *Physiological Basis of Ventilatory Support,* J.J. Marini and A.S. Slutsky (eds.), New York: Marcel Dekker, pp. 177-208, 1998.

[9] Loring, S.H. and Mead, J. "Abdominal muscle use during quiet breathing and hyperpnea in uninformed subjects." *J. Applied Physiol: Respirat. Environ. Exercise Physiol.*, 52(3): 700-704, 1982.

[10] Rahn, H., Otis, A.B., Chadwick, L.E. and Fenn, W.O. "The pressure-volume diagram of the thorax and lung." *Am. J. Physiol.* 146: 161-178, 1946.

[11] Rothenberg, M. "A new inverse-filtering technique for deriving the glottal airflow waveform during voicing." *J. Acous. Soc. Am.*, 89: 1777-1781, 1973.

[12] Slifka, J. *Respiratory Constraints on Speech Production at Prosodic Boundaries.* Ph.D. Thesis, Massachusetts Institute of Technology, 2000.

[13] Slifka, J. "Respiratory constraints on speech production: Starting an utterance." *J. Acous. Soc. Am.* 114: 3343-3353, 2003.

[14] Van den Berg, J. "Direct and indirect determination of mean subglottal pressure." *Folia Phoniatrica* 8: 1-24, 1956.

[15] Weismer, G. "Speech breathing: Contemporary views and findings," In *Speech Science*, R.G. Daniloff (ed.), San Diego: College Hill Press, pp. 47-72, 1985.

[16] Wohl, M., Turner, J. and Mead, J. "Static volume-pressure curves of cog lungs - in vivo and in vitro." *J. Applied Physiol.* 24(3): 348-354, 1968.

Dynamics of Speech Production and Perception
P. Divenyi et al. (Eds.)
IOS Press, 2006

Speech Gestures by Deduction, Gesture Production and Gesture Perception

René CARRÉ
Laboratoire Dynamique du Language
Université Lyon 2
Lyon, France

Abstract. The objective of the chapter is to derive, from a tube 18 cm in length, an acoustic production system well adapted for communication needs according to principles: the shape of the acoustic tube must be deformed so that the acoustic contrast is always "sufficient" or "maximum" between the sounds it produces, the smallest possible area deformations lead to the largest possible formant variations (minimum of energy principle). The deformations so obtained can be represented by a limited number of commands (called "speech gestural deformations" or "speech distinctive gestures") summarized within the Distinctive Region Model. It can be observed that the dynamic of the model is consistent with the speech production system. Most importantly, the simulations predict the vowel triangle which has the largest possible area that can be obtained with an acoustic tube of fixed length. The deductive approach also allows us to infer standard places of articulation for vowels and consonants and thereby identify the primary physical underpinnings of phonological distinctions. This approach predicts vocalic systems and the role of F3 in the /d, g/ distinction. Using sequential and/or parallel (coproduced) combinations of distinctive gestures, V_1V_2 and V_1CV_2 utterances are easily generated. Perception of gesture combinations indicates that, in VV and VCV utterances, a surprisingly high degree of perceptual invariance can be achieved despite relatively large variations of gesture characteristics, such as gesture asynchrony, duration, and movement trajectory.

Keywords. Speech production, speech gestures, vowel space, formant transitions

Introduction

In vision, the importance of dynamics (kinematics) for an analytic account of how we recognize movement is well known. Consider, for example a person's hand (=the subject) moving to grasp an object. If we view this movement as an integrated, unitary event that is perceived as such, all possible variants of the task must be part of its repertoire of forms, both produced and perceived, thus necessitating an enormous event memory bank. By contrast, if the complex task is viewed in terms of its component gestures both its production and its perception can be reduced to two elementary primitives, one gesture to reach the object, one to grasp it. Note that, if such elementary components exist, they must be autonomous – or else the complex task reverts to an integral unitary event.

Assuming then that our example represents a complex task consisting of two component gestures, its perception raises three main points: (i) the manner of coordination of the different articulators (here, arm and hand) participating in the realization of each gesture is generally not perceived; (ii) the gestures are identified in the course of their realization before the task is completed; (iii) within certain limits and under certain constraints, the range of durations, velocities, and relative phases of the component gestures may be quite large, without significantly changing the percept of the total movement. For example, the grasping gesture may start either before the reaching gesture is complete, or after the object has been reached. In the latter case, the two gestures are realized sequentially, that is, in series. In the former case, the two gestures are realized in parallel, i.e., they are co-produced, and presumably co-perceived, with a certain freedom of phasing, movement, and duration without any change in the effectiveness of perception of the task.

One advantage of performing the two gestures in parallel is that the duration of the task can be reduced. Moreover, the observed movement is relative because the observer, analyzing the task, is able automatically to take into account any displacement of the subject with respect to the object to be reached. Thus, regardless of whether the subject is moving or stationary, the perception of an arm reaching toward an object remains the same because the information is encoded as the difference between successive states of the arm gesture alone: the information lies in the dynamics. To be easily perceived, the complex task or its gestural components should not be apprehended as a succession of static parameters, each characterized in absolute coordinates; rather, the observer needs to attend only to variations between states: the coding is then efficient, requiring a minimum amount of information (as in delta modulation).

Similarly, a spoken utterance is the acoustic result of gestural movements deforming the vocal tract shape. We hypothesize that the mechanisms underlying perception of speech gestures are the same, in principle, as those underlying visual perception of gestures. In speech production, the light source lighting the hand movement is replaced by the vocal source. Speech is structured by the acoustic properties of the vocal tract. Several elementary gestures, to be characterized, are at the origin of this structuration -- gestures of the tongue, the lips, the velum, the larynx. These gestures too may be realized in parallel, with acoustic consequences observable throughout the duration of a syllable and possibly beyond [13]. In the case of reduction [23], or hypo-speech [24] gestures do not reach fixed static targets, but we assume that there is sufficient information in the signal to allow recovery of the original intention.

The main purpose of this chapter is to characterize the production and perception of speech gestures. As a first step, we will present a study aimed at determining the duration of gestures, followed by a sketch of a theory of gestures. In the final part, we test the theory in two perceptual experiments.

1. The Syllable: A Dynamic Unit of Gestural Coproduction

Both theories of coarticulation and empirical observations reported by several researchers lead to the hypothesis that the unit of speech programming may be the syllable, a cohesive unit of coproduced gestures, as schematized in Figure 1 [6] [22][28][12][1][20][16][19][3][17][14]. At the abstract level, a CV syllable (CV2) is

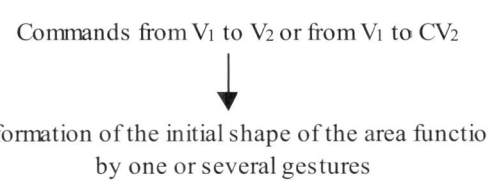

Figure 1. Gestural syllabic coproduction model.

represented in terms of gestures intended to deform the shape of the vocal tract. At the peripheral level, the gestures start from a preceding vowel configuration (V1).

To develop this hypothesis, we rely on Fowler's analysis [17] of the two main theories of coarticulation currently available, feature spreading and coproduction. The former is purely abstract and offers no account of the actual process of coarticulation. The latter, by contrast, as proposed by Kozhevnikov and Chistovich [22] is a process of syllabic coproduction in which a CV sequence is produced as a unit, the consonant gesture and the vowel gesture being realized at the same time. This means that, at any given instant the signal carries information on both vowel and consonant in parallel (for more on coproduction, see Fowler [15][17]). Indeed, Öhman [28] observed that, in V_1CV_2 production, the C-V_2 transitions are affected by the first vowel V_1 and, reciprocally, V_1-C transitions are affected by the final vowel V_2. To explain these observations, he proposed a model in which the observed formant transitions are determined by superimposing local perturbations, caused by consonant articulation, on baseline V_1-V_2 transitions: consonant and vowel are coproduced. If we adopt gestures, that is, linguistic actions in the vocal tract [2], to describe vowels and consonants, syllables are then a process of "gestural coproduction". Recalling our earlier comments on visual perception of movement, we conclude that coproduction theory offered a more coherent and empirically valid account of the CV syllable than the purely abstract theory of feature spreading.

The proposed realization of a CV2 syllable starting from a preceding vowel V1 is shown in Figure 2. Here we have chosen a V2 formed by two gestures, a lip gesture and a tongue gesture. Deformation of the initial V1 shape of the vocal tract area function is then effected by the three gestures of the syllabic command executed in parallel. As in the optically specified movements of hand and arm in our example above and as in articulatory phonology [4], the effects of the gestural commands on the area function are not necessarily in phase, nor of the same duration or movement. Indeed, the realizations of the gestures as more or less orthogonal primitives are independent of each other. The relation between intention and the real physical domain of the vocal tract is direct (without the cognitive mediation of translation theories [18]).

According to our hypothesis, the same set of initial abstract planned commands (starting at time 0) will evoke gestures whose effect on the area function can have a variety of different manifestations in the time domain on different occasions, such as different temporal durations, movement patterns and intergestural phasing. Such differences can be attributed either to specific articulatory constraints or to speaker variability, or to both. In any case, the existence of any abstract representation means that the corresponding action must be detectable in the signal.

Between the abstract syllabic command (at time 0) and the corresponding actions there is a time delay. At the global action stage, the syllable begins with the vg_1 gesture, as shown in Figure 2. If we take the beginning of the syllable to coincide with the onset

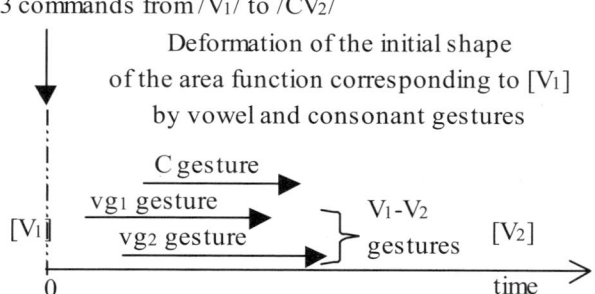

Figure 2. Gestural syllabic coproduction of /V_1-CV_2/. From gestural abstract commands to corresponding gestural deformations of the vocal tract in the time domain.

of consonantal closure, V_2 is anticipated because the acoustic effect of the gesture vg_1 is already observable in the preceding syllable (in V_1). At the signal stage, the acoustic effect of gestures can be delayed by articulatory to acoustic non-linearities: For example, the acoustic effects of a lip gesture are proportionately greater for small lip areas than for large lip areas. In our model, at the abstract level, the beginning of the syllable includes what is generally referred to as anticipation. With such a model, the transition V1C can be altered by the vowel V2 as a function of gestural phasing. Accordingly, a production model that takes more than a syllable into account, such as the V1CV2 type of model proposed by Kent [20], is not necessary to explain V1C alteration. Moreover, if the realization of one component gesture of a syllable is not completed by the beginning of the realization of the following syllable, then gestural reduction occurs. The proposed command model inherently integrates coarticulation, coproduction, and reduction phenomena. All these phenomena, it is hypothesized, originate at the level of gestural realization. Within such a modeling, the acoustic effects due to gestural reduction are not systematically centralized.

Assuming that the purpose of a speech gesture is to generate an acoustic perturbation, we may reasonably suppose that the tools used to deform the area function (i.e., the articulators) should be well adapted for the task. Here, for the sake of simplicity, we focus on deformation gestures that are well adapted for generating specific acoustic perturbations, without taking account of possible articulatory constraints. Note, however that syllabic gestural coproduction with parallel gestures can be transformed into a serial process, if the gestural commands are incompatible at the articulatory level (giving rise to incompatible acoustic effects!). For example, to produce [ida], the [d] occlusion at the front of the vocal tract would have to be realized at the same time as the [a] constriction at the back of the vocal tract. In such a case, Kozhevnikov and Chistovich [22] suggest the consonant gesture is realized before the vowel gesture. We could also realize first, the beginning of the vowel gesture, then the consonant gesture, and at last, the gesture from the end of the consonant to the vowel.

We now have to define the real, physical characteristics of gestures.

2. Modeling Speech Gestures

Our purpose now is to describe the characteristic properties of gestural deformations of the vocal tract. These gestures must be well adapted for acoustic communication: gestural deformations of the vocal tract shape must provide audible and pseudo-orthogonal acoustic consequences, and they must be realized with a minimum of deformation. Since speech has to be heard, speech gestures are actions on the area function of the vocal tract with acoustic goals. Accordingly instead of defining gestures in articulatory terms, we prefer an alternative approach, namely, to define gestures deductively on an acoustic tube. Our purpose is to derive, from a tube 18 cm in length, distinctive gestural deformations of the tube shape, for an efficient acoustic communication system, without invoking any knowledge of human speech production.

Before embarking on such an endeavor, we must decide what principles should constrain the development of such a system.

- Acoustic communication can operate in a noisy environment. Thus, it appears reasonable to assume that, for communication to be possible, the shape of the acoustic tube must be deformed so that the acoustic contrast is always "sufficient" or "maximum" between the sounds it produces, according to the level of noise. Formants, because they carry maximum relative spectral energy, may be regarded as the prime representatives of acoustic differences between sounds.

- To achieve the acoustic contrast efficiently, we assume that the tube has to be deformed at points where the smallest possible area deformations lead to the largest possible formant variations.

Deformations with these characteristics can be represented by a limited number of commands summarized in the Distinctive Region Model (DRM) [26][7]. Because these specific deformations give rise to distinctive acoustic variations usable for acoustic communication, they are called "acoustic distinctive gestures" or "acoustic gestural deformations". The antisymmetrical behavior of the model leads to complex deformations: for example, a tongue gesture effected by a front constriction is associated with an increase in back cavity volume and vice-versa [25]. Indeed, we can deduce, from the physical properties of any acoustic tube, an 'acoustic phonology' in terms of dynamic

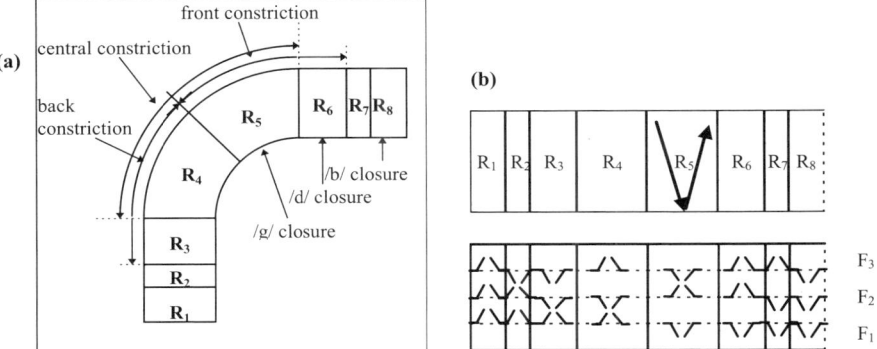

Figure 3. (a) Scheme of the distinctive region model with its 8 regions; (b) Formant transition behavior for its uniform configuration in the case of region closing-opening: the 8 combinations of falling and rising transitions are obtained (pseudo-orthogonality of the model).

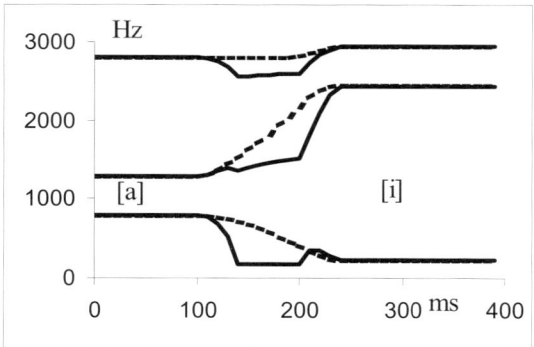

Figure 4. [ai] (dotted line) and [abi] (bold line) production by superposition of the [ai] vowel gesture and the [b] consonant gesture.

gestural deformations. This result provides theoretical support for the articulatory pho-nology of Browman and Goldstein [5].

When three formants are taken into account in the deductive process, eight regions are obtained as shown in Figure 3(a), representing an uniform tube closed at one end and open at the other. The formant variations obtained by closing and opening the tube in each region are schematized in Figure 3(b). All possible combinations of formant rises and falls are obtained, demonstrating the pseudo-orthogonality of the model.

Figure 4 compares the acoustic production model with the speech production sys-tem. Evidently, the dynamic properties of the DRM are consistent with the facts of speech production. R1 corresponds to the laryngeal cavity, regions R3, R4, R5, and R6 to the tongue, R8 to the lips. The vowel triangle, and the vowel and consonant places of articulation are automatically deduced [7]. Two important conclusions follow from the model:

1. the neutral configuration (corresponding to a uniform tube) plays a central role as a point of reference [10];
2. as far as formant frequencies are concerned speech phonology originates in the "acoustic phonology" intrinsic to an acoustic tube.

The gestural syllabic coproduction hypothesis was adopted to build a speech pro-duction model. Using serial and/or parallel (coproduced) combination of distinctive ges-tures, V_1V_2 and V_1CV_2 utterances were generated. Figure 5 shows the formant frequencies in the time domain for the production of [ai] and [abi] by, respectively, one vowel gesture (from V1 to V2) and the same vowel gesture associated with a consonant gesture. These two gestures are identically phased with respect to V1 and have the same duration. As in Öhman's data [28], information for the second vowel appears at the end of the first one and vice versa : in [abi] production, all formant transitions at the end of the vowel [a] point ahead to [i], and all formant transition at the beginning of [i] point back to [a].

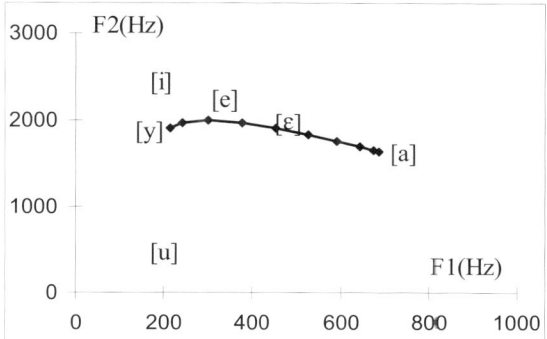

Figure 5. F_1-F_2 plane representation of the [aya] transition. Note that the trajectory from [a] points first to [i] before turning toward [y].

3. Perception of Speech Gestures

Using serial and/or parallel (coproduced) combinations of parameters, V_1V_2 and V_1CV_2 utterances were synthesized and presented for judgement in several experiments. Perception of gestural combinations remained remarkably invariant despite considerable variations in the duration, phasing and movement of the coproduced gestures [6][9][8]. Such results demonstrate the invariant properties of distinctive gestures no less than the variability of their realization in the time domain; gestural parameters are not fixed at constant intrinsic values, but can vary at the peripheral level as necessary to reproduce (and explain) the phenomena of coproduction. This point complements Fowler's view [16] on theories of extrinsic timing. A large range of variability is a necessary condition of speech communication between speakers, as it is of a child's acquisition of phonetic categories. Variability may also be central to the process of phonological sound changes: for example with variations in gestural phasing, new acoustic segment markers may arise and generate new phonetic categories [6].

Here, we wish to recall two perceptual experiments with results important to the present argument: one on the perceptual role of the shape of the trajectory in the case of [aya] production [9], and the other on the role of the neutral vocal tract configuration in the perception of plosives [10].

3.1 Experiment 1. Perception of [aya]

Using the DRM, [aya] was synthesized with the two gestural commands: tongue constriction and lip rounding, strictly synchronized. The F_1-F_2 trajectory corresponding to [aya] is illustrated in Figure 6. Notice that the acoustic effect of lip rounding (manifest as a drop in F_1 and F_2) occurs later than that of the lingual constriction (manifest as a drop in F_1 and a rise in F_2). In natural speech, the trajectory is typically straight, an effect, it would seem, of labial anticipation [11]. Indeed, if we simulate an anticipatory labial gesture with the DRM, the resulting trajectory is straight. Thus, the acoustic effect of lip rounding is late (at a labial cross-section of between 2.3 cm^2 and 0.5 cm^2) and labial anticipation generally observed in speech may occur to compensate for the acoustic delay. The [aya] transition was considered an appropriate stimulus to study the per-

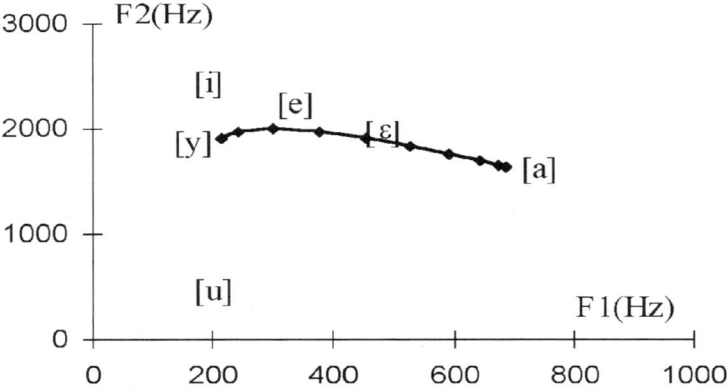

Figure 6. F_1-F_2 plane representation of the [aya] transition. Note that the trajectory from [a] points first to [i] before turning toward [y].

ception of curved trajectories generated by a composite gesture. The main results of this experiment [9] showed that merely reaching the target [y] was insufficient to generate a definite /aya/ percept; in order for that to happen, [y] had to be present as a *steady-state* vowel for a duration longer than 30 ms. When the duration of the steady state [y] was shorter than 30 ms, /i/ rather than /y/ was perceived, presumably because the trajectory points to [i] over much of its length; if the trajectory was a straight line from [a] to [y], the percept was always /aya/. In other words, unless the transition halted at [y] and remained there for a minimum duration (30 ms), the lip rounding gesture that distinguishes /i/ from /y/ was ignored. This finding strongly suggests that vowel-to-vowel transitions are governed by temporal integration of the trajectory vectors in the F_1-F_2 plane: Evidently, some perceptual mechanism *calculates the time average* of the *length* and *direction* of formant trajectories (by definition, time-varying) and *predicts the target* of the trajectory, even if it is not actually reached.

3.2 Experiment 2. Production and Perception of Neutral-C-Neutral

The pseudo-orthogonal formant transition generated by DRM around the neutral position (Figure 3) has consequences for the perception of plosive consonants and for the role of F_3 in the coronal/velar distinction. Perceptual tests were set up to study the role of the second and third formant transitions at the boundaries between /b, d, g/ in the context of surrounding neutral vowels. For the neutral vowel, F_1=500, F_2=1500, F_3=2500 Hz (higher formants F_4, F_5, etc. were not used). Formant transitions were linear with symmetrical offsets and onsets. For F_1, the endpoints were always –3 Barks from the first formant of the neutral position. For F_2 and F_3, the endpoints were –1.5, –0.75, 0, 0.75, 1.5 Barks around the neutral positions. 25 different synthetic items were obtained with a formant synthesizer and used for the perception tests (Figure 7). The subjects had to choose among /b/, /d/ and /g/ (forced choice).

The results are given in Figure 8 in the F_2-F_3 plane [10]. The 25 items are represented by different symbols, depending on the dominant labeling response. Decreasing F_2 and F_3 (corresponding to closing R8) leads to a /b/ percept (square); increasing F_2 and F_3 (closing R6) leads to a /d/ percept (diamond); increasing F_2 and decreasing F_3 (clos-

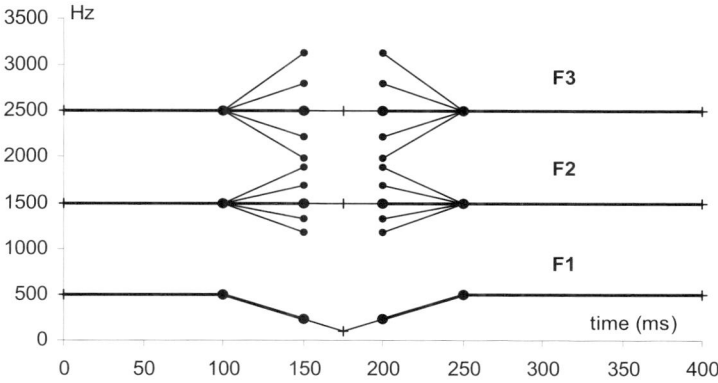

Figure 7. /əCə/ formant transitions in the time domain.

ing R5) leads to a /g/ percept (triangle). $F_2 = 1500Hz$ corresponds to the boundary between R6 and R7; $F_3 = 2500Hz$ corresponds to the boundary between R5 and R6 or R7 and R8. The percept obtained for a decrease of F_2 and an increase of F_3 (corresponding to R7) is not clear. In such a case, the large formant variations imposed symmetrically are probably impossible to reach with an acoustic tube. The large circle represents F_2 and F_3 for the second neutral vowel (corresponding in this case to the uniform tube). The results of the perception tests are in full agreement with the prediction: three main categories corresponding to 3 different combinations of falling/rising F_2, F_3 formant transitions are obtained.

Our results suggest that perceptual identification of plosives can be carried out very simply as a function of formant transitions rising or falling around the neutral baseline. Taking the neutral vocal tract configuration as a reference for decoding transitional cues simplifies phonemic categorization. The neutral configuration is specific to speech: it corresponds to a uniform tube in production and to the approximate mean formant val-

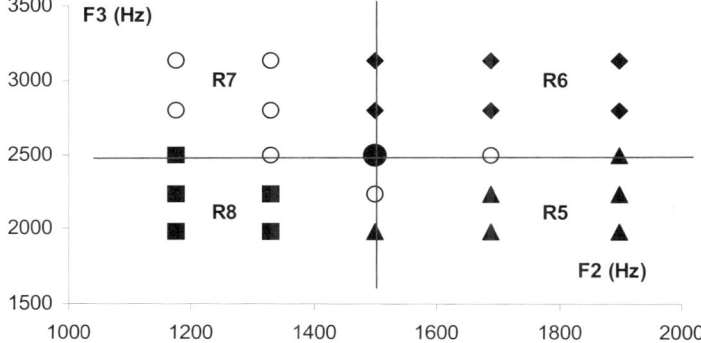

Figure 8. /əCə/ results in the F2-F3 plane. Filled symbols correspond to stimuli for which there were at least responses 70% in favor of one category. Small circles correspond to less than 70%. The horizontal and vertical lines correspond respectively to flat F_3 and F_2 transitions. Decreasing F_2 and F_3 (corresponding to closing R8) leads to a dominant /b/ percept (represented by a square); increasing F_2 and F_3 (corresponding to closing R6) leads to a dominant /d/ percept (diamond); increasing F_2 and decreasing F_3 (corresponding to closing R5) leads to a dominant /g/ percept (triangle).

ues of the vowel triangle in perception. The neutral configuration also facilitates phoneme identification in reduce speech.

4. Conclusions

This chapter has outlined a theoretical approach to speech production and perception that assumes "no mismatch between knowledge and action" [17]. Knowledge is the result of action including evolutionary adaptation. Actions derives not only from perceptual and articulatory experience per se, but also from an intimate knowledge of the physical properties of an acoustic tube as embodied in the vocal tract, that has permitted humans to discover the optimal use of such a tube. Indeed, the deductive approach shows that the actual, empirical actions in the vocal tract are acoustically optimal for communication: there are no "articulatory constraints". Why? Additional experiments have to be undertaken to determine whether this apparently acoustically optimal speech communication system reflects adaptations specialized for communication. In other words, has the system evolved in response to selective pressures for efficient communication (as predicted by an ecological point of view [29])?

Our approach is basically dynamic (or kinematic): (i) gestures are defined in the time domain; (ii) speech is a dynamic process of coproducing gestures in parallel; (iii) the form of an action or gestural trajectory is a variation from its point of origin; (iv) the direction of gestures (in the F_1, F_2, F_3 plane) is more important than the static targets to be reached. Vowel reduction [23], hyper- and hypo-production phenomena [24] can be easily represented in terms of gestures.

In this approach, the role of the neutral configuration is central to the speech mode. The variations are around the neutral, defined as a uniform tube with its corresponding formant frequencies. The neutral seems to be the best point of reference for observing formant frequency variations for identification.

If the speech communication system can be deduced from the natural, fixed properties of an acoustic tube, then the system supports a "single-strong theory" based on the dynamic properties of the vocal tract. We do not have to accept the premises of a "double-weak theory", postulating that neither the production system nor the perception system can fully explain the speech communication process [27][21].

Acknowledgements

My thanks to Pierre Divenyi, Björn Lindblom, Rudolph Sock, Michael Studdert-Kennedy and Willy Serniclaes for instructive comments, discussions and encouragement. The work was supported by "The Cognitique Program: Language et Cognition n° 41" of the French Research Ministry.

References

[1] Benguerel, A. and Cowan, H. "Coarticulation of upper lip protrusion in French." *Phonetica* 30: 41-55, 1974.
[2] Browman, C. and Goldstein, L. "Towards an articulatory phonology." In C. Ewan and J. Anderson, eds., *Phonology yearbook*, (Cambridge University Press, Cambridge) pp. 219-252., 1986.
[3] Browman, C.P. and Goldstein, L. "Some notes on syllable structure in articulatory phonology." *Phonetica* 45: 140-155, 1988.

[4]   Browman, C.P. and Goldstein, L. "Articulatory gestures as phonological units." *Phonology* 6: 201-252, 1989.

[5]   Browman, C.P. and Goldstein, L. "Gestural specification using dynamically-defined articulatory gestures." *J. Phonetics* 18: 299-320, 1990.

[6]   Carré, R. "Perception of coproduced speech gestures." *Proc. 14th Int. Cong. Phonetic Sciences*, pp. 643-646, 1999.

[7]   Carré, R. "From acoustic tube to speech production." *Speech Communication*, 42: 227-240, 2004.

[8]   Carré, R., Ainsworth, W.A., Jospa, P., Maeda, S. and Pasdeloup, V. "Perception of vowel-to-vowel transitions with different formant trajectories." *Phonetica* 58: 163-178, 2001.

[9]   Carré, R. and Divenyi, P. "Modeling and perception of 'gesture reduction'." *Phonetica* 57: 152-169, 2000.

[10] Carré, R., Liénard, J.S., Marsico, E. and Serniclaes, W. "On the role of the 'schwa' in the perception of plosive consonants." In *Proc. Int. Cong. Speech Language Processing*, pp. 1681-1684, 2002.

[11] Carré, R. and Mrayati, M. "Vowel-vowel trajectories and region modeling." *J. Phonetics* 19: 433-443, 1991.

[12] Daniloff, R. and Hammarberg, R. "On defining coarticulation." *J. Phonetics* 1: 239-248, 1973.

[13] Fant, G. *Speech Sounds and Features*. Cambridge, MA: MIT Press, 1973.

[14] Farnetani, E. and Recasens, D. "Coarticulation models in recent speech production theories." In *Coarticulation Theory, Data and Techniques*, W. J. Hardcastle and N. Hewlett (eds.), Crambridge: Cambridge University Press, 1999.

[15] Fowler, C. *Timing Control in Speech Production*. Bloomington, IN: Indiana University Linguistics Club, 1977.

[16] Fowler, C. "Coarticulation and theories of extrinsic timing." *J. Phonetics* 8: 113-133, 1980.

[17] Fowler, C.A. "Phonological and articulatory characteristics of spoken language." *Haskins Laboratory Status Report on Speech Research* SR-109/110: 1-12, 1992.

[18] Fowler, C.A., Rubin, P., Remez, R. and Turvey, M.T. "Implications for speech production of the general theory of action." In S*peech Production I: Speech and Talk*, B. Butterworth (ed.), London: Academic Press, pp. 373-420, 1980.

[19] Keating, P. "The window model of coarticulation: Articulatory evidence." *UCLA Working Papers in Phonetics* 69: 3-29, 1988.

[20] Kent, R.D. and Minifie, F.D. "Coarticulation in recent speech production models." *J. Phonetics* 5: 115-133, 1977.

[21] Kluender, K.R. and Lotto, A.J. "Virtues and perils of an empiricist approach to speech perception." *J. Acoust. Soc. Am.* 105: 503-511, 1999.

[22] Kozhevnikov, V.A. and Chistovich, L.A. *Speech, Articulation and Perception. JPRS-30543*. NTIS, US Dept. of Commerce, 1965.

[23] Lindblom, B. "Spectrographic study of vowel reduction." *J. Acoust. Soc. Am.* 35: 1773-1781, 1963.

[24] Lindblom, B. "Explaining phonetic variation: a sketch of the H and H theory." In *Speech Production and Speech Modelling*, A. Marchal and W.J. Hardcastle (eds.), Dordrecht: Kluwer, pp. 403-439, 1990.

[25] Mattingly, I.G. "The global character of phonetic gesture." *J. Phonetics* 18: 445-452, 1990.

[26] Mrayati, M., Carré, R. and Guérin, B. "Distinctive region and modes: A new theory of speech production." *Speech Communication* 7: 257-286, 1988.

[27] Nearey, T.M. "Speech perception as pattern recognition." *J. Acoust. Soc. Am.* 101: 3241-3254, 1997.

[28] Öhman, S. "Coarticulation in VCV utterances: spectrographic measurements." *J. Acoust. Soc. Am.* 39: 151-168, 1966.

[29] Shepard, R.N. "Ecological constraints on internal representation: Resonant kinematics of perceiving, imagining, thinking and dreaming." *Psychological Review* 91: 417-447, 1984.

Dynamics of Speech Production and Perception
P. Divenyi et al. (Eds.)
IOS Press, 2006

Speech Dynamics: Acoustic Manifestations and Perceptual Consequences

Louis C.W. POLS and R.J.J.H. van SON
Institute of Phonetic Sciences
Amsterdam Center for Language and Communication
Amsterdam, The Netherlands

Abstract. Speech is generally considered to be an efficient way of communication between humans, and will hopefully play that same role in the future for communication between humans and machines as well. This efficiency in communication is achieved via a balancing act in which at least the following elements are involved: (1) the lexical and grammatical structure of the message, (2) the way this message is articulated, leading to a dynamic acoustic signal, (3) the characteristics of the communication channel between speaker and listener, and (4) the way this speech signal is perceived and interpreted by the listener. This chapter concentrates on the dynamic spectro-temporal characteristics of natural speech and on the way such natural speech, or simplified speech-like, signals are perceived. Dynamic speech signal characteristics are both studied in carefully designed test sentences as well as in large, annotated and searchable, speech corpora with a variety of speech. From actual spectro-temporal measurements we try to model vowel and consonant reduction, coarticulation, effects of word stress and speaking rate on formant contours, contextual durational variability, prominence, etc. The more speech-like the signal is (on a continuum from a tone sweep to a multi-formant /ba/-like stimulus) the less sensitive listeners appear to be to dynamic speech characteristics such as formant transitions (in terms of just noticeable differences). It also became clear that the (local and wider) context in which speech fragments and speech-like stimuli are presented, plays an important role on the performance of the listeners. Likewise does the actual task for the listener (be it same-different paired comparison, ABX discrimination (X being either A or B), or phoneme or word identification) substantially influence his/her performance.

Keywords. Speech dynamics, local context, efficiency, vowel and consonant reduction, formant sweeps

Introduction

Speech is generally considered to be an efficient way of communication between humans, and will hopefully play that same role in the future for communication between humans and machines as well. This efficiency in communication is achieved via a balancing act in which at least the following elements are involved:

- the lexical and grammatical structure of the message;

- the way this message is articulated, leading to a dynamic acoustic signal;
- the characteristics of the communication channel between speaker and listener;
- the way this speech signal is perceived and interpreted by the listener.

This chapter will concentrate on the dynamic spectro-temporal characteristics of natural speech and on the way such natural speech, or simplified speech-like, signals are perceived. Dynamic speech signal characteristics are both studied in carefully designed test sentences as well as in large, annotated and searchable, speech corpora with a variety of speech. From actual spectro-temporal measurements we try to model vowel and consonant reduction, coarticulation, effects of word stress and speaking rate on formant contours, contextual durational variability, prominence, etc.

The more speech-like the signal is (on a continuum from a tone sweep to a multi-formant /ba/-like stimulus) the less sensitive listeners appear to be to dynamic speech characteristics such as formant transitions (in terms of just noticeable differences). It also became clear that the (local and wider) context in which speech fragments and speech-like stimuli are presented, plays an important role on the performance of the listeners. Likewise does the actual task for the listener (be it same-different paired comparison, ABX discrimination (X being either A or B), or phoneme or word identification) substantially influence his/her performance.

1. Dynamic Spectro-Temporal Characteristics of Natural Speech

Because of articulatory efficiency it is understandable that natural speech is more a continuum of overlapping events than a concatenation of discrete events [2]. Whether this is also beneficial for the listener is one of the topics in the second half of this paper. The dynamicity of speech manifests itself in many different ways, such as:

- the deletion (in pronunciation) of phonemes, syllables, and words, such as the pronunciation of Dutch /Ams@dAm/ rather than /Amst@rdAm/, or /brEm/ for the first part of 'bread and butter' (see also [5]);
- the insertion of phonemes to ease pronunciation, such as in Dutch /du-w-@n/ for 'doe een (do one)', or /di-j-@n/ for 'die een (that one)';
- the almost complete lack of clear word boundary manifestations in conversational speech, compared to the highly functional and visible white space between words in printed text;
- the substantial amount of within and between word coarticulation, assimilation, and degemination, as is for instance clear in the pronunciation of Dutch 'is zichtbaar (is visible)' as /IsIxbar/ rather than as /Is/ /zIxtbar/;
- the existence of vowel and consonant reduction, which is most apparent in not clearly articulated (=sloppy) speech and in unstressed syllables.

Apart from efficiency in articulation, there are various other factors that influence dynamicity, such as speaker idiosyncrasy, speaking style (clear vs. sloppy; hyper vs. hypo) and speaking rate. We are most interested in the acoustic manifestations of these dynamic spectro-temporal phenomena, such as in pitch, loudness, and formant contours in (preferably segmented and labelled) speech. In order to study (the variation in) these

Condition	Number of vowel items	Static (1 frame) % correct	Dynamic (3 frames) % correct
Original	35,385 438 x 13 x (1...25)	59.3	66.9
Speaker normalized	35,385	62.2	69.2
V centers	5,374 438 speakers x 13 vowels	78.9	90.1
Speaker normalized	5,374 438 x 13	87.9	94.5

Table 1. Percentage correct vowel classification of the TIMIT data set using discriminant functions and static or dynamic spectral information. The 4 conditions reflect the use of speaker normalization and/or vowel clustering. For more details, see [21].

contours, one has to measure, stylize, curve fit, and/or mathematically model them in such predefined segments. See for instance Pols and van Son [12] in which either a fixed number of 16 points per (vowel) segment is used to describe formant contours, or 5 fourth-order (Legendre) polynomials. This allows a comparison between normal and fast-rate speech, or between stressed and unstressed syllables. One of the most important conclusions of that study was that rate changes in vowel duration did not change the amount of vowel undershoot, thus indicating an active control of articulation speed, at least for the trained speaker that was studied here.

In Weenink [21] one can find a very straightforward illustration of the efficiency in using a simplified form of dynamic information (rather than static information) for vowel recognition in the TIMIT database. All 10 training and test sentences of all 438 male speakers were used, resulting in 35,385 (hand-labeled) vowel segments, that were spectrally analyzed, using a one-Bark bandfilter analysis of 18 filters (1 bark spaced as well as 1 bark bandwidth). Each bandfilter spectrum was intensity normalized. Three 25-ms frames per segment were used: one central frame, as well as the frames 25 ms to the left and to the right of that central frame. Table 1 shows the results of a discriminant analysis to classify 13 monophthongal vowel categories, using static (1 frame) or dynamic (3 frames) information. Under all 4 conditions (related to using speaker normalization and/or vowel clustering as well) the dynamic results are always substantially better than the static results. Huang [6] found similar results.

Van Bergem [1] showed that acoustic vowel reduction is a function of (experimentally controlled) sentence accent, word stress and word class (in words like 'can', 'candy', 'canteen'). He also analyzed, and then modelled, the coarticulatory effects on the schwa in nonsense words of the type $C_1 @ C_2 V$ and $V C_1 @ C_2$. The schwa appeared NOT to be a centralized vowel but something that is completely assimilated with its phonemic context.

Only after averaging the results over all contexts, one returns to the more commonly known picture of a schwa being a centralized vowel.

Later on van Son and Pols [15] tried to model *consonant* reduction as well. For that purpose 791 comparable VCV-segments were isolated from 20 min. of spontaneous speech and from that same text read aloud. Various aspects of vowel and consonant reduction could be identified, that can perhaps be summarized in the following way:

- in spontaneous speech (compared to read speech) there is a decrease in articulation speed, leading to lower F2-slope differences;

- any vowel reduction seems to be mirrored by a comparable change in the consonant, thus suggesting that vowel onsets and targets change in concert;
- in spontaneous speech there is a decrease in vocal and articulatory effort, resulting in shorter vowels and consonants and in a lower center-of-gravity (COG, first spectral moment).

The above-mentioned studies of van Son and van Bergem were successful, partly because they analyzed material in a carefully designed database. Nowadays it is more and more customary to rely on (annotated) large speech corpora, of which TIMIT is small by present standards. In our own institute, the IFA-corpus is a good medium-size example [17]. It contains about 5.5 hours of speech from 4 male and 4 female speakers of various styles, from informal speech to read texts, and individual sentences, words and syllables. These about 50 K words are segmented and labeled at the phoneme level. The audio files, the annotations, as well as the metadata are accessible in a relational database. Questions can be asked like, what percentage of -en endings in Dutch verbs and nouns (such as in 'geven', to give and 'bomen', trees) are realized as /-@n/ rather than as /-@/? This percentage appears to grow from 0.3% in informal speech to 77% in read sentences. The IFA-corpus is also used to provide Dutch input to the INTAS 915 project about "Spontaneous speech of typologically unrelated languages Russian, Finnish and Dutch: Comparison of phonetic properties". For some preliminary results, see [3].

The 10-million words Spoken Dutch Corpus (CGN) contains much more material (1,000 hrs of speech) from many different speakers under a variety of styles including telephone speech, but contains less varied material from a single speaker. After its completion at the end of 2003, it will be fully transcribed at the level of orthography, part-of-speech, and lemmas, and partly transcribed at the phonemic, prosodic and syntactic level [10]. In the DARPA community one sees now the next level of speech collection, namely so-called 'found' speech, such as Broadcast News [4]. This material is collected for other purposes, but appears to be useful for training and testing automatic speech recognition and creates other scientific challenges and resources.

Above we briefly mentioned some spectro-temporal phenomena related to vowel and consonant reduction. Meanwhile we extended this work by incorporating also the concept of *efficiency* in speech production [18]. Our claim is that the organization of spoken utterances is such that more speaking effort is directed towards important speech parts than towards redundant parts. In order to test this we have to define a measure for the importance of a segment. Based on a model of incremental phoneme-by-phoneme word recognition [9], the importance of a segment is defined as its contribution to word disambiguation. More specifically, the importance of a specific segment for word recognition is defined as the reduction in the number of words in a large corpus (CELEX) that fit the preceding word-onset by adding the target phoneme as a constraint. For example, to determine the importance of the vowel /o/ in the word /bom/ (English 'tree'), we determine how many of the words that start with /b/ have /o/ as their second phoneme. This reduction in the ambiguity is then expressed as the information I_s (in bits) contributed by the vowel /o/ of /bom/. To incorporate also the average influence of the local context on the predictability of a target word, we adapt the CELEX word counts using the context distinctiveness [8] of the target word. For more details see van Son and Pols [19]. By dividing the data into quasi-uniform subsets that are uniform with respect to all relevant factors, we could show for (a subset of) the speech material in the IFA corpus that some 90% of the total variance in I_S could be accounted for by the following factors: phoneme position, phoneme identity, word length in syllables, prominence, lexical syllable stress, length of consonant clusters, syllable part (onset, kernel, or coda), word position in the sentence, and syllable position in the word. The two first factors are most important and account for 81% of the variance already. If we do a similar factorial analysis on acoustic reduction factors such as phoneme duration or Center of Gravity, interestingly enough we find a similar ordering of the factors. These (weak) positive correlations between I_S and acoustic reduction are evidence for our tendency as language user toward greater efficiency.

2. Perception of Speech Dynamics

In his interesting new book about the intelligent ear, Plomp [13] emphasizes the fact that several biases have affected the history of (speech and) hearing research. They can be summarized as follows:

- a dominance of the use of sinusoidal tones as stimuli;
- a preference for the microscopic approach (e.g. phoneme discrimination rather than intelligibility);
- an emphasis on psychological rather than cognitive aspects of hearing;
- the use of clean stimuli in the laboratory, rather than the acoustic reality of the outside world with its disruptive sounds.

Concerning these biases there seems to be a clear parallel between hearing research (or psychoacoustics) and speech research. We know much more about the perception of simple stationary signals than about (spectro-temporally) complex and dynamic signals. Handbooks tell us something about the detection threshold and the just-noticeable-difference for pitch,

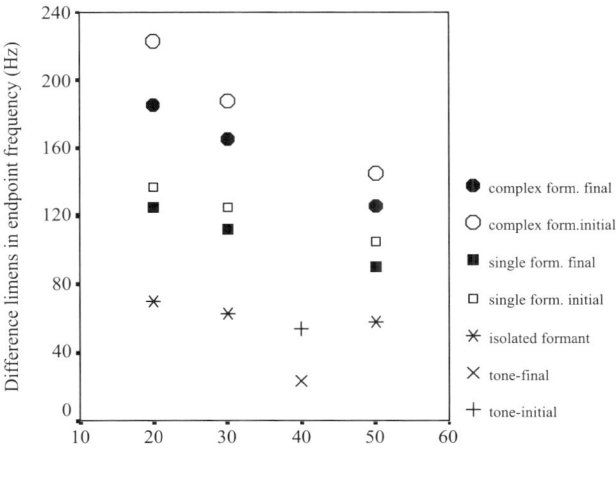

Figure 1. Difference limens in endpoint frequency for various initial and final tone sweeps, single-formant sweeps, and complex formant sweeps. For more details see [23].

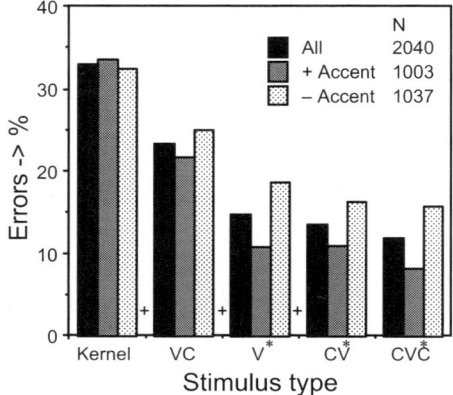

Figure 2. Error rates of *vowel* identification for the various stimulus types. Given are the results for all tokens pooled ("All") as well as for vowels with and without sentence accent separately (+ and – Accent respectively). Long-short vowel errors were ignored, i.e., /A/-/a:/ and /O/-/o:/ confusions in our experiment. Chance response levels would result in 86% errors and a $\log_2$ perplexity of 2.93 bits. +: p0.01, McNemar's test, two tailed between "All" categories. *: χ^2 12, $v = 1$, p0.01, between + and – Accent.

loudness, timbre, and direction of pure tones and sometimes of single-formant stationary periodic signals, but very little about the perception of speech-like formant transitions [11].

2.1 Perception of speech-like tone and formant sweeps

That is why van Wieringen [22] started her thesis project on this topic, see also van Wieringen and Pols [23]. Her most intriguing results (see Figure 1), in our opinion, indicate that sensitivity (in terms of difference limen [DL] in endpoint frequency) decreases the more complex, the more speech-like, the /ba/- and /ab/-type stimuli get! This means that DL is larger for complex multi-formant stimuli than for simple single-formant or sweep-tone stimuli. Furthermore it appeared that DL is larger for shorter transitions (20 ms) than for longer transitions (50 ms), and larger for initial than for final transitions. She used synthetic /ab/- and /bu/-like signals, but later also natural, truncated stimuli. The lesser sensitivity for more

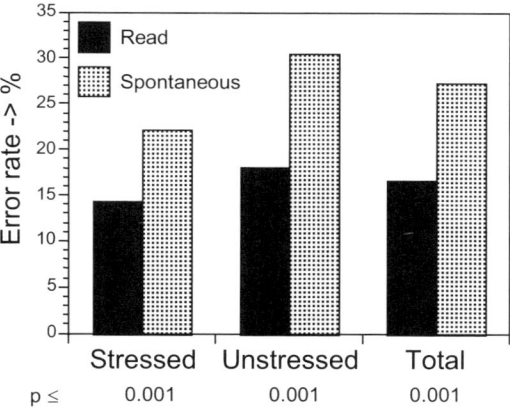

Figure 3. Mean error rate for consonants. For more details see text.

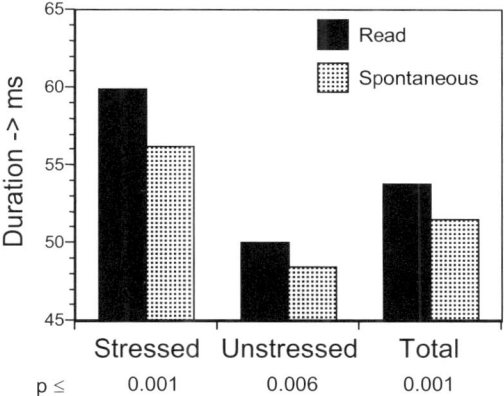

Figure 4. Mean consonant duration identification for 791 VCV pairs from spontaneous and read speech of one male speaker.

complex, more speech-like stimuli, may actually help us to survive in the real world with highly variable speech input. With an analytic hearing we would have to interpret lots of variability that is most probably not very relevant for phoneme categorization.

2.2 Speech identification as a function of context, speaking style, reduction and noise

Rather than discrimination, van Son studied vowel identification with and without (synthetic) formant transitions with a variable frequency range, both symmetric as well as with onglide or offglide only [12]. Under these experimental conditions there was no indication of perceptual overshoot caused by these transitions [7]. Actually there was much more evidence for an averaging behavior of the trailing part of the formant track. In a subsequent study he took 120 CVC speech fragments from a long text reading and presented truncated segments for vowel and consonant identification [16]. The truncated

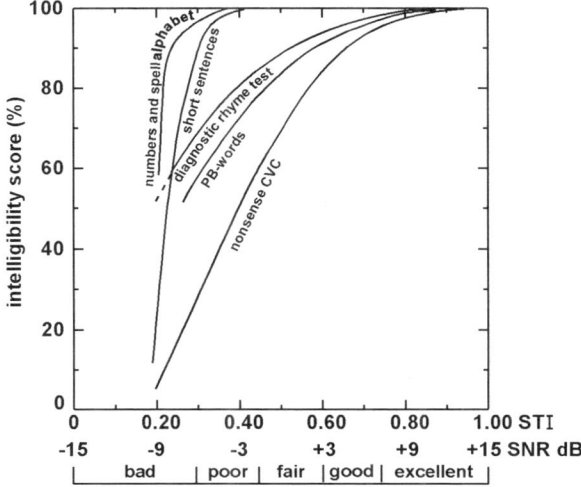

Figure 5. Speech intelligibility for various text types, as a function of the masking noise level.

condition	M1	M2	F1	F2	Average
isolated vowels%	95.2	88.9	88.0	86.4	89.6
(3 sets per speaker)ASC	433	404	447	634	480
words %	88.1	78.8	84.9	85.3	84.3
(5 sets per speaker)ASC	406	320	374	529	407
unstr., free conv.%	31.2	28.7	33.3	38.9	33.0
(10 sets per speaker)ASC	174	119	209	255	189

Table 2. Average percentage correct identification by 100 Dutch listeners of isolated vowel segments, from 2 male and 2 female speakers, extracted under 3 different conditions. The Acoustic System Contrast (ASC) is also presented as a measure of the total variance in the log F1 - log F2 space. For more details see [8].

segments varied from the 50 ms vowel kernel only, to the full CVC segment. As can be seen in Figure 2, it is clear that any addition was beneficial for vowel identification, but the left context was more beneficial than the right context. There was also a context effect (not shown), in the sense that consonant and vowel identification was significantly better when also the other member of the CV-pair was correctly identified. Phoneme identification also differs substantially for speech segments taken from either spontaneous or read speech, and likewise differs for stressed and unstressed syllables.

Van Son and Pols [14] present some interesting results for the, so far not very well defined, phenomenon of *consonant reduction*. Spontaneous speech of one trained male Dutch speaker was collected first, after which this speaker also read aloud that same text. Next, from these two speech fragments 791 comparable pairs of VCV segments (both stressed and unstressed) were extracted and presented to subjects for consonant identification. The mean error rate over 22 subjects (see Figure 3) clearly shows that more intervocalic consonants were misidentified in segments taken from spontaneous speech than from read speech, whereas also unstressed segments cause more errors than stressed segments. This reduction in consonant identification is also clearly reflected in the amount of acoustic consonant reduction. Figure 4 illustrates this acoustic reduction in the form of shorter consonant durations, but similar effects were found for other attributes of acoustic consonant reduction, such as lower Center of Gravity, smaller intervocalic sound energy differences, shorter formant distances of the adjacent vowels, and larger differences of F2 slopes. For more details, see van Son and Pols [14][15].

Above we emphasized the effect of the presence of local context, likewise there is also ample evidence for the effect of lack of context. Take for instance the interesting data of Koopmans-van Beinum [8]. She compared vowel identification for vowel segments taken from three different conditions: isolated vowels, isolated words, and vowels taken from unstressed syllables in free conversation. The average intelligibility of the 12 different Dutch vowels reduced from 89.6, to 84.3, and to 33.0%, respectively, in accordance with the reduction in vowel contrast (a measure for the total variance in the two-formant vowel space), see Table 2. One must realize of course that in their original context all vowels were perfectly well understandable!

The effect of context on intelligibility can also be nicely illustrated by measuring the speech intelligibility in masking noise for various text types. This psychometric function, going from zero intelligibility at low signal-to-noise levels to 100% intelligibility at high SNR, is much steeper for highly predictable material like the spelling alphabet, than for highly unpredictable material like CVC nonsense words, see Figure 5 taken from Steeneken [20].

3. Discussion

In this short contribution we were only able to present some examples in the fascinating field of the acoustic manifestations of speech dynamics and their perceptual consequences. It will be clear that, mainly because of articulatory efficiency, dynamic rather than stationary signals are the norm. Methods are gradually being developed to measure, stylize and model the spectro-temporal variation in the speech signal. There appears to be substantial reduction, both at the vowel and the consonant level, in conversational speech, but there is also a tendency for efficiency, in such a way that more speaking effort is directed towards important speech parts than towards redundant parts. Our perceptual system is very well capable of properly interpreting these dynamic events, but here also efficiency is apparent. The detailed and analytic mode of listening for simple stimuli changes into more global listening where context and redundancy become much more important.

References

[1] Bergem, D. van. *Acoustic and Lexical Vowel Reduction*. Ph. D. Thesis, University of Amsterdam, IFOTT 16, 1995.
[2] Carré, R. "Speech gestures by deduction, gesture production, and gesture perception." Chapter 5 in this volume, 2006.
[3] De Silva, V., Iivonen, A., Bondarko, L.V., Pols, L.C.W. and INTAS 915 partners. "Common and language-dependent phonetic differences between read and spontaneous speech in Russian, Finnish and Dutch." *Proc. Int. Cong. Phon. Sci.*, 2003.
[4] Graff, D. "An overview of Broadcast News corpora." *Speech Communication* 37: 15-26, 2002.
[5] Greenberg, S. "The role of temporal dynamics in understanding spoken language." *In this volume*, 2006.
[6] Huang, C.B. *An Acoustic and Perceptual Study of Vowel Formant Trajectories in American English*. MIT RLE Technical Report No. 563, 1991.
[7] Lindblom, B.E.F. and Studdert-Kennedy, M. "On the role of formant transitions in vowel recognition." *J. Acoust. Soc. Am.* 42: 830-843, 1967.
[8] Koopmans-van Beinum, F.J. *Vowel contrast reduction. An acoustic and perceptual study of Dutch vowels in various speech conditions*. Ph. D. thesis, University of Amsterdam, 1980.
[9] McDonald, S.C. and Shillcock, R.C. "Rethinking the word frequency effect: The neglected role of distributional information in lexical processing." *Lang. Speech* 44: 295-323, 2001.
[10] Norris, D., McQueen, J.M. and Cutler, A. "Merging information in speech recognition: Feedback is never necessary." *Behavior. Brain Sci.* 23: 299-325, 2000.
[11] Oostdijk, N., Goedertier, W., Van Eynde, F., Boves, L., Martens, J.-P., Moortgat, M. and Baayen, H. "Experiences from the Spoken Dutch Corpus project." *Proc. LREC*, 340-347, 2002.
[12] Pols, L.C.W. "Psycho-acoustics and speech perception." In: *Computational Models of Speech Pattern Processing*, K. Ponting (ed.), Berlin: Springer Verlag, pp. 10-17, 1998.
[13] Pols, L.C.W. and Son, R.J.J.H. van. "Acoustics and perception of dynamic vowel segments." *Speech Communication* 13: 135-147, 1993.
[14] Plomp, R. *The Intelligent Ear. On the Nature of Sound Perception*. Mahwah, NJ: Erlbaum, 2002.
[15] Son, R.J.J.H. van and Pols, L.C.W. "The correlation between consonant identification and the amount of acoustic consonant reduction." *Proc. Eurospeech,* pp. 2135-2138, 1997.
[16] Son, R.J.J.H. van and Pols, L.C.W. "An acoustic description of consonant reduction." *Speech Communication* 28: 125-140, 1999.

[17] Son, R.J.J.H. van and Pols, L.C.W. "Perisegmental speech improves consonant and vowel identification." *Speech Communication* 29: 1-22, 1999.

[18] Son, R.J.J.H. van and Pols, L.C.W. "Structure and access of the open source IFA-corpus." *Proc. IRCS Workshop on Linguistic Databases*, pp. 245-253, 2001.

[19] Son, R.J.J.H. van and Pols, L.C.W. "An acoustic model of communicative efficiency in consonants and vowels taking into account context distinctiveness." *Proc. Int. Cong. Phon. Sci.,* pp. 2141-2144, 2003.

[20] Son, R.J.J.H. van and Pols, L.C.W. "Information structure and efficiency in speech production." *Proc. Eurospeech,* pp. 769-772, 2003.

[21] Steeneken, H.J.M. *On Measuring and Predicting Speech Intelligibility.* Ph. D. thesis, University of Amsterdam, 1992.

[22] Weenink, D. "Vowel normalizations with the TIMIT acoustic phonetic speech corpus." *Proc. Institute of Phonetic Sciences* 24: 117-123, 2001.

[23] Wieringen, A. van. *Perceiving Dynamic Speechlike Sounds: Psycho-acoustics and Speech Perception,* Ph.D. thesis, University of Amsterdam, 1995.

[24] Wieringen, A. van and Pols, L.C.W. "Discrimination of short and rapid speechlike transitions." *Acta Acoustica* 84(3): 520-528, 1998.

Perceptual Dynamics of Speech

Dynamics of Speech Production and Perception
P. Divenyi et al. (Eds.)
IOS Press, 2006

Perceptual Dynamics of Speech

Pierre DIVENYI

Speech and Hearing Research
Veterans Affairs Medical Center
and
East Bay Institute for Research and Education
Martinez, California USA

In the previous section, we were shown the importance, and consequences, of considering the dynamic processes behind speech production. But, in order for verbal communication to occur, the perceptual mechanisms responsible for decoding the speech signal must also take into consideration its dynamically changing nature. Some of the chapters in that section, for example those by Björn Lindblom *et al.* (Chapter 1), René Carré (Chapter 5), and Louis Pols and Rob van Son (Chapter 6), used perception data as a way to verify production dynamics and, as a results, showed perceptual consequences of the dynamic processes of speech production. The seven chapters in the present section unveil perceptual aspects of the time-varying acoustic signal that speech represents. They all support the argument that viewing speech as it evolves over time is indispensable for understanding how it is even possible for the casual listener to comprehend everyday speech – speech by talkers of different dialects, speech distorted by noise or reverberation, speech transmitted often imperfectly over telephone, television, or radio. Indeed, speech intelligibility has been reported by a great number of researchers to be extremely robust. But, as demonstrated in the chapter by Steve Greenberg *et al.* (Chapter 13), without considering the dynamic fluctuations of speech with regard to amplitude, phase, and frequency, this robustness cannot be explained. These fluctuations represent modulations of amplitude, phase, and frequency in the speech signal that the auditory system detects and interprets. The chapters in this section throw light on different aspects of these modulations.

Most apparent among the modulations are the continuous changes in the amplitude envelope of speech; these amplitude modulations (AM) break the speech flow into syllables – segments that Kozhevnikov and Chistovich [3] were among the first to recognize as the basic units of speech. This syllabic segmentation explains the language-independent 4-Hz mean of the modulation spectrum amplitude shown in the chapter by Greenberg et al. What these authors also find is that the high-frequency region of the speech spectrum has a second, 15- to 25-Hz modulation spectral peak that can account for sub-syllabic segmentation, such as between syllable onset and syllable coda consonants and the vowel in the syllable nucleus. Although the consonant-vowel (CV) and vowel-consonant (VC) transitions do produce envelope changes in separate frequency bands, they signal changes in the vocal tract resonance pattern and thus generate rapid (20- to 50-ms) formant glides: frequency-modulation (FM) sweeps the percept of which, in the second- and third-formant (F2 and F3) ranges, approaches that of sinusoidal glides. We know that these glides represent important cues for consonant and also vowel identification (see Carré's chapter). However, although we can view these increasing or decreasing monotonic FMs as dynamic changes in the frequency domain, they also represent volley-like short-duration amplitude envelope increases across frequency channels – i.e., patterns of AM. These volleys can be simulated in a manner analogous to two successive light flashes giving the percept of a motion between them (called the phi-phenomenon), demonstrated in the chapters by Valentina Lublinskaja *et al.* and by Larry Feth *et al.* (Chapters 7 and 8). As these authors show, the identity of a consonant can be established from sparse spectral representation of a transition as long as its time course between the endpoints is similar to that of a transition in real speech. It is as if the auditory system does not care about the details of the spectral profile and performs a running weighted-averaging, or spectral center-of-gravity (c-o-g) computation, across the active frequency channels, no matter how sparsely represented they are. The paucity of the necessary spectral information (i.e., the number of channels needed) is also stressed in Chapter 13 by Steve Greenberg *et al.* – showing that intelligibility can be achieved through spectral "slits" – and in Chapter 9 by Georg Meyer *et al.* – showing that the absence of sufficient energy to create a formant is interpreted by the listener as a spectral zero (that is, a nasality cue) following an instantaneous transition.

But does this *"trompe-l'oeuil"* (or rather *"trompe-l'oreille"*) mean that sparse c-o-g transitions are perceptually indistinguishable from either a sweep across all adjacent frequencies of an auditory filter bank or a sinusoidal glide? Larry Feth *et al.* experimentally show that this is not the case: a listener is quite able to tell which type of transition is presented and, although a sinusoidal glide in one ear will be fused with a steady-state vowel in the same or the other ear to evoke the percept of a CV syllable, the glide is still clearly audible. This is new proof of the existence of "duplex perception" [4], which is also reinforced by a result reported in the Georg Meyer *et al.* chapter: the perception of a VC sound's formant dynamics can be reinforced or weakened by a synchronous, but spectrally disconnected sinusoidal glide, depending on the direction of that glide alone.

The presence of a rapid frequency transition, in addition to conferring phonetic identity to speech sounds, also helps localizing the its source in the horizontal plane, as Chapter 11 by Rich Stern *et al.* shows. Without the amplitude and frequency modulations in the speech signal the listener would find it more difficult to segregate a target talker's speech from the babble produced by voices of a crowd – a task that is known to become harder as we age [5], just as the ability to localize sounds does [1]. Temporal resolution of slow AM and FM changes in speech is also important for segregating even as few as two sources, as shown in Chapter 10 by Pierre Divenyi, and this ability is also diminished in older listeners.

Chapter 12 by Richard Turner *et al.* presents another interesting dimension of perceptual speech dynamics. It appears that temporal processing in the ear, in addition to the short-term analysis used to extract periodicity information for pitch and the long-term analysis to extract syllabic and subsyllabic segments, also keeps track of the duration and shape of resonance patterns inside each separate auditory channel. That information is indispensable for characterizing the speaker's gender, age, and size – in other words, the speaker's identity – and offers an explanation of why different formant values across men, women, and children are yet understood as belonging to the same vowel.

The chapters in this section thus constitute pieces of a hitherto little explored edifice: speech as a flow of amplitude- and frequency-modulated signal with multiple but well-circumscribed ranges of modulation frequencies. If adopted by the speech research community, an integrated view of these multi-tier modulation processes (as proposed by Greenberg [2]) should find diverse uses in speech and hearing aid technology and would also represent a belated recognition to the Leningrad group's, and especially Ludmilla Chistovich's, vision.

References

[1] Abel, S.M., Giguere, C., Consoli, A., and Papsin, B.C. (2000). The effect of aging on horizontal plane sound localization, *J Acoust Soc Am*, 108 (2), 743-52.

[2] Greenberg, S. (2006). A multi-tier framework for understanding spoken language, in *Listening to Speech: An Auditory Perspective*, Greenberg, S. and Ainsworth, W., Editors, Lawrence Erlbaum Associates: Mahwah, NJ, pp. 412-425.

[3] Kozhevnikov, V.A. and Chistovich, L.A. (1965). Speech, articulation, and perception. NTIS, US Dept. of Commerce.

[4] Liberman, A.M., Isenberg, D., and Rakerd, B. (1981). Duplex perception of cues for stop consonants: Evidence for a phonetic mode, *PP*, 30, 133-143.

[5] Snell, K.B., Mapes, F.M., Hickman, E.D., and Frisina, D.R. (2002). Word recognition in competing babble and the effects of age, temporal processing, and absolute sensitivity, *J Acoust Soc Am*, 112 (2), 720-7.

Dynamics of Speech Production and Perception
P. Divenyi et al. (Eds.)
IOS Press, 2006

Auditory Perception and Processing of Amplitude Modulation in Speech-like Signals: Legacy of The Chistovich–Kozhevnikov Group

Valentina V. LUBLINSKAJA[1], Jaan ROSS[2] and Elena V. OGORODNIKOVA[1]
[1]Pavlov Institute of Physiology
Russian Academy of Sciences, St. Petersburg , Russia
[2]Department of Arts
University of Tartu, Tartu, Estonia
and Estonian Academy of Music and Theatre, Tallinn, Estonia

Abstract. Research into the auditory perception of speech signals has been carried out in two main directions by the Chistovich-Kozhevnikov group in St. Petersburg (Leningrad): modeling of the peripheral auditory analysis and experimental research of how the peripheral auditory representation is processed on the central auditory levels. The main assumptions for those studies were, first, that the output of peripheral auditory analysis represents a sequence of prominent features and events in a speech flow and, second, that the most important role of the central analysis is the allocation and processing of those features and events. A model of processing of the amplitude envelope in speech signals has been developed, in order to extract the so-called on- and off-events. According to the model, positive and negative markers are localized at precisely the time were the model detects amplitude increases and decreases in any of the frequency channels. Experimental evidence about perception of speech-like signals with step-like formant amplitude jumps is presented in the paper. It demonstrates how listeners use those amplitude jumps at different frequencies to attribute a specific phoneme quality of consonants, and how an abrupt change in the amplitude of one of the formants may influence a perceived quality of a following vowel. An attempt is made to interpret the above results on the basis of short-time peripheral adaptation. The important role of auditory processing of amplitude modulation in speech signals are discussed.

Keywords. Amplitude modulation, auditory processing, syllables

Introduction

Research into auditory perception of speech signals has been carried out in two main directions by the Chistovich-Kozhevnikov group in St. Petersburg (Leningrad): modeling of peripheral auditory analysis, and experimental research into how the peripheral auditory representation is processed at central auditory levels. The main assumptions of those studies were, first, that the output of peripheral auditory analysis represents a sequence of prominent features and events in running speech and, second, that the most important role of the central analyzer is the allocation and processing of those features and events. A model for processing the amplitude envelope in speech signals has been developed, in order to extract what we call the on- and off-events. According to the model, positive and negative markers are localized at precisely the time when the model detects amplitude increases and decreases in any of the frequency channels. Experimental results for perception of speech-like signals with step-like formant amplitude jumps are presented in this paper. These results demonstrate how listeners use those amplitude jumps at different frequencies to attribute a specific phoneme quality of [m] or [l] to a consonant, and how an abrupt change in the amplitude of one of the formants may influence the perceived quality of a following vowel. We attempt to interpret these results on the basis of short-time peripheral adaptation.

1.   A Brief History and the General Approach to Research

In the late 1950s, Ludmilla Chistovich and Valery Kozhevnikov organized a young research group in Leningrad. The group started to work on the production and auditory perception of speech signals, following methodological principles which were very different from the approach in traditional physiology of that time. First, computers and information theory were penetrating into all spheres of science and technology, so it was no surprise that the new group adopted a rather technological vision of speech perception, using metaphors which originated from information theory. To a certain extent, those early developments were stimulated by advanced engineering in the area which is now known as speech technology. It happened that at the same time in Leningrad, a group of engineers headed by the talented expert Leopold Warshawski were working on the construction of the voice coder, or vocoder. This group exhibited interest in the processing of speech signals by the human auditory system because they believed that discovering those mechanisms could help them solve technological problems in the field of speech recognition.

   Research by the Chistovich-Kozhevnikov group started with an assumption that the auditory system and the brain represent a highly organized, automatic system carrying out computational and logical operations in order to process speech. If this is true, studies would reveal the algorithms of these operations as well as their function. Today the above assumption does not seem odd to anybody. The modeling of speech processing and speech production now constitutes two extensive areas in speech research. Some members of the European research community who created anthropomorphic models of speech processing used the ideas from the computational theory formulated by Marr [22] for visual perception (for example, see [2][33]). The Chistovich-Kozhevnikov group had advocated the computational theory of speech processing even before the Marr's book was published. As Chistovich ([4], p. 67) has written, "we believe in our group that the only way to describe human speech is to describe not the perception itself but the artificial speech understanding system that is most compatible with the experimental data obtained in speech perception research."

   From the moment of their foundation there were two formally separate laboratories, headed by Chistovich and Kozhevnikov, respectively, at the Pavlov Institute of Physiology; however, they actually worked together as a single group. After Kozhevnikov's unfortunate death in 1982 the two laboratories were united into one that continued working under supervision of Chistovich. After her retirement in 1986, a small research group of five persons remained. This group still attempts to follow the general direction of research which was initially set by Kozhevnikov and Chistovich. This group's studies include experiments on the effects of the spectral center-of-gravity with dynamic signals [19] and perception of frequency-localized on-events in speech-like sounds, which will be reported in the present paper. In recent years new research has started on children's perception of degraded speech [21] and on speech perception by patients with cochlear implants [15].

Initially, the group (of which the first author was a member) considered their main task to be the study of speech production. This direction followed the motor theory of speech perception [6] which postulated that, in order to recognize speech, it was necessary to transform the auditory images of speech signals back to articulatory commands. A set of transducers for continuous recording of articulatory and acoustic parameters of fluent speech was developed as a tool for the study of the articulatory phenomena that underlie their acoustic manifestations [7].

The possibility of representing speech flow by a sequence of discrete responses from the articulatory transducers that reflect the phonemic attributes of speech seemed to be a tempting idea for constructing a vocoder. The transfer of discrete signals requires a much narrower bandwidth of a transmitting channel than the transfer of analogue signals, and the group got to work building such a device. Although we never constructed an actual vocoder, the use of transducers allowed us to investigate the dynamics of the speech production process. As a result, we obtained a number of interesting new results. In particular, the articulatory gestures underlying the effect of coarticulation were established for the pronunciation of phoneme sequences. These data allowed us to formulate a hypothesis about a serial-parallel scheme of articulatory programming, which we called the comb model [6]. Later Ohala further developed and tested this model [27].

Interesting and important data were obtained by the method called shadowing, which requires rapid repetition of syllables presented to a listener. Results revealed processing and information accumulation mechanisms which precede phonemic decisions. Subsequently, Marslen-Wilson [23] used this method in developing the cohorts' theory, which is related to lexical analysis.

The general theoretical principles of, and major results obtained by, the Chistovich–Kozhevnikov group were published in the former Soviet Union in two monographs: Chistovich, Kozhevnikov et al. [6], and Chistovich et al. [9]. The 1965 book [6] has been translated into English. Papers by Pickett [29] and Porter [30] also contain a detailed survey and discussion of the group's work from its beginning until 1985.

Studies of auditory perception of speech signals followed two distinct paths in the group from the mid-1960s. One path was the modeling of the peripheral auditory analyzer, which has been accomplished via perception experiments, as well as via representations of the speech signal at the output of the peripheral auditory system. Another research focus has been the processing of the peripheral image by the central auditory system at stages prior to phonemic interpretation. It should be noted that studies in this second direction remain at the center of research up to the present day.

A great deal of psychoacoustic research with speech and speech-like stimuli has allowed us to establish that the output of the auditory analyzer, the dynamic "auditory spectrogram," reflects a time sequence of prominent features and events (which are

understood as quick changes) in running speech. We hypothesized that the main function of central processing is to allocate and analyze those prominent features and events.
We modeled this function to be carried out in a set of processing blocks working in parallel. Some blocks are thought to react only to the fast intensity and frequency changes
of spectral components. Other blocks may deal with stationary portions of a speech signal (i.e., with those constant in time) in which certain prominent features are allocated
and analyzed. As a rough approximation, operation of those two types of blocks can be
considered equivalent to two types of neural reactions: phasic ones, which respond only
to the onset and offset of a stimulus, and tonic ones, which keep responding for the
whole duration of a stimulus. The two types of neural responses have been observed in
almost all parts of the central auditory pathways (see the review in [11]).

This idea was accepted and further developed elsewhere, in particular by the Grenoble group [34]. An extensive series of psychoacoustic experiments and modeling was
devoted to auditory processing of the spectral envelope and to the phonemic interpretation of the speech signal. Results of those experiments included new findings on the
detection of formants and formant transitions, vowel categorization, the "spectral center-of-gravity" theory, temporal accumulation of spectral shape, etc. Chistovich [5] presented a review of this work.

Another series of experiments targeted the central auditory processing of amplitude
modulation (AM) in speech and speech-like signals. This work is the main topic of the
present paper because the principles of AM processing can perhaps reflect the dynamics
of speech perception in the best possible way. A review of this topic can be found in
Sorin [37] and a detailed survey of the work on amplitude modulation in Porter [30].
This paper will concentrate on the work carried out after 1985.

2. Model of Auditory Processing of the Amplitude Envelope

The most well-known and frequently simulated AM events are the onset and offset of a
segment, or simply on- and off-events. At the end of the 1970s, Kozhevnikov and his
colleagues developed the model of processing amplitude envelopes in the frequency
channels of the auditory spectral analyzer. It is known as the Detection of Amplitude
Irregularities (DAI) model. The simulation of auditory processing of on- and off-events
has been rather active in the last decade as, for example, in the work of the Grenoble and
Sheffield groups [34][3].

The first version of the model was built as an analog device [16] and later was
implemented on a digital computer [42][40]. A linear spectral analyzer consisting of
128 frequency channels carried out the first processing stage with the filters' frequency
tuning characteristics close to the characteristics of the basilar membrane and first-order
auditory neurons. The signals in each channel were half-wave rectified and compressed.
The front-end also included non-linear blocks simulating two-tone suppression (lateral
inhibition) and short-term adaptation. As a result, a time-frequency display was com-
piled, which we call the dynamic auditory spectrogram. It served as an input for the DAI
model, consisting of three bandpass filters with central frequencies equal to 4, 25, and
75 Hz. When the output of the envelope filter exceeded some fixed positive threshold,
an on-marker was triggered, while crossing the negative threshold gave rise to an off-
marker.

The choice of filter characteristics was based on the results of experiments described by Chistovich et al. ([9], p. 146). These results showed that sequences of periodic sinusoidal amplitude modulation near 4 Hz were perceived as sequences of CV-syllables consisting of a stop consonant and a vowel. At a higher frequency of 25 Hz, the same signal was still perceived as a CV-syllable but instead of a stop, the consonant acquired the quality of [r]. At even higher rate of repetition of about 75 Hz the sequence lost its syllable-like character and gave way to a sensation of roughness. These observations were in general agreement with well-known psychoacoustic data showing that the auditory perception of amplitude modulation depends upon the rate of modulation. According to Terhardt [41], rapid amplitude modulation of signals (from 50 to 100 Hz) can elicit judgments of roughness which vary with the rate and depth of modulation. Slower rates of AM (approximately 4 Hz) can result in a perception described as the fluctuation of salience [12].

It is possible to see the positive markers as an approximate equivalent to the on-responses and the negative markers as an equivalent to the off-responses. In this way, the signal is represented by positive and negative markers from each of the three band-pass filters for every frequency channel. This kind of image consists of elementary AM-events, called primitives. At the next stage of processing, coherent configurations of this image are analyzed to form more complex events. What are the characteristics of such coherent configurations, how are they formed, and what function do they perform?

According to one hypothesis, the auditory system conducts spatial summation (along the frequency axis) of on- and off-responses arising synchronously in time. This assumption is based on psychoacoustic data showing a reduction in the thresholds for detecting amplitude irregularities in a compound signal depending on the number of irregularity–inducing components [32][17][43]. As a rule, auditory processing models for amplitude irregularities include summation across the full frequency range of synchronous local on- and off-responses as an unavoidable computational requirement [33][3]. A similar procedure was included in the DAI model [40]. As a result, a single response is formed at a given moment in time. This is considered the most reliable cue for segmenting speech flow.

This procedure results in marked sequences of intervals, which are a precondition for measuring their duration. In the early work by Chistovich et al. ([9], p. 152) it was shown that vowel-like sounds with a complex stationary spectrum were perceived as syllables if a rapid amplitude jump occurred in the signal some time after its onset. If the amplitude was increased as a result of the jump, the sound was perceived as a CV-syllable, and conversely, if the amplitude was decreased, the sound was perceived as a VC-syllable. In the case of CV-syllables, the duration of the first signal segment with lower amplitude was shown to influence the quality of the perceived consonant in the quasi-syllable: It was perceived as a voiced stop if the duration of the initial segment was less than 30 ms, and it was perceived as a nasal if duration of the initial segment was more than 30 ms. This indicates that the temporal location of the on- and off-events is analyzed during auditory processing of speech signals and, moreover, that it can be used for phonemic interpretation of the signal.

However, the available evidence suggests that the auditory system is not indifferent to the frequency location of the neural on-responses when it measures segment duration. This has been demonstrated by data concerning auditory segregation or grouping of subsequent sound streams [1]. A number of experimental results suggest that duration mea-

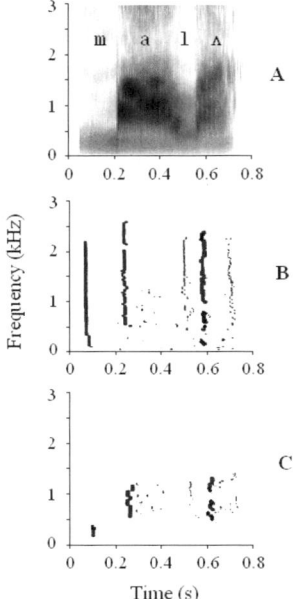

Figure 1. Spectrogram of the Russian word [malʌ] (top) and the DAI model's responses to the same word
with two settings for the threshold parameters (middle and bottom).

surement appears to be possible only for those temporal intervals which are framed with
markers emerging in the same frequency channels [17].

   In the DAI model, different configurations of the marks localized with respect to the
frequency axis can be obtained by selecting different threshold parameters. Figure 1
shows the model's response, with the filter cutoff set to 25 Hz, to a natural speech signal
(the Russian word *malo* [malʌ] "small") for two modes of the threshold setting. The top
panel shows the output of the first level of the model, the spectral analyzer. The middle
panel shows output of the model with the thresholds selected to make the maximum
number of channels respond. It can be seen in the middle panel that on-marks which
correspond to the beginning of vowels and off-marks which correspond to their end
form contours in the shape of vertical lines. The bottom panel shows the distribution of
markers obtained when the thresholds were set 20 dB above the preceding ones. In this
case, the vertical lines along the frequency axis have more local character.

3. Perception of Frequency Localization of On-Events

Although the auditory system has been shown to detect AM-events in areas localized
with respect to frequency [25], it is not clear whether a listener is aware of the frequency
of these areas, or whether the frequency-localized on-events contribute to phonetic
interpretation of the speech signal. Investigations of listeners' use of acoustical cues in
speech suggest that the temporal pattern of on-events in the frequency channels can
serve as a useful cue for phonemic identification, in particular, for fricatives or nasal
consonants in a syllable [38]. Use of the local frequency range of on-responses as a pho-

netic cue has been stressed by Delgutte [10]. In his model, responses from two frequency ranges were summed, the limit between them was set to 0.8 kHz, and information at higher frequencies was associated with stop consonants while information at lower frequencies was associated with vowels.

The question of whether it is possible to use the local frequency range of on- or off-events as a phonetic cue for phonemic interpretation could be answered by experimental evidence. Namely, in speech recognition, the phonemic decision-makers are able to react differentially to the frequency location of the amplitude irregularities. The first attempt to demonstrate this was made by experiments with synthesized two-formant vowel-like signals in which the amplitude of the first formant changed abruptly several dozen milliseconds after the onset [20]. Results of this study, however, did not permit us to answer the question definitively. In the present paper, we will describe additional experiments aimed at showing the effect of frequency localized on-events on a phonetic interpretation of speech signals.

3.1 Method and stimuli

Listeners were asked to identify synthesized speech-like stimuli. The stimuli were vowel-like sounds consisting of "formant impulses" (short tonal impulses with a triangular envelope shape, which approximate the output of a bandpass filter tuned to a frequency of F_1, F_2 or F_3). A more detailed description of the stimulus generation is presented by Chistovich and Ogorodnikova [8]. Three-formant sounds were used for the experiment. A three-formant impulse was synthesized by adding the waveforms of the F_1, F_2 and F_3 impulses with equal coefficients. The impulse duration was 10 ms, which corresponds to a fundamental frequency of 100 Hz. The stimuli contained 25 formant impulses, so that the total duration of a stimulus was 250 ms The frequencies of the formants were chosen in order to make the stimuli similar to the vowel [a], as well as making the distances between the formants approximately equal to each other on the bark scale: $F_1 = 0.6$ kHz, $F_2 = 1.2$ kHz, and $F_3 = 2.2$ kHz. The signals were synthesized at a sampling frequency of 20 kHz and a low-pass filter cut-off of 10 kHz, using a 12-bit digital-to-analog converter.

Three types of stimuli were used in the experiments:

1. The amplitude of one of the formants (F_1, F_2, or F_3) or of all three formants (F_1, F_2, and F_3) was attenuated during the initial 80 ms of the sound. The amount of attenuation could vary from zero to 40 dB compared to the initial level. As a result we obtain four versions of quasi-syllables: for three versions, the on-event is located in one of three possible frequency regions. In the fourth version, the on-event appears simultaneously in all three regions. Figure 2 shows the spectrograms for all four versions of quasi-syllables. They illustrate temporal changes in formant amplitudes while formant frequencies remain unchanged.

2. Stationary vowel-like stimuli with constant formant amplitudes during the whole stimulus duration.

3. Stationary vowel-like stimuli with the same formant frequencies, as in the previous stimuli, but with attenuation of the amplitudes for pairs of formants (F_1 and F_3, or F_1 and F_2) during the whole duration. The amount of attenuation could vary over the same range as for the quasi-syllables.

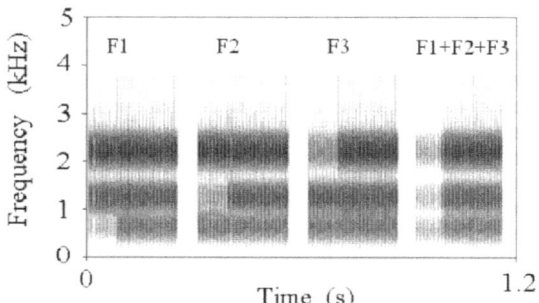

Figure 2. Spectrograms of stimuli in the experiment with attenuation, during the initial segment of sound, of one or several maxima in the spectrum. In the stimuli from left to right, either F_1, F_2, F_3, or all three formants are attenuated, respectively.

3.2 Listeners and procedure

Nine people with normal hearing participated in the experiments. They were asked to identify each stimulus as a vowel, as a syllable consisting of a consonant following a vowel, or as a vowel with some irregularity. The stimuli were presented monaurally via high-quality TDS-5 headphones. The intensity of the stimuli was in the range 60-77 dB SL.

3.3 Results

The experiment was organized into two series. In the first series, stimulus types 1 and 2 were used, while in the second series stimulus types 2 and 3 were used. It should be emphasized that the frequencies of the formants did not vary in any of the cases, so that there were *no* frequency transitions in the stimuli.

Results of the first series are shown in Figure 3, which presents the identification data in relation to the formant amplitudes of the stimuli. The data were pooled for all levels of amplitude attenuation during the initial segment of the sound. Responses are grouped into the following categories:

1. A vowel (of whatever phonetic quality). The stimuli were most often identified as [a] but responses [e], [i], [o] and [y] also occurred. All responses consisting only of a vowel were combined into a single category represented as a V in the leftmost column of Figure 3.

2. A vowel (of whatever phonetic quality) with some amplitude irregularity, indicated as V~ in Figure 3.

3. A syllable consisting of an initial consonant [l] followed by a vowel [a], indicated as LA.

4. A syllable consisting of a consonant [m] and a vowel [a] indicated as MA.

5. A syllable [na], indicated as NA.

Figure 3 demonstrates that the stationary, vowel-like stimuli were mostly identified as vowels, while the stimuli with an amplitude jump after the initial 80 ms of the sound were perceived as syllables. The quality of a consonant in the perceived syllable seems to

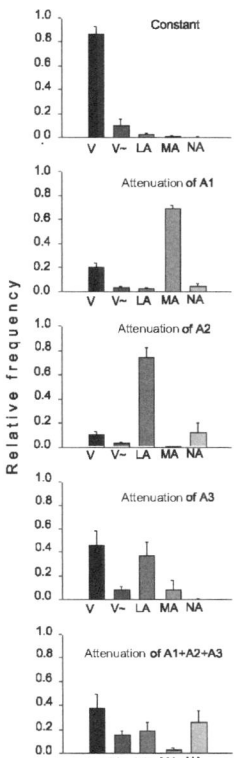

Figure 3. Distribution of responses in the identification experiment. The panels represent, from top to bottom, responses to the stimuli with no amplitude attenuation; attenuation of F_1, F_2, or F_3; or of all three formants in the spectrum, respectively. The columns indicate proportions of identification of the stimuli as a vowel, a vowel with amplitude irregularity, or a syllable [la], [ma] or [na].

be determined by the frequency position of the amplitude jump. Attenuation of F_1 results in identification of the syllable as [ma], and attenuation of F_2 leads to identification as [la]. Attenuation of F_3 results in a more heterogeneous distribution of responses which are divided between a vowel and the [la]-syllable. The widest dispersion of responses was observed for stimuli with the amplitudes of all three formants attenuated at the beginning of the sound.

Analysis of variance (MANOVA) across the stimuli and across the response categories indicated a strong effect of the formant frequency on the identification results, as averaged over subjects [F $(20,120) = 11.39$; p < 0.001]. There were only small variations for separate categories of responses (mean errors) among the subjects. This shows that the results are sufficiently homogeneous. The experimental data confirmed our predictions of the DAI model: listeners used on-responses integrated across a wide frequency range as a boundary between consonant and vowel, and they used on-responses localized in a narrow frequency band as a cue for the phonemic interpretation of consonants.

In the first series of experiments we noticed that attenuating the amplitude of one, or more, formants had an effect on the identification of the quality of the second segment (i.e., the vowel) in a quasi-syllable, despite its spectral position remaining constant for

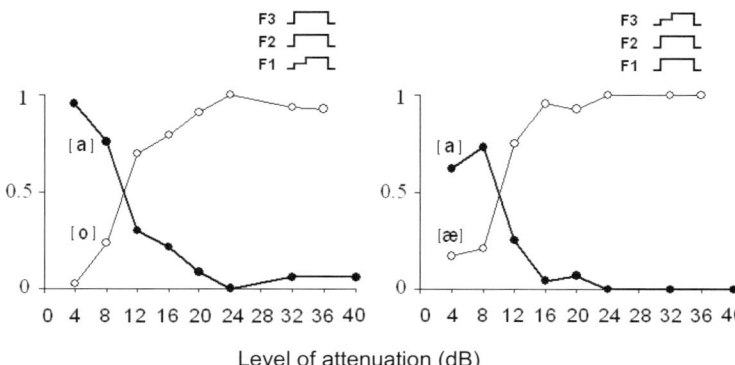

Figure 4. Identification of quasi-vowels depending upon the size of amplitude attenuation of the spectral maxima. The left panel represents the distribution of the most prominent response categories when F_1
has been attenuated and the right panel the distribution of prominent responses with an attenuated
F_3. Data are averaged for five subjects.

all categories of stimuli. This effect was observed for only five listeners. Results of the
vowel identification by these subjects depended on the amount of amplitude attenuation
of a formant. Figure 4 presents the average data for the five listeners. The sounds with
the least attenuation of F_1 during their initial portion were mostly identified as [a], while
the sounds with a greater level of attenuation of F_1 were identified as [o] (left panel).
The sounds with less attenuation of F_3 were mostly identified as [a] too, but with an
increase in of the amount of attenuation, the responses became dominated by the [æ]
vowel (right panel).

We have tried to explain this result as an effect of short-term peripheral adaptation
on the spectral envelope of the stimuli. It is likely that during the second segment of the
stimulus, the intensity of that formant which was attenuated during the first segment
will be amplified as compared to the two adjacent formants. This redistribution of the
amplitude relationship among the three formants may account for the change in vowel
quality. The influence of previous context on phoneme identification, due to the effect
of short-term adaptation, has been investigated by Mushnikov and Chistovich [26] and
later by Lacerda and Moreira [18].

It would be possible to check this assumption if we compared the identification of
stationary vowels with two formant amplitudes attenuated for their whole duration, with
the identification of quasi-syllables with the remaining single formant amplitude attenuated for the initial segment. If the identification results for the two types of stimuli were
similar to each other, then the short-term adaptation mechanism may be accountable for
the observed vowel quality change. In the second series of experiments, the amplitude
of F_2 or F_3 was attenuated from 4 to 24 dB during the initial segment of a quasi-syllable.
The amplitudes of F_1 and F_3, or F_1 and F_2, were attenuated by the same amount during
the whole vowel-like sounds. The stimuli were synthesized and the experimental methods were similar to the first experimental series.

Figure 5 presents the identification results for quasi-syllables, with the amplitude of
F_1 attenuated during the initial segment, and the identification results for quasi-vowels,
with the amplitudes of F_2 and F_3 attenuated with respect to that of F_1 during the whole
duration. It can be seen that the responses of the listeners are dominated by [o] for both

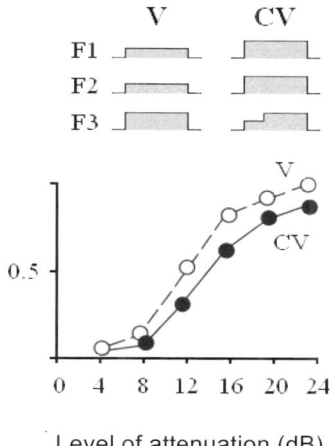

Figure 5. Identification of the vowel [o] with vowel-like stimuli (open circles) and syllable-like stimuli (filled circles) depending on the size of amplitude attenuation. F_1 and F_2 were attenuated for the whole duration of a stimulus in a quasi-vowel and F_3 was attenuated for the initial segment of a stimulus in a quasi-syllable.

the quasi-syllables and quasi-vowels when the amount of attenuation exceeds approximately 12 dB. The two response curves are remarkably similar.

Furthermore, we have calculated the spectral envelopes for both quasi-syllables and quasi-vowels according to the model of auditory processing described above, varying the size of the time averaging window. Figure 6 presents the output of the auditory processing model for a quasi-syllable and a quasi-vowel, with a time window of 40 ms. In the upper panel, the spectral envelope is presented for 40 ms from the beginning of the second segment in a quasi-syllable, after F_1 has been attenuated by 20 dB during the first segment of the same quasi-syllable. In the lower panel, the spectral envelope is presented for a segment from a quasi-vowel with both F_2 and F_3 attenuated by 16 dB during the whole sound. Both stimuli have been identified as [o] by a majority of the listeners. The two curves in Figure 6 are remarkably similar.

3.4 Discussion and conclusions

The experiments with synthetic quasi-syllables have confirmed that the phoneme interpreter seems to be aware not only of cues for spectral changes in some plosive consonants but also of the frequency localization of the most prominent amplitude change in the spectrum. It is possible that under normal (acoustic) listening conditions, when speech possesses all necessary spectral attributes, many of the described AM-events do not participate in the recognition process. It is difficult, however, to deny the primary role of on- and off-events in the formation of internal representations for the rhythm of utterances even under normal circumstances. When listeners' spectral analyzers fail, they may resort to the AM characteristics, not only for the perception of rhythm, but also for phonemic analysis.

For the last several decades, interest in the principles and mechanisms of auditory processing of temporal modulation in speech has increased. Although this issue has not been completely overlooked in recent years (e.g. [28][14][30][35]), it has been at least

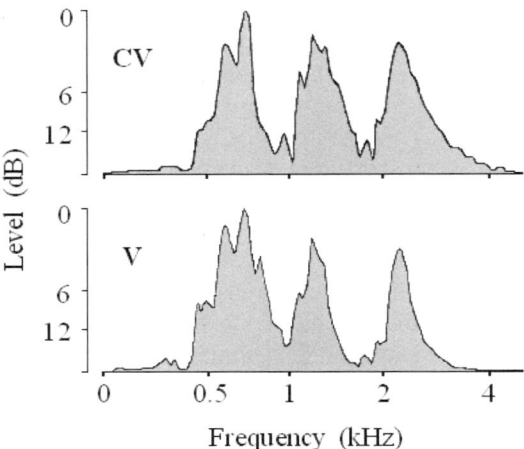

Figure 6. Auditory spectra of the syllable-like stimuli (CV) or vowel-like stimuli (V) which were identified in similar ways.

overshadowed by the more popular view that spectral analysis is the most important operation in phonetic interpretation of speech sounds. This view, in turn, stems from a belief that auditory recognition is based on the "beneficial attributes" which remain time–invariant for the majority of conditions. The remaining acoustical features which do not belong to these beneficial attributes were considered redundant from the point of view of speech perception. It is becoming increasingly clear these days, however, that the so-called secondary attributes of speech signals are in fact not redundant, but provide a description necessary for speech recognition when the primary beneficial attributes are distorted or absent. Discussion of this problem can be found elsewhere in the present volume [24]. A significant contribution to understanding the significance of AM attributes in speech perception has been made by Shannon et al. [36]. They have demonstrated that under conditions where only a minimal amount of spectral information is available to the listener, speech recognition is still possible on the basis of temporal cues. Further, Stickney and Assmann [39] showed that temporal information in a limited spectral range can provide a listener with highly intelligible speech, and that intelligibility may be influenced by specific localization of the frequency range. These facts have special importance for comprehending how speech perception is accomplished by people who use cochlear implant devices. It is well known that a cochlear implant processor can transmit spectral information to the central level of the auditory system using only a limited number of frequency channels.

The work reported in this paper presents evidence of the possibility of using temporal envelope characteristics in different frequency channels for recognizing speech signals, without necessarily specifying exactly which features participate in what kind of phonemic interpretation. The results of our experiments point to the resources that may be used in speech perception, including the AM processing, under conditions where only limited spectral information is present. We observed changes in phoneme identification in quasi-vowels and in quasi-syllables depending on the formant frequencies and the degree of their amplitude attenuation. Our data can be interpreted as a result of a short-term adaptation mechanism, in which the amplitude of an attenuated formant is increased in the initial part of the segment following attenuation. This explanation is related to Repp's [31] conception of the role of short-term adaptation in perceiving contrasts between [m] and [n]. He claims that enhanced place cues in higher formant transitions at vowel onset may result from energy attenuation in the region of the first formant.

This explanation based on short-term adaptation, however, contradicts the conclusion of Chistovich [5] that listeners accumulate information about spectral envelope for the whole duration of a vowel. It is possible that in addition to short-term peripheral adaptation, another neural mechanism is active on a longer time scale. Delgutte et al. [11] presented data indicating that some neurons in the central auditory system are specialized for adapting to the influence of the longer context than during the short-term peripheral adaptation. There are also data suggesting that amplitude modulation is detected and analyzed in the auditory system not only in the separate frequency channels but also between them. Research on the "center-of-gravity" effect demonstrates that listeners perceive dynamic redistribution of energy between successive frequency channels in a way similar to how they perceive changes of spectral maxima in time [19][13]. All this permits us to agree with Repp ([31], p. 1536) that "the internal representation of the auditory signal from which phonetic information is derived, particularly at points following rapid spectral change, is, therefore, different from the one visible in a spectrogram or oscillogram."

Acknowledgements

We are very grateful to our colleagues and friends Elvira Stoliarova for processing the stimuli in the auditory model, to the late Tasia Malinnikova for her extensive help in the preparation of the stimuli and in conducting the experiments, and to Elena Vershinina for her help in the statistical analysis of data.

References

[1]   Bregman, A.S. "How does physiology support auditory scene analysis?" In *Auditory Physiology and Perception*, Y. Cazals (ed.) New York: Oxford, pp. 417-427, 1992.

[2]   Brown, G.J., and Cook, M.P. "Modeling modulation maps in the higher auditory system." *Brit. J. Audiol.* 24: 5-6, 1990.

[3]   Brown, G. J. *Computational Auditory Scene Analysis: A Representational Approach.* Doctoral Thesis, Department of Computer Science, University of Sheffield, 1992.

[4]   Chistovich, L. A. "Auditory processing of speech." *Language and Speech* 23: 67-73, 1980.

[5]   Chistovich, L. A. "Central auditory processing of peripheral vowel spectra." *J. Acoust. Soc. Am.* 77: 789-805, 1985.

[6]   Chistovich, L. A., Kozhevnikov, V. A., Aljakrinskij, V. V., Bondarko, L. V., Goluzina, A. G., Klaas, Ju. A., Kuzmin, Ju. I., Lisenko, D. M., Lubliskaja, V. V., Fiodorova, N. A., Shupljakov, V. S. and Shupljakova, R. M. *Rech: articuljacija i vosprijatie (Speech: Articulation and Perception).* Leningrad: Nauka, 1965. [Russian]

[7]   Chistovich, L. A. and Kozhevnikov, V. A. *Speech: Articulation and Perception.* US Dept. of Commerce, JPRS: 30, 543, Washington, 1965. [English translation of [6]].

[8]   Chistovich, L. A. and Ogorodnikova, E. A. "Temporal processing of spectral data in vowel perception." *Speech Communication* 1: 45-55, 1982.

[9]   Chistovich, L. A., Ventsov, A. V., Granstrem, M. P., Zhukov, S. Ja., Zhukova, M. G., Karnickaja, E. G., Kozhevnikov, V. A., Lisenko, D. M., Fiodorova, N. A., Haavel, P. H., Chistovich, I. A. and Shupljakov, V. S. *Fisiologija rechi. Vosprijatie rechi chelovekom (Speech Physiology. Speech Perception).* Leningrad: Nauka, 1976. [Russian]

[10] Delgutte, B. "Preliminary analysis of French stop consonants with a model of the peripheral auditory system," in *CNET* (Lannion), vol. 7, pp. 3-24, 1981/1982/1983.
[11] Delgutte, B., Hammond, B. M., Kalluri, S. K, Litvak, L. M., and Cariani, P. A. "Neural encoding of temporal envelope and temporal interactions in speech." *Proc. ESCA Workshop on the Auditory Basis of Speech Perception*, 1996.
[12] Fastl, H. "Fluctuation strength and temporal masking patterns of amplitude-modulated of broadband noise." *Hear. Res.* 8: 59-69, 1982.
[13] Feth, L. L., Fox, R. A., Jacewicz, E., and Iyer, N. "Dynamic center-of-gravity effects in consonant-vowel transitions." Chapter 9 in this volume, 2006.
[14] Kay, R. H. "Hearing of modulation in sounds." *Physiol. Rev.* 62: 894-975, 1982.
[15] Koroleva, I. V., Lublinskaja, V. V., Stoljarova, E. I. and Jagunova, E. V. "Invariant perception of speech stimuli in cochlear implanted patients." *Proc. 25th World Congress* Int. Assoc. Logoped. an Phoniatr., pp. 105-109, 2001.
[16] Kozhevnikov, V. A., Drozdova, N. E. and Stoljarova, E.I. "The application of analog models of some auditory mechanisms for speech signal processing," In *Netherlands Phonetic Archives. In Honor of Ilse Lehiste.* pp. 151-159, 1987.
[17] Green, D. M., and Forrest, T. G. "Temporal gaps in noise and sinusoids." *J. Acoust. Soc. Am.* 86: 961-970, 1989.
[18] Lacerda, F., and Moreira, H. O. "How does peripheral auditory system represent formant transitions? A psychophysical approach." In *The Representation of Speech in the Peripheral Auditory System,* R.C. Carlson and B. Granström (eds.) Amsterdam, pp. 89-94., 1982.
[19] Lublinskaja, V. V. "The "center of gravity" effect in dynamics." *Proc. ESCA Workshop on the Auditory Basis of Speech Perception,* pp. 102-105, 1996.
[20] Lublinskaja, V.V., Stoljarova, E.I., and Zhukov, S.Ja. "The study of auditory detection of jump of formant frequency and amplitude as a consonant." *Proc. 11th Int. Cong. Phon. Sci..* Vol. 3, pp. 190-193, 1987.
[21] Lublinskaja, V.V., Koroleva, I.V., Kornev, A.N. and Iagunova, E.V. "Perception of noised words by normal children and children with speech and language impairments." *Proc. 5th European Conference on Speech Communication and Technology,* pp. 2491-2494, 1997.
[22] Marr, D. *Vision.* San Francisco: W. H. Freeman, 1982.
[23] Marslen-Wilson, W. D. "Speech shadowing and speech comprehension," *Speech Communication* 4, 55-74, 1985.
[24] Meyer, G., Harding, S. and Perez, E. "Multi-resolution analysis in speech perception." In this volume, 2006.
[25] Möller, A. R. *Auditory Physiology.* New York: Academic Press, 1983.
[26] Mushnikov, V. N. and Chistovich, L. A. "Projavlenie adaptacii pri vosprijatii reche-podobnyh stimulov (The adaptation phenomenon in the perception of speech-like stimuli) In *Teorii i metody issledovanija vosprijatija rechevyh signalov.* Leningrad, pp. 51-62, 1971. [Russian]
[27] Ohala, J. J. "The temporal regulation of speech." In *Auditory Analysis and Perception of Speech,* G. Fant and M.A.A. Tatham (eds.). New York: Academic Press, pp. 431-464, 1975.
[28] Plomp, R. "The role of modulation in hearing," In *Hearing: Physiological Bases and Psychophysics.* Berlin: Springer Verlag, pp. 270-276, 1983.
[29] Pickett, J. M. "Shadows, echoes and auditory analysis of speech." *Speech Communication* 4, 19-30, 1985.
[30] Porter, R.J. "Pavlov Institute research in speech perception: Finding phonetic messages in modulations." *Speech Communication* 4: 31-39, 1985.
[31] Repp, B.H. On the possible role of auditory short-term adaptation in perception of the prevocalic [m]-[n] contrast." *J. Acoust. Soc. Am.* 82: 1525-1538, 1987.
[32] Rodionov, V. D., Carré, R. and Kozhevnikov, V. A. "Obedinenie informacii o kratkovremennyh izmenenijah ogibajushih signalov v razlichnyh chastotnyh kanalah (Integration of short-term changes of signals envelope under different frequency channels)." *Fiziologija cheloveka* 2:1021-1027, 1976. [Russian]
[33] Schwartz, J.L. and Escudier, P. "Integration for extraction: what speech perception researchers can learn from Gibson and Marr." *Proc. 12th Int. Cong. Phon. Sci.* Vol. 1, pp. 68-72, 1991.

[34] Schwartz, J. L., Beautemps, D., Arrouas, Y. and Escudier, P. "Auditory analysis of speech gestures." In *The Auditory Processing of Speech*, M. E. H. Schouten (ed.), Berlin: Mouton de Gruyter, pp. 239-252, 1992.

[35] Shannon, R. V., Zeng, F. G. and Wygonski, J. "Speech recognition using only temporal cues," in *The Auditory Processing of Speech*, M. E. H. Schouten, ed. Mouton de Gruyter, Berlin, New York, pp. 263-274, 1992.

[36] Shannon, R.V., Zeng, F.G., Kamath, V., Wygonski, J. and Ekelid, M. "Speech recognition with primarily temporal cues." *Science* 270: 303-304, 1995.

[37] Sorin, C. "Bibliography [of Lyudmila Chistovich]." *Speech Communication* 4: 9-12, 1985.

[38] Stevens, K.N. "Evidence for the role of acoustic boundaries in the perception of speech sounds."*Speech Comm. Group Working Paper.* Res. Lab. Electronics, MIT, Vol. 4, pp. 1-13, 1984.

[39] Stickney, G. S., and Assmann, P. F. "Acoustic and linguistic factors in the perception of bandpass filtered speech," *J. Acoust. Soc. Am.* 109, 1157-1165, 2001.

[40] Stoljarova, E. I. "The functional model of auditory segmentation." *Proc. 12th Int. Cong. Phon. Sci.* Vol. 3, pp. 398-401, 1991.

[41] Terhardt, E. "On the perception of periodic sound fluctuations (roughness)." *Acustica* 30: 201-213, 1974.

[42] Ventsov, A.V., Zotova, E. N. and Stoljarova, E. I. "Programmnyj compleks dlja issledovanija rechevyh signalov (The software for the study of speech signals)." *Proc. 15th Workshop on Automatic Recognition of Auditory Images*, pp. 188-189, 1989. [Russian]

[43] Yost, W.A. and Sheft, S. "Across-critical-band processing of amplitude-modulated tones," *J. Acoust. Soc. Am.* 85: 848-857, 1989.

Dynamics of Speech Production and Perception
P. Divenyi et al. (Eds.)
IOS Press, 2006

Dynamic Center-of-Gravity Effects in Consonant-Vowel Transitions

Lawrence L. FETH, Robert A. FOX, Ewa JACEWICZ and Nandini IYER
Department of Speech and Hearing Science
The Ohio State University
Columbus, Ohio, USA

Abstract. Lublinskaja (1996) has reported that dynamic changes in the spectral center-of-gravity (c-o-g) in selected Russian vowels led to changes in vowel identification. Movement of the c-o-g was effected by simultaneous amplitude modulation of two formants placed at the end points of the desired frequency transition. Experiment 1 of the present study explored whether c-o-g effects extend into the processing of consonant-vowel transitions in /da/-/ga/. Three different stimulus sets were synthesized in which the F_3 transition was a formant, a frequency modulated (FM) tone, or a Virtual Frequency (VF) glide. Listeners' identification of /da/ or /ga/ was not affected by changing the means by which spectral changes were made to F_3. Experiment 2 examined whether subjects could identify the type of F_3 transition in /da/ (formant, FM tone, VF glide) after a short training period. Responses did not differ with the transition type, thus, processing of transition information does not depend on the method used to elicit the perception of a frequency change. Experiment 3 was conducted to eliminate a possible confounding of transition cues in the VF stimuli used in Experiments 1 and 2 and to test listener performance in a dichotic listening condition. The results indicate that the dynamic c-o-g effect is evident in identification of English CV's just as it was for Russian vowels. The results lend support to the proposition that neural activity rather than signal energy is summed in the spectral integration process.

Keywords. Spectral integration, center-gravity-effect, virtual frequency glide

Introduction

When two formant peaks of a vowel are close in frequency, their combined energy leads to a percept much like that of a single formant peak. This phenomenon has been variously called spectral integration, formant averaging, or the center-of-gravity (c-o-g) effect. Chistovich and Lublinskaja [3][2] have suggested that the frequency separation between the formants and the relative amplitude of the formant peaks are important factors in spectral integration. A recent review of this topic may be found in Xu *et al*. [13].

Lublinskaja [8] demonstrated spectral integration for speech sounds in which the spectral centroid was changed dynamically. She asked listeners to identify three-formant synthetic Russian vowels in which F_2 and F_3 were modulated so that as the amplitude of one formant increased over time, the amplitude of the other decreased. When the amplitude of F_2 decreased while the amplitude of F_3 increased, the resulting percept was phonetically categorized as similar to a two-formant diphthongal vowel with a rising F_2. Conversely, when the amplitude of F_2 increased as that of F_3 decreased over time, listeners categorized the signal as similar to a two-formant diphthongal vowel with a falling F_2. Lublinskaja reported that the ability of listeners to identify these sounds was limited to critical separations between F_2 and F_3 of roughly 4.3 Bark (or 6 ERBu).[1]

Anantharaman [1] investigated spectral integration for dynamic sinusoidal signals suggested by the results reported by Lublinskaja. He generated two-component signals called virtual frequency (VF) glides. The amplitudes of the tones were modulated so that the intensity of one tone (usually the higher frequency component) increased while that of the other (lower frequency component) decreased. The changes in amplitude gave rise to the perception of a changing pitch, similar to that of a frequency modulated (FM) tone. Anantharaman's results show that listeners can match the rate of frequency transition in a virtual glide to the rate of change of an FM glide. These results were used to extend the Perceptual Centroid Model that had been previously applied to static signals. Further, he found that the dynamic c-o-g effect extended to at least 5.6 Bark (8 ERBu) and, thus, far exceeded the frequency separation reported by Lublinskaja.

Iyer [6] further investigated the processing of VF signals in temporal acuity and temporal masking experiments. The goal was to determine what is integrated in the "spectral integration" process. If the process is mediated near the periphery, signal energy may be the variable of interest; however, at more central locations the signal is represented by patterns of neural activity. Listener performance in a step- vs. linear glide discrimination task [9] was compared for FM and VF signals. Just-discriminable step durations were measured for three conditions: type of signal (FM and VF), center frequency (1000 and 4000 Hz), and frequency separation (2, 5, and 8 ERBu). The just discriminable step was found to be approximately 10 ms for both signal types at 1 kHz at 5- and 8 ERBu separations. All estimates were higher at 2 ERB (approximately 14 to 19 ms) and the 4 kHz result at 8 ERBu was about 12 ms. Iyer offers plausible explanations for the differences from Madden and Feth [9] and, in general, concludes that the temporal acuity task indicates that both FM and VF signals undergo similar processing in the auditory nervous system.

Using FM and VF glides as maskers for brief tones located at the center frequency of the glide led Iyer to very different results. When the probe was placed near the onset or the end of either masker, results were predictable from the power spectrum model of masking [11]. However, when the probe was placed at the temporal center of the glide signal, the shift in threshold was very different for the FM and VF maskers. As expected, the FM glide increased the threshold of the probe by approximately 30 dB for all three frequency separations. While there was substantial masking by the VF signal at 2 ERBu, there was much less at 5 ERBu and almost none at 8 ERBu. Thus, FM and VF signals are processed quite differently at the level of the inner ear, where direct masking effects are assumed to be mediated.

The large difference between masking produced by equivalent VF and FM maskers indicates that, at the periphery, the representation of these two signals is quite different. However, the similarity of temporal acuity results leads us to infer that they are represented by similar neural activity patterns higher in the central auditory system. Thus, the locus of spectral summation must be higher in the central auditory system. Said another way, it is neural activity, rather than signal energy, that is summed in this spectral integration process.

The study reported here addresses the phonetic processing of VF signals for consonant-vowel (CV) transitions in /da/ and /ga/. It builds on the work reported by Lublinskaja [8] and replicated by Iyer *et al.* [7]. The main question is whether VF and FM transitions are processed in a way that makes them perceptually equivalent to that of a synthetic formant transition. If so, then we may conclude that when neural activity moves from one frequency location to another, the percept will be the same for a variety of stimulus configurations.

Extending the investigation of the dynamic c-o-g effect observed in diphthongal vowels to CV transitions is dictated by the dynamics of speech and the role that amplitude changes may play in addition to frequency changes in processing of larger units of speech. Selecting /da/ and /ga/ as CV units for the present investigation is particularly well-suited because the direction of F_3 transition has shown to differentiate /da/ from /ga/ perceptually in three-formant synthetic approximations of the syllables [4][10][12]. The auditory distinction between /da/ and /ga/ is determined by the slope of the transition at the onset of the third formant (F_3): a rising transition specifies /g/ and a falling transition leads to the percept of /d/. Replacing the F_3 transition with an FM- or VF-glide should not cause a change in the perception of syllables as /da/ or /ga/ in response to either stimulus type. Furthermore, if the synthetic CV's are well-matched, listeners may not be able to easily discern the type of the transition.

1. Method

1.1 Subjects

There were 13 listeners in Experiment 1, 11 listeners in Experiment 2, and 8 listeners in Experiment 3. Some individuals participated in all three experiments, some in two of the three and a few participated in only one of them. All were native speakers of American English and were graduate students or research affiliates at The Ohio State University. All subjects reported normal hearing.

1.2 Stimuli

The test signals consisted of synthesized versions of the consonant-vowel (CV) tokens of /da/ and /ga/ based on those described in Fox *et al.* [4]. A 'base' token (the CV base) was generated at a sampling rate of 10 kHz using the parallel version of the Klatt synthesizer. It consisted of a 50-ms transition portion and a 200-ms steady-state portion. The transition portion consisted of F_1 and F_2 only, whereas the steady-state portion contained the first three formants of the vowel. For the F_1 transition, the initial frequency was 279 Hz and the final was 765 Hz. For the F_2 transition, the frequencies were 1650 Hz and 1230 Hz, respectively. The final frequency of both formants in the transition portion of the CV base corresponded to the frequencies of the steady-state portion. Fundamental frequency changed linearly from 120 Hz to 110 Hz. The base token did not contain a stop release burst.

Three types of F_3 transitions were added to the CV base to obtain three different continua: (a) Klatt-synthesized formant transition, (b) FM glide, and (c) VF glide. These parameters were changed for Experiment 3 for reasons discussed below. For the first continuum, the F_3 transitions were generated using the Klatt synthesizer. The final frequency of F_3 was 2527 Hz, which also corresponded to the F_3 frequency of the steady-state portion. The initial frequency of F_3 transitions ranged from 2018-2818 Hz in 80-Hz steps, creating an 11-step continuum.

For the second continuum, the F_3 transition was replaced by an FM glide, which had the same parameters (i.e., duration, and initial and final frequencies) as the Klatt-generated formant transition. The FM glides were generated in Matlab 5.3 and added to the base signal. The initial frequency of the glides was changed in 80-Hz steps to obtain an 11-step continuum.

For the third continuum, a VF glide was generated by simultaneously modulating the amplitudes of two fixed-frequency tones. For Experiments 1 and 2, the frequencies of the tones corresponded to the initial and final frequencies of the Klatt-synthesized F_3 transitions. Since the final frequency of the synthesized F_3 transitions was always 2527 Hz, the frequency of one of the tones in the VF glide was always 2527 Hz. The frequency of the other tone was varied in 80-Hz steps to obtain an 11-step continuum. In order to achieve a rising F_3 transition (as in /ga/), the relative amplitude of the lower frequency was 14 dB more intense; over time, the amplitude of the lower frequency decreased, while that of the higher frequency increased, until the higher frequency was 14 dB more intense at the end. The amplitude differences created an effect of c-o-g "movement" over the 50 ms transition portion. A downward F_3 transition (as in /da/) was obtained by reversing the amplitude modulations. Similarly, the relative amplitudes of the two tones changed over a 14-dB range. The virtual glides were generated and added to the CV base using Matlab 5.3. The amplitudes of the FM glides and the VF glides were adjusted so that the rms amplitude of the transition portion matched the rms amplitude of the Klatt-synthesized tokens.

For Experiment 3, the frequencies of the tones were fixed at the initial and final frequencies of the Klatt-synthesized F_3 transitions (2018 Hz and 2658 Hz, respectively). To produce a rising VF glide, the amplitude of the 2018 Hz tone decreased linearly over the 50 ms duration as the amplitude of the 2658 Hz tone increased. For a falling VF glide, the amplitude of the higher frequency tone declined as the lower frequency tone increased in amplitude. Initial and final amplitudes were chosen to make the signal c-o-g traverse the desired frequency range for each of the 8 tokens generated. The virtual glides were generated and added to the CV base using Matlab 5.3. The amplitudes of these VF glides were adjusted so that the rms amplitude of the transition portion matched the rms amplitude of the Klatt-synthesized tokens.

Experiment 3 was conducted several months after the first two experiments in order to minimize possible confounding in the VF signals used for the first two experiments. Because the frequency of the lower tone in the VF pair was changed for each token in Experiment 1, it was suggested that listeners might base their identification on the locus of that tone even if no formant-like transition was produced by the amplitude modulations.

Figure 1 displays spectrograms of the three token types for /ga/. The top panel (a) shows the full CV. In the lower panels, the F_3 transition has been isolated and displayed in a separate channel: (b) the Klatt-synthesized F_3 transition, (c) the FM glide, and (d) the VF glide. For the dichotic presentations in Experiment 3, the second channel was delivered to the earphone contra-lateral to the one containing the CV-base signal. Signals were played at a 10 kHz sampling rate, via the TDT system II, with low-pass filtering at 5 kHz.

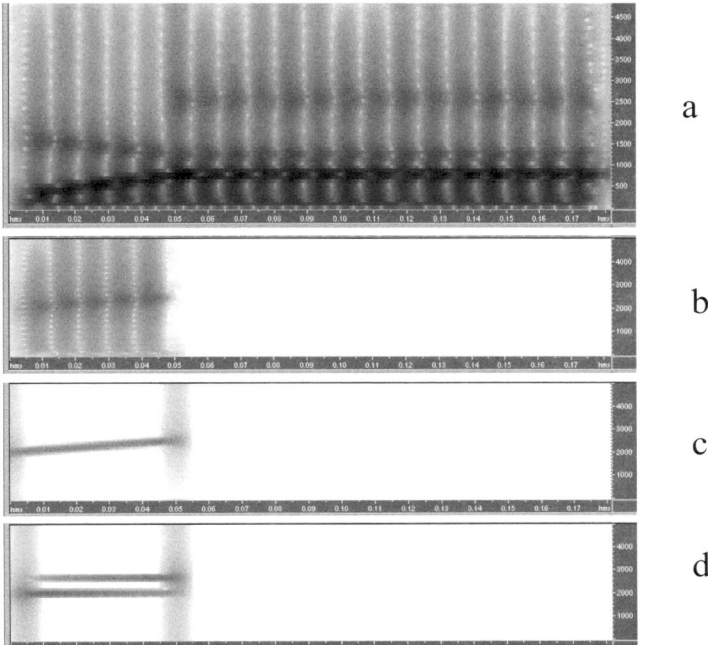

Figure 1. Spectrograms of the synthetic speech stimuli used in the experiments. Panel (a) displays the base Klatt-synthesized /ga/ CV. Notice the "missing" F_3 transition. The Klatt-synthesized F_3 transition alone is shown in panel (b). Panel (c) shows a frequency-modulated tone substituted for the formant on FM trials, and panel (d) shows a virtual frequency transition used in VF trials.

1.3 Procedure

For Experiments 1 and 2, signals were presented monaurally via Sennheiser HD 580 headphones to a subject seated in a sound-attenuating booth. In Experiment 1, a single-interval 2-AFC identification task was used with the response choices /da/ and /ga/ displayed on the computer screen. Subjects were asked to indicate whether they heard a /da/ or a /ga/ for each token presented. There were 660 stimuli presented randomly in 3 experimental blocks (3 transition types x 11 tokens x 20 repetitions). In Experiment 2, subjects responded in a single-interval, 3-AFC identification task indicating whether the token of /da/ they heard was generated with a Klatt formant transition (K), an FM Tone transition (T), or a VF transition (V). The three choices (K, T, or V) were displayed on the screen. Here, 120 stimuli were presented in one block (4 /da/-tokens, 3 transition types x 10 repetitions). Subjects were trained prior to the task by listening to 80 trials of /da/-tokens blocked by each transition type and presented in the following order: Klatt-synthesized formant transition, FM transition, and VF transition.

For Experiment 3, signals were presented binaurally via Sennheiser HD 580 headphones to a subject seated in a sound-attenuating room. The response task was identical to that used in Experiment 1. Half of the presentations were diotic (same signal to both ears). For the other half of the blocks of trials, the CV base signal was delivered to one ear and the Klatt, FM or VF transition was delivered to the contra-lateral ear. Six of the eight tokens were presented 20 times each in diotic and dichotic listening conditions. Results are averaged over the eight subjects.

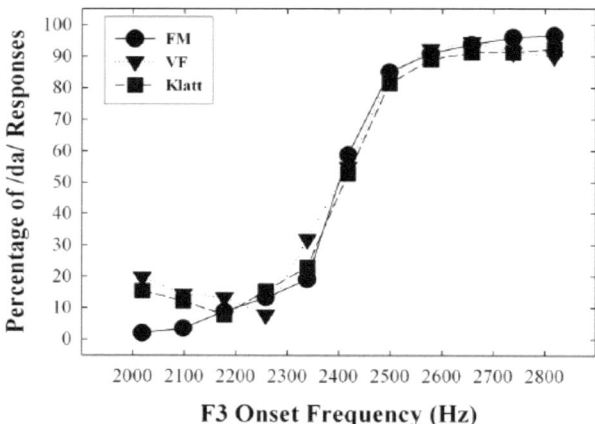

Figure 2. Identification functions for the CV stimuli presented in Experiment 1. Squares denote Klatt transitions; circles represent FM transitions; and inverted triangles are plotted for VF transitions. Results are averaged for 13 listeners.

2. Results

Figure 2 presents the averaged identification functions for 13 subjects in Experiment 1. The abscissa shows starting frequency for the F_3 formant transition. Each datum corresponds to a point on the 11-step /ga/ - /da/ continuum. The ordinate is percentage of /da/ identifications. Thus, the lowest starting frequency was rarely identified as a /da/ sound while the highest one was most often labeled as /da/. Squares represent the Klatt-synthesized transition; circles represent the FM tone transitions; and inverted triangles represent VF glide transitions.

The identification data were analyzed in two separate ways. First, the total number of /ga/ responses (summed across all 11 steps) for each subject were analyzed using a repeated-measures analysis of variance with the factor stimulus type (Klatt, FM glide, VF glide).

There was no significant effect of stimulus type ($F[2,24] = 2.726$, $p > .08$). Second, the category boundaries were analyzed in the same manner. The category boundary (the 50% cross-over point) for each subject for each stimulus type was calculated using PROBIT analysis. Again, there was no significant effect of stimulus type ($F[2,24] = 0.026$, $p > .90$). Both results appear to support the claim that the precise manner in which perceived frequency changes in the F_3 transition were elicited did not affect the phonetic category of the stimulus.

Experiment 2 examined whether listeners can identify the F_3 transition type (Klatt, FM glide, VF glide) after a short training in responding to each stimulus type. The last four tokens on the 11-step continuum with a gradually falling F_3 transition were selected for identification as /da/. Identifications averaged over 11 subjects reached 37% correct for the Klatt-synthesized transition, for the FM glide 32.3% correct, and for the VF glide 32% correct. Since chance performance equals 33.3%, the results indicate that the subjects did not differentiate between the transition type in their identifications of the stimuli as /da/. Results are shown in Table 1.

Stimulus/ Response	FM	VF	KL
FM	32.3	29.3	28.9
VF	34.3	32.0	34.1
KL	33.4	38.2	37.0

Table 1. Results of Experiment 2. Averaged performance for 11 subjects using the last four tokens of the continuum. Listeners were asked to identify the type of transition: Klatt-synthesized (KL), Virtual Frequency (VF), or Frequency modulated tone (FM). Entries are the percentage of responses for each stimulus type.

Experiment 3 was conducted to investigate the possibility that identification of a CV with the VF glide substituted for F_3 could have been cued by the difference in the frequency of the lower tone. Recall that the lower frequency for each virtual glide was changed to produce the F_3 "virtual" transition in the signals used in Experiments 1 and 2. For Experiment 3, the frequency of the lower tone was fixed, and the virtual transition was generated solely by changing the depth of amplitude modulations imposed on the tone pair. Signals representing six of the first eight steps (steps 1,2,4,5,7,8) in the original 11-step /da/ - /ga/ continuum were used in this experiment. For the diotic listening condition, only FM and VF transitions were tested since there was such good agreement between the Klatt signals and the FM transition signals in the earlier tests. Eight listeners heard 20 repetitions of each token in both diotic and dichotic listening modes. Results are shown in Figure 3 (a – diotic; b – dichotic). The psychometric functions plot the percentage of /da/ responses for each token averaged over eight listeners. For the diotic condition, the identification function for the FM transition is very similar to that shown in Figure 2, but the function for the VF transition is shifted to the left in frequency. The slope of the VF ID function is also less steep than that of the FM signals.

The /da/-/ga/ category boundaries (representing the 50% cross-over point) for the tone and virtual glide continua were calculated for each subject using PROBIT analysis. These boundaries were then analyzed using a within-subject analysis of variance. Results showed a significant difference in the category boundaries between the two stimulus sets [$F(7,1)=39.2$, $p<.001$, $\eta = 0.85$]. The mean category boundaries for the tone and virtual glide continua were 2346 Hz (= 38.5) and 2185 Hz (= 37.5), respectively.

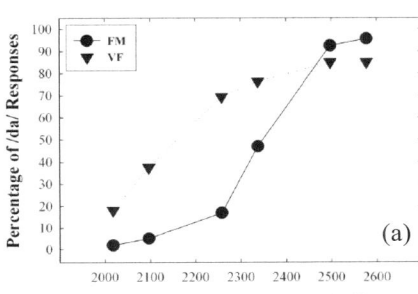
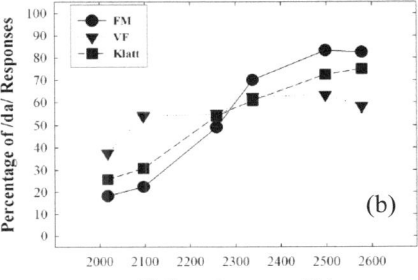

Figure 3. Identification functions for the CV stimuli presented in Experiment 3. Only FM and VF transitions were tested in the diotic (a) listening condition. Klatt, FM, and VF transitions were used in the dichotic (b) listening condition. Symbols are the same as in Figure 2.

For the dichotic listening condition, the three ID functions are shown in Figure 3b. The coordinates are the same as those for Figure 3a. Here, the slope of the function for FM transitions is steeper than that for the Klatt-synthesized transition, and the function for the VF transition is much flatter.

3. Discussion

This study addressed the question of whether VF and FM CV transitions are processed in a way that makes them perceptually equal to that of a synthetic formant transition. F_3 transitions in a /da/ - /ga/ continuum were replaced by FM and VF glides, respectively. Results from Experiment 1 showed no significant difference in the identification responses as a function of stimulus type. Similarity in perception and processing of VF and FM signals has been manifested in the phonetic processing of a CV unit, whose identification as /da/ or /ga/ was affected only by the direction of F_3 transition and not by the means by which the dynamic information was delivered to the listener's central nervous system. This shows that phonetic processing as well as interpretation of transitional information are independent of method used to elicit perception of frequency change. Or, how "excitation" is moved from one place to another has little effect on the listener's identification of the CV.

The third experiment was conducted to account for possible confounding in the VF transitions used in the first experiment. In addition, a dichotic listening condition patterned after Whalen and Liberman [12] was added. The identification function for VF transitions was shifted to the left of that for the FM (and Klatt) transitions. This may reflect a small bias in the calculation of the dynamic center-of-gravity for each token and require some minor modifications to the Perceptual Centroid Model. Listeners do hear the stimuli as belonging to the /da/ - /ga/ continuum. The effect is further diminished in the dichotic condition, where the FM transitions produce greater differences between the end points of the continuum than the original Klatt-synthesized signals. Clearly, further work is needed before we can assert that there is no difference in processing of VF, FM and Klatt-synthesized CV sounds.

Experiment 2 was conducted to ensure that perception of frequency change was not a consequence of presenting all three token types in the same experimental block for a phonetic identification as /da/ or /ga/. It could be argued that the nature of the task provided details which otherwise would not come into play in processing a particular type of F_3 transition. The listeners were asked to respond directly to the type of the transition after a reasonable amount of practice with each token type, ignoring the phonetic content of the syllable /da/. The results showed that listeners could not differentiate between the type of transition, not being able to indicate whether they heard a synthetic Klatt-version, an FM glide-version, or a VF glide-version of the transition in /da/. This implies that the dynamic character of F_3 transitions take perceptual precedence over the amount of information about the transition itself, be it frequency change of a formant, frequency change of a tone, or amplitude modulation of a signal. These details tend to be ignored if they do not contribute crucially to the identity of a phonetic unit.

Results from these experiments indicate the importance of dynamic information in speech processing. Extending the investigation of the c-o-g effect observed in diphthongal vowels to CV transitions revealed that the dynamic change caused by amplitude modulation is a phenomenon comparable to a frequency change. This "virtual" frequency change is processed similarly in acoustic and speech signals and the processing occurs more centrally along the auditory system.

Acknowledgments

This work was supported by a grant from The Ohio State University, College of Social and Behavioral Sciences to L. L. Feth and an INRS Award from NIH to R. A. Fox.

Note

1. Estimates of the width of the peripheral auditory filter, once known as the critical bandwidth, were initially given in units named "Barks," based primarily on work done in Zwicker's laboratory. More recent work, characterized by that from the laboratories of Patterson and Moore in Cambridge, has shown that the earlier estimates were systematically wider than now thought. The more recent unit for this estimate of auditory filter width is commonly called the Equivalent Rectangular Bandwidth unit, or ERBu. The original 3.5 Bark noted by Chistovitch and Lublinskaja [3] is approximately equal to 5 ERBu. Chapter 10 in Hartmann's book [5] has a discussion of the historical and technical details.

References

[1] Anantharaman, J.N. *A dynamic multi-channel perceptual spectral-centroid model for the processing of speech and other complex sounds.* Doctoral dissertation, The Ohio State University, Columbus, OH, 1998.

[2] Chistovich, L.A. "Central auditory processing of peripheral vowel spectra." *J. Acoust. Soc. Am.* 77: 789-804, 1985.

[3] Chistovich, L.A. and Lublinskaja, V.V. "The 'center of gravity' effect in vowel spectra and critical distance between formants: Psychoacoustical study of perception of vowel-like stimuli." *Hearing Research* 1: 185- 195, 1979.

[4] Fox, R.A., Gokcen, J. and Wagner, S. "Neurophysiological and behavioral evidence for a phonetic processor." *Proc. Chicago Linguistic Society's Thirty-third Meeting,* Vol. 33-2, pp. 311-332, 1997.

[5] Hartmann, W.M. *Signals, Sound and Sensation.* Woodbury, NY: American Institute of Physics, 1997.

[6] Iyer, N. *Temporal Resolution and Masking Patterns Using Frequency Modulated and Virtual Frequency Signals.* Doctoral dissertation, The Ohio State University, Columbus, OH, 2001.

[7] Iyer, N., Jacewicz, E., Feth, L.L. and Fox, R.A. "Center of gravity effects in the perception of virtual formant transitions." *J. Acoust. Soc. Am.* 109: 2294, 2001.

[8] Lublinskaja, V.V. "The 'center of gravity' effect in dynamics." *Proc. Workshop Auditory Basis of Speech Perception,* pp. 102-105, 1996.

[9] Madden, J.P. and Feth, L.L. "Temporal resolution in normal-hearing and hearing-impaired listeners using frequency-modulated stimuli." *J. Speech Hearing Research* 35: 436-442, 1992.

[10] Mann, V.A. and Liberman, A.M. "Some differences between phonetic and auditory modes of perception." *Cognition* 14: 211-235, 1983.

[11] Patterson, R.D. and Moore, B.C.J. "Auditory filters and excitation patterns as representations of frequency resolution." In *Frequency Selectivity in Hearing,* B.C.J. Moore (ed.), London: Academic Press, 1986.

[12] Whalen, D. and Liberman, A.M. "Speech perception takes precedence over non speech perception." *Science* 237: 169-171, 1987.

[13] Xu, Q., Jacewicz, E., Feth, L.L., and Krishnamurthy, A.K. "Bandwidth of spectral resolution for two-formant synthetic vowels and two-tone complex signals." *J. Acoust. Soc. Amer.* 115: 1653-1664, 2004.

Dynamics of Speech Production and Perception
P. Divenyi et al. (Eds.)
IOS Press, 2006

Multi-Resolution Analysis in Speech Perception

Georg F. MEYER[1], Sue HARDING[2] and Elvira PEREZ[1]
[1]*Centre for Cognitive Neuroscience, School of Psychology,*
Liverpool University, Liverpool, UK
[2]*Department of Computer Science*
University of Sheffield, Sheffield, UK

Abstract. It is tempting to think of speech perception as a single, perhaps highly specific, processing module defined by a single set of constraints, such as the spatio-temporal resultion of the underlying analysis. We present a series of experiments that exploit a duplex stimulus to support our argument that speech perception requires analysis at different spectro-temporal scales. Auditory scene analysis, which is essential for segregating target speech sounds from competing background noises, requires analysis and processing at a fine spectral and temporal scale to exploit features such as pitch differences between target and competing sounds or small differences in the onset times of the elements making up an auditory scene. It is therefore not surprising that analysis is carried out in a high-resolution representation. Speech pattern matching, on the other hand, requires significant generalisation to allow the acoustical speech signal to be mapped into invariant representations. The pattern matching, for instance, should be independent of the speech pitch and discount fine differences in formant trajectories imposed by co-articulation or speaker differences. We show that frequency modulated sines (chirps) that are presented in the position where normal formant transitions between vowels and nasals would be expected change the speech percept independent of their slope even though the chirps are clearly segregated into a separate (duplex) percept and differences between the chirps can be identified. While our data is consistent with the view that there are specific representations or processing modules for different auditory analysis tasks, we do not feel that our data supports the case for a specific biological module that uses speech gestures as an underlying representation. We argue that the different behaviour is consistent with the different processing requirement of different auditory tasks, specifically that high-resolution processing is necessary for the segregation of speech from background noise while a low-resolution representation is much more suitable for speech pattern matching. We show that frequency modulated sines (chirps) that are presented in the position where normal formant transitions between vowels and nasals would be expected change the speech percept independent of their slope even though the chirps are clearly segregated into a separate (duplex) percept and differences between the chirps can be identified. While our data is consistent with the view that there are specific representations or processing modules for different auditory analysis tasks, we do not feel that our data supports the case for a specific biological module that uses speech gestures as an underlying representation. We argue that the different behaviour is consistent with the different processing requirement of different auditory tasks, specifically that high-resolution processing is necessary for the segregation of speech from background noise while a low-resolution representation is much more suitable for speech pattern matching.

Keywords. Speech perception, pattern matching, frequency modulation

Introduction

The aim of this chapter is to present a case for thinking of speech perception not as a single unified process, but as a set of interdependent modules, that each utilise representations that are optimised for their specific role. In terms of the dynamics of speech perception we argue that there is not "one set of speech dynamics" but multiple sets of task-specific dynamic constraints that define our perception of speech.

The argument we present is based on a set of experiments that exercise two different aspects of speech perception: perceptual organisation and speech pattern matching. We show that the perception of synthetic vowel-nasal stimuli changes if a frequency modulated sine is presented in the position where a formant transition would be expected. The stimulus leads to a duplex percept; that is the listener hears a speech signal that incorporates the chirp, as well as hearing a chirp as a separate auditory object. When the direction of the chirps is manipulated to be consistent and inconsistent with normal formant transitions, listeners are able to differentiate the chirps, but report the same effect on speech perception. We interpret this finding as evidence that the spectro-temporal resolution used for speech pattern matching is much lower than that available for auditory scene analysis and argue that this is consistent with the specific processing requirements for the two tasks.

Perceptual Organisation and Speech Pattern Matching

A fundamental assumption of the argument presented here is that speech pattern matching and the processes involved in the perceptual organisation of complex sound environment are separate processes. This view is supported by a wealth of theoretical argument (e.g. [5][7]) and experimental evidence (e.g. [21][22]). We will briefly review the relevant literature.

Human communication almost always takes place in a background of noise and it is therefore perhaps not surprising that listeners are remarkably good at recognising speech sounds in the presence of other signals (review, [3]). A theoretical framework that seeks to explain this robustness is Auditory Scene Analysis (ASA, [5]). In analogy to a visual scene, an auditory scene is proposed that contains features with properties, such as continuity in time, a given spatial sound source location, or a fit into a given harmonic structure. The underlying assumption is that all features that share common properties derive from a single sound source and can be separated into perceptual streams without recourse to high level knowledge. This perceptual organisation process requires a) the segregation of signal components into separate representations and b) the grouping of components that are likely to derive from a single source into an information stream. Primitive signal descriptors, such as the signal fundamental frequency (F0), source location, or spectro-temporal features can be used as the basis of heuristic processes that perform this operation (e.g. [5][7]).

An important observation at this point is that the cues for perceptual organisation rely on the *fine detail* of the representation, such as the F0 for pitch based segregation, interaural level or time differences for localisation cues, or exact formant position or timing for continuity grouping.

A particular challenge for speech recognition is the variability between speakers as well as the context dependency of individual tokens produced by single speakers. The variation of formant frequencies across speakers, for instance, is discussed by Patterson *et al.* (this volume) who propose an algorithm that claims to remove this vocal tract variability. Formant frequencies show variation across speakers because of their vocal tract length dependency; they also vary across languages because they are adjusted such that the relationship between the vowels in terms of their acoustic distance from one another is similar [13][16]. They are also changed by context; in particular, when coarticulated with consonants, transitions from the consonant to the vowel do not always reach the formant frequencies found when the vowels are spoken in isolation [16][19][Carre's chapter in this volume]. The variability of human speech production requires robust pattern matching during recognition which may explain why synthetic speech, such as the stimuli used in the experiments described here, are perceived as plausible speech sounds. Further evidence for the robustness of speech pattern matching comes from studies investigating speech perception in noise or the perception of distorted speech.

Perceptual data based on highly abstract synthetic stimuli that are nevertheless perceived as speech may be taken as evidence that speech perception takes precedence over auditory scene analysis (e.g. [22]) or that auditory scene analysis principles do not apply to low-level features of speech (e.g. [18]). The arguments for or against this viewpoint are very well rehearsed (e.g. [4][7]), but the important consideration for the purposes of our argument is that there is no question that speech perception is robust to a much greater extent than scene analysis would predict. For our argument it is important to note that speech pattern matching is largely unaffected by variations in speaker pitch, speaker position, amplitude of the signal and the precise spectro-temporal shape of the signal – in fact speech recognition would not be possible if the pattern matching could not deal with this variability.

We therefore argue that the fine detail that is essential for perceptual organisation would hinder speech pattern matching and therefore a signal representation that codes much broader and more invariant features is essential. On this basis we argue that speech perception depends on the interaction of multiple complementary representations.

1. Methods

We report on a series of speech perception experiments that share a common experimental design and very similar stimuli. The aspects common to all experiments are described in this section.

All speech stimuli used in the experiments described in this paper were synthesised using a parallel version of the Klatt [12] synthesiser. The syllables consisted of a vowel preceding a nasal /m/ or /n/.

The nasals /n/ and /m/ have common formants at 250 Hz and 2000 Hz. The distinguishing feature is that the /n/ has a nasal zero at 1000Hz while the /m/ has a formant in this position, Figure 1.

The vowels used in this study were chosen so that their first and third formants could be fixed while the second formant could range from 800-2000Hz, so that it would coincide with the second formant of both the /m/ and the /n/ prototype. A continuum of vowels ranging from /o/ (F_2 at 370 Hz) to /e/ (F_2 at 2700 Hz) was used in the experiments. The signals were sampled at 20 kHz and a resolution of 16 bits and presented

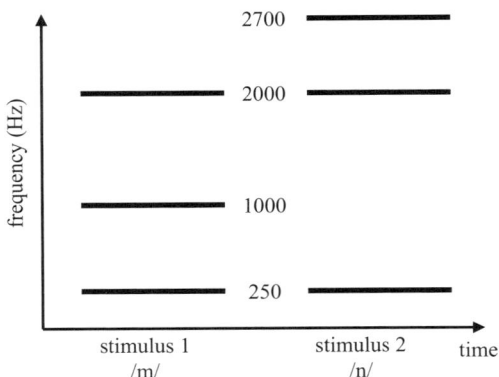

Figure 1. Schematic diagram of the formant positions of the nasal prototypes.

using a Terratec EWS64XL sound card (synthesizer signal path) and Sennheiser HD 480-II headphones in a quiet room.

Subjects were asked to identify the nasal in a forced choice paradigm. All experiments were self-paced and subjects were allowed to adjust the signals to comfortable levels. The participants in this study were staff and students of the Institute of Phonetics, Saarbrücken University, and of the Department of Psychology, Liverpool University. All participants reported normal hearing. Each subject took part in two separate sessions.

2. Baseline Experiments

We present the results obtained in a number of experiments. Two of them are baseline data and a further experiment was designed to show multi-resolution processing in the auditory system. The baseline data is discussed in this section. The first experiment demonstrates that the perceived identity of a nasal in vowel-nasal complexes depends on the second formant of the vowel if there are no formant transitions between the vowel and the nasal. Experiment two shows that linear formant transitions of 5ms duration are sufficient to overcome the perceptual changes seen in experiment one. Experiments three and four attempt to answer the question of whether the spectral or temporal fine structure of the transitions between vowel and nasal are important to the percept – we show that they are not.

2.1 Experiment 1: Perception of synthetic vowel-nasal syllables without formant transitions

2.1.1 Experimental Design

Each experiment consisted of 140 intervals where VC syllables were played in a random sequence.

The second formant for the vowel was varied in steps of 200 Hz between 800 Hz and 2000 Hz. In half of the trials the vowel preceded the nasal prototype for /m/ (Figure 1) in the other half the prototype for /n/ was presented. The signal contained instanta-

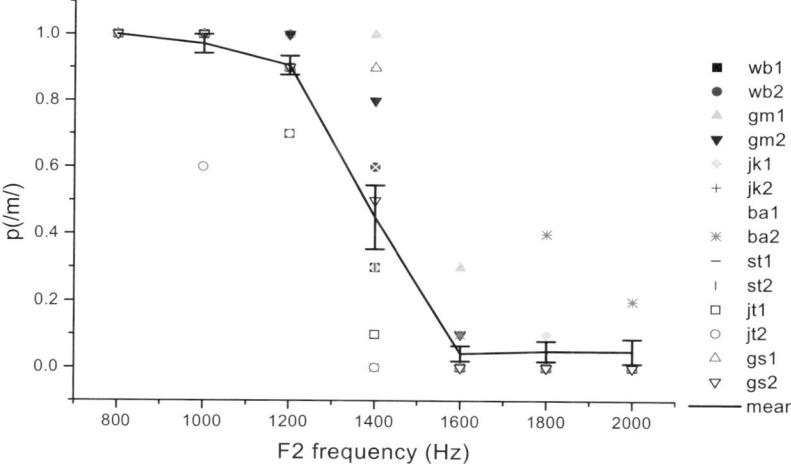

Figure 2. Probability of subject hearing /m/ in a vowel-consonant pair where the second formant of the vowel was varied between 800 Hz and 2000 Hz. The spectrum of the consonant was that for /m/. Above a vowel F_2 of 1600 Hz more than 95% of subject responses were /n/. The error bars are standard errors (SE). The numbers "1" and "2" after each subject's initials designates the listening session.

neous transitions between the vowel and nasal formant positions and amplitudes. The pitch of the signals was static at 100 Hz. Each random sequence contained ten examples of the 14 stimulus configurations.

After each signal presentation subjects were asked to judge whether the consonant sounded more like an /n/ or an /m/ by pressing the appropriate button on a computer graphical user interface. Subjects were instructed that the vowel preceding the nasal was not relevant.

2.1.2 Results

Subject responses for the vowels preceding the synthetic /m/ are shown in Figure 2. The probability of a subject responding with /m/ is plotted against the vowel F_2 frequency. All subjects hear the nasal /m/ when it precedes the vowel /o/ (F_2 at 800Hz) in 100% of all trials; if the vowel F_2 lies at 2 kHz (/e/) subjects consistently (95% of all responses) report hearing the nasal /n/, although the spectrum of the nasal presented has not changed in any way.

$$y = \frac{A_1 - A_2}{1 + (x - x_0)^p} + A_2 \tag{1}$$

A logistic curve, Equation 1, was fitted to the data to estimate the threshold point, x_0. The resultant parameter values are: $A_1 = 0.9766 \pm 0.03$, $A_2 = 0.034 \pm 0.03$, $x_0 = 1382 \pm 14.8$ Hz and $p = 21.03 \pm 6.38$. The χ^2 value is 0.002.

A similar effect can be demonstrated if a synthetic /n/ follows the vowels, Figure 3. Here the subjects are more likely to report hearing an /m/ for vowels with F_2 values at or below 1 kHz while the /n/ is always reported if the vowel F_2 lies at or above 1800Hz. A

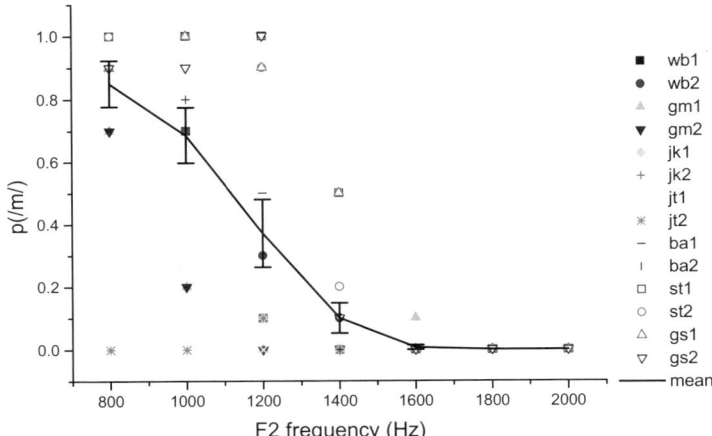

Figure 3. Probablility of subject hearing /m/ in a vowel-consonant pair where the second formant of the vowel was varied between 800 Hz and 2000 Hz. The spectrum of the consonant was that for /n/. Above a vowel F_2 of 1400 Hz more than 90% of subject responses were /n/. The error bars are standard errors (SE).

logistic curve fit produced the following parameter values: $A_1 = 0.867 \pm 0.08$, $A_2 = -0.01 \pm 0.04$, $x_0 = 1162 \pm 42.26$ Hz and $p = 9.62 \pm 3.05$, with a χ^2 value of 0.053.

Both curves show a clear F_2 dependent switch in the identity of the perceived nasal. Subjects report hearing an /m/ for low vowel F_2 values which changes into an /n/ as the vowel F_2 increases.

2.1.3 Discussion

We show that the second formant in a vowel preceding a nasal can change the perceived identify of this nasal from /m/ to /n/ and vice versa. It is well known that the nasals /m/ and /n/ are difficult to recognise if no context is provided to the listeners (e.g. [1][11]); a possible explanation for the switch in the percept might be that the two synthetic stimuli are inherently ambiguous. We feel that ambiguity alone does not explain the results for two reasons. The first reason is that all subjects achieved recognition rates greater than 80% for 300 ms long steady state synthetic nasals in isolation in an initial experiment. The second reason is that the category boundaries shown in figures two and three are different for the two nasals; if the stimuli were merely ambiguous the same boundaries would have been expected.

Auditory scene analysis may provide another possible intuitive framework explaining the perceptual organisation underlying the change in the percept: If the nasal spectrum is that of the /m/ prototype, and the vowel is /e/ then the second formant of the /e/ and the third formant of the /m/ are both at 2 kHz. If some low-level perceptual process were to link formants by proximity in time and frequency space, the obvious link to make would be the two formants at 2 kHz and probably also the first formants at 375 Hz (/e/) and 250 Hz (/m/). This configuration would leave nothing to link the second formant of the /m/ to. A 'scene analyser' may conclude that the formant is some extraneous sound that is not part of the percept and put it into another perceptual stream. The two remaining formants of the /m/ are those of the /n/. The nasal zero of the /n/ would be expected in the position of the /m/ F_2, which also would be consistent because the energy in this position has been assigned to a separate perceptual stream.

The vowel formant frequency where the switch from an /m/ to an /n/ percept takes place is at 1382 Hz. If this frequency is expressed in ERBs, a psychophysically moti-vated frequency scale that takes the non-linear frequency spacing of the auditory system into account [17], then the threshold lies almost exactly on the mid-point between the two formant frequencies of the nasal. The midpoint between F_2 and F_3 of the /m/ lies at 18.11 ERB, the threshold at 17.88 ERB. A process that simply associated each formant with the closest (in ERB space) preceding or succeeding formant (proximity grouping) would explain the perceptual data well.

While the argument advanced above sounds attractive, it is not entirely convincing – a key assumption of the ASA approach is that the signal is segregated and different streams should be heard as separate signals. A vowel with a high second formant that is followed by the nasal prototype /m/ should therefore result in a simultaneous percept of /en/ and a second stream that corresponds to the orphaned second formant of the /m/ prototype. In reality subjects cannot hear a second signal.

While this observation is not enough to discount proximity grouping, more evi-dence against this theory is provided by experiments where the nasal prototype is /n/: The first observation is that the category boundary for experiments using the /n/ proto-type lies much lower, at 1162 Hz or 16.48 ERB, but still 25% above the mid-point of the two first formants of the /n/ (13.21 ERB). More importantly, the simple explanation that energy may be moved into another perceptual stream is no longer possible because in this configuration the nasal /n/ does not have any energy at 1 kHz, where it would be expected for the /m/. Indeed the ASA model would have to be extended to allow the generation of formant representations that are not present in the stimulus to explain the perceptual data by proximity grouping of formants.

This means that an explanation proposing the use of formant structure as the basis for perceptual organisation of these stimuli is difficult to justify.

2.2 Experiment 2: Perception of synthetic vowel-nasal syllables with formant transitions

The previous experiment shows that a vowel preceding a nasal can change the percep-tion of the nasal. We assume that the effect is due to the absence of formant transitions rather than some artefact in the synthesis. If natural formant transitions are present then the perception of the nasals should not be influenced by the preceding vowel. The experiment serves two purposes:

1. to show that the introduction of transitions removes the influence of the pre-ceding vowel from the nasal perception, and
2. to establish what range of transition durations are permissible for this purpose.

2.2.1 Experimental Design

The experimental design was identical to that described for experiment one with the fol-lowing differences. The nasal prototype for /m/ is perceived as an /n/ if it is preceded by a vowel with high second formant frequencies; for low second formant values the vowel

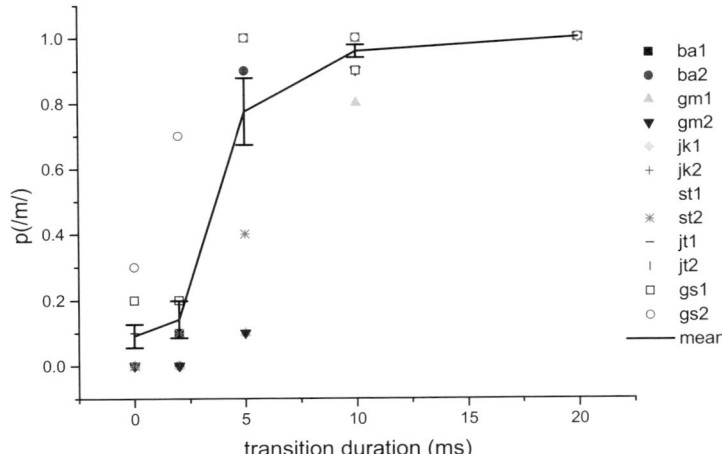

Figure 4. Probability of subject judging stimulus to be /em/ against transition duration for the synthetic /em/
sound. If no or very short transitions between the steady state vowel and nasal segment are used,
subjects report hearing /em/ in only 9.1% (no transition) or 14.1% (2ms transition) of trials; for transitions of 10 ms or more subjects report hearing /em/ in more than 95% of the trials. The continuous
line is mean subject data; error bars indicate standard error.

is perceived as an /m/. The stimuli used in this experiment therefore all use the /m/ nasal
prototype and the vowel /e/ with a second formant that coincides with the third formant
of the nasal at 2 kHz. Linear transitions between the two steady state segments were
introduced with durations of 0, 2, 5, 10 and 20 ms. The synthesizer used frames of 1 ms
duration to allow formant transitions to be generated that were shorter than a glottal
period. The formant frequencies and amplitudes were interpolated linearly between the
start and end point of the formant transition over the duration.

Subjects were asked to judge whether the nasal component of the signal sounded
more like an /n/ or /m/. Each subject completed two experimental runs with 100 intervals each.

2.2.2 Transition duration changes the percept

Figure 4 shows the subject data as a scatter plot; the mean and standard error values are
superimposed on the data. The introduction of transitions into the stimulus changes the
percept from an /en/ to /em/ as would be expected. If no transitions are present 9.16%
(SE 3.5%) of the subjects' judgements are /en/ while for 20ms transitions 100% (SE
0%) of the judgements are /em/. A logistic curve fit (eqn 1) through the combined subject response data was used to estimate the threshold value at 5.08 ms (SE=0.04 ms)
with a χ^2 value of 0.117.

2.2.3 Discussion

The introduction of transitions between vowel and nasal makes the identity of the nasal
consistent with the percept heard when the nasals are presented in isolation. This is consistent with the view that the change in percept found in experiment one is caused by the
absence of formant transitions. This does not mean that formants are tracked for percep-

tual organisation – in fact we argue that the data we show is inconsistent with the notion that formants are tracked to provide continuity cues, which would explain the perceptual data.

Our argument is based on the length of the 'formant transitions' required to have an effect on the percept. We were surprised to see that 'formant transitions' of just 5 ms duration are sufficient to change the percept from /en/ to /em/. The signals were synthesized at a f_0 of 100 Hz so that the shortest effective transitions were less than a glottal period in duration. A transition between 2 kHz and 1 kHz, as used in the experiments, would therefore be almost indistinguishable from a transition going in the opposite direction.

3. Experiment 3: Evidence for Multi-Resolution Analysis

The previous two experiments show that context governs the perception of nasals. Nasals, which are reliably identified in isolation, change their perceived identity if they are preceded by certain vowels (experiment 1) and change back to their original identity if very short transitions between vowel and nasal are introduced (experiment 2). These changes are unlikely to be caused by perceptual organisation processes that use formant proximity or continuity for the reasons discussed earlier. A possible explanation for the perceptual changes would be a pattern matching process that a) takes context into account to explain the data shown in experiment one, and b) does not carry out a detailed analysis of the fine spectral structure of the stimuli to account for the fact that formant transitions as short as 5 ms are sufficient to change the percept.

The experiment described below was designed to test the hypothesis that speech perception processes are unable to use fine detail, as is suggested by the very short transitions seen to have an effect in experiment two. Rather than using formant transitions we decided to introduce frequency modulated pure tones (chirps) at the position where natural signals would have formant transitions. If speech pattern matching depends on fine detail then these signals, which differ fundamentally from the structure of speech sounds, should not make a difference to the percept, while they should be included in the percept if only a coarse signal representation is used for pattern matching. We used chirps following the expected formant transition between 2 kHz and 1 kHz but also ran conditions where the chirps run in the opposite direction. If a coarse representation is used for pattern matching then the direction of the frequency modulation should have little effect for short duration chirps but should become increasingly more obvious as the duration of the chirps increases.

3.1 Experimental Design

The signal used in the experiment was the synthetic /em/ stimulus discussed in the previous sections. A frequency modulated pure tone with RMS energy 36 dB below that of the vowel-nasal syllable was added. The duration of the chirp was set to 5,10,20 and 40 ms; a control condition without the chirp (labelled 0 ms) was also used. The amplitude of the chirps was modulated with a raised cosine window over the full duration of the chirp.

In addition to chirps that were designed to coincide with an expected F_2 transition,

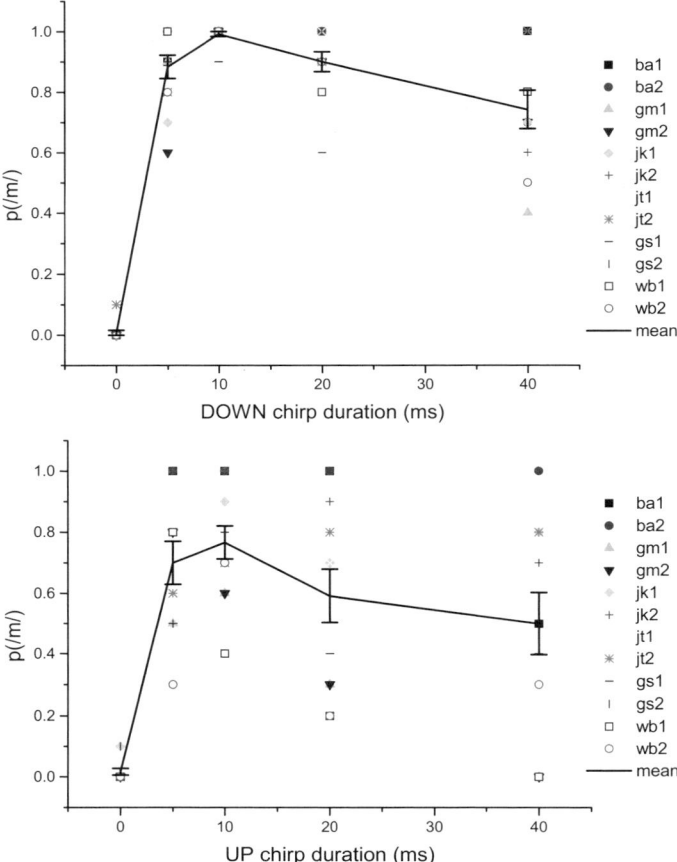

Figure 5. Effect of the introduction of a frequency modulated sine wave that changes from 2 kHz to 1 kHz,
with the duration shown, on the probability of subjects hearing /em/.

i.e. falling from 2 kHz to 1 kHz (down-chirp), a set of chirps going in the opposite direction, rising from 1 kHz to 2 kHz (up-chirp) were used.

Each of six subjects was presented with 20 repetitions of each condition in a semi-random sequence as above and asked to indicate whether the signal sounded more like an /em/ or an /en/.

3.2 Addition of chirps changes the percept

The response data shown in Figure 5 clearly show that the introduction of the chirps has an effect on the perceived identity of the nasal. This change is predicted by the hypothesis that speech pattern matching is based on relatively coarse representations. For chirps that follow the trajectory of the expected formant transitions more than 80% of the stimuli were reported to be heard as /em/ provided the duration of the chirp was between 5 ms and 20 ms. If no transitions or chirps are placed between the vowel and nasal, /em/ is heard in only 0.8% of trials; a 10 ms chirp, in contrast, causes subjects to identify the stimulus as /em/ in 99% of the trials. As the chirp duration increases further the probability of hearing /em/ reduces to 74%. For chirps that run in the opposite direction to the expected formant transition the effect is less pronounced but follows a very similar pattern. Here the majority of stimuli containing chirps going between 1 kHz and 2 kHz were identified as /em/. In the control position and for chirps of 40 ms duration the majority of stimuli were identified as /en/.

The stimuli in the experiment were chosen to provide salient cues for auditory scene analysis. If auditory scene analysis is carried out, then the chirps should be audible as secondary sounds to the subjects. All subjects report hearing the speech syllable *plus* a chirp but are unable to say exactly where in the stimulus the chirp occurs. This is entirely consistent with the notion that auditory scene analysis is carried out.

A possible explanation for the similar effect of the upward and downward chirps might be that listeners are unable to hear a difference between the signals. To test this hypothesis listeners were asked in a separate experiment to identify the chirps as moving up or down. The stimuli used in the experiment were identical to those used in the nasal identification task. Four out of five subjects were able to identify well in excess of 90% of the chirps after only a single training session. A striking finding was that on debriefing most subjects reported finding it very difficult to switch their attention from the speech identification to the chirp identification task, which in our view further suggests that multiple processes are active in evaluating the stimuli.

3.3 Discussion

Chirps of 5 ms duration, independent of their direction, are apparently integrated seamlessly into the speech signal and change the percept from /en/ to /em/. For longer duration the direction of the chirp matters but for chirp durations up to 20ms the majority of stimuli are still heard as /em/, independent of the direction of the chirp, although a significant difference between the up and down-swept chirp exists. For 40 ms upward chirps the percept reverts back to an /en/ in 50% of the trials. In spite of the seamless integration of the chirps into the speech percept, they are simultaneously segregated from the speech signals and heard by the listeners as secondary sounds. While listeners are unable to identify exactly where in the speech sounds the chirps occur, the majority are able to identify the direction of the frequency modulation.

4. Conclusion

We show clear context dependent effects in the perception of synthetic nasal sounds. We argue that an explanation based on perceptual organisation by formant structure is unlikely. Formant proximity explains the category change seen for the /m/ prototype when it is preceded by vowels with high second formant frequencies but the expected concomitant perceptual segregation of the second formant of the nasal is not reported by subjects. Perceptual organisation by formant proximity is even less likely for the stimuli using the /n/ prototype, which is heard as /m/ for vowels with low F_2 values. A formant based approach would have to postulate the internal generation of a second formant around 1 kHz that is not present in the stimulus. Continuity based perceptual organisation seems unlikely for the stimuli that contained explicit formant transitions because the effects of the formant transitions are seen for transition durations of 5 ms. These formant transitions complete within half a glottal period so that the signal contains minimal cues for the transition direction. This finding is confirmed by the studies reported in experiment three which showed that the addition of frequency modulated tones in place of formant transitions have the same effect as the formant transitions. This effect is seen whether the chirp direction is consistent or inconsistent with the expected formant transition in the stimulus.

The chirp not only influences speech perception but is simultaneously heard as a secondary sound which subjects find hard to localise relative to the timing of the speech signal, showing that perceptual organisation by auditory scene analysis is carried out. Subjects are able to discriminate between upward and downward chirps even for the shortest chirp durations tested.

The data suggest that at least two systems are active when subjects hear the chirp stimuli:

1. a module for speech pattern matching that does not differentiate formant transitions from chirps in either direction, which suggests that speech pattern matching uses a very coarse internal representation, and

2. a module for auditory scene analysis, which identifies (but does not segregate!) the chirp in the speech signal. This type of processing requires a very high definition representation.

We argue that two complementary representations are necessary for the specific processing carried out in the two 'modules'. Auditory scene analysis has previously been shown to exploit low-level features, such as the fundamental frequency or fine timing cues to segregate sounds into separate streams. Low-level segregation requires very high resolution processing but also uses exactly the types of cues that are most likely to be highly variable within and across speakers such as the F_0 or fine timing cues. For pattern matching, representations that use invariant signal descriptors are much more useful; examples are gross spectral shape or secondary invariant representations (see Patterson *et al.* this volume).

The view that separate modules are involved in speech perception is not new and is well represented by Liberman [14] in his argument that 'speech is special'. Liberman presented the single formant transition that causes a difference in the /da/ and /ga/ percept to one ear and the remainder of the stimulus to the other ear. Rather than hearing the stimuli as a chirp in one ear and an ambiguous stop in the other, subjects hear a clear speech signal that includes the formant transition as well as a chirp appropriate to the isolated formant transition.

Our stimuli – and our conclusions – differ in a number of important points. Liberman's key finding was that the 'phonetic' module seemed to be independent of perceptual modules (the sound localisation module) when presented with speech signals that contained conflicting segregation cues.

We provide further evidence that shows a duplex effect for monaural stimuli but – more importantly – we show that the processing constraints differ for the perceptual and phonetic modules. The phonetic module appears to be blind to the precise nature of the chirps added to our speech signals: the simple frequency modulated tones we used are fundamentally different from isolated formant transitions but are still integrated into the speech percept. Perceptual modules, in contrast, clearly represent fine detail of the acoustic signals because subjects can differentiate between upward and downward chirps in a chirp identification task. We argue that the different dynamic constraints seen in the modules are a necessary reflection of their specific specialisations.

We do not share the view of Liberman and Mattingly [15] who argue for a specialised biological module that detects the intended gestures of the speaker forming the basis of phonetic categories. An alternative account for the data is that the 'phonetic module' is a pattern matching system that is specifically adapted to deal with the variability that is introduced by different speakers, speaking style or coarticulation and that – because of this specialisation – ignores fine detail.

Our data shows that perceptual organisation based on ASA processes that exploit formant proximity or continuity is unlikely, so that an interpretation that posits a special (and separate) module for speech perception may seem to be an appropriate conclusion. It would however be hard to reconcile this view with what we know about speech perception in adverse conditions (review: [3]) as well as our knowledge on the perceptual organisation of simple stimuli, such as those by Bregman and co-workers in his seminal studies [5].

We propose an alternative view that assumes closely integrated perceptual (low level segregation) and phonetic (schema or pattern matching) processing stages. We suggest that the role of the perceptual stage is not the segregation of auditory scenes into multiple representations that can be attended in turn, but as a stage that carries out a high resolution analysis and informs the pattern matching stage of any aspects of the signal that warrant closer attention. The pattern matching stage could then look at the joint probability of all possible interpretations of a complex scene rather than relying on early selection of streams by a scene analysis stage. A probabilistic framework would explain much of the perceptual data and would allow the reconciliation of experimental results that would appear to be contradictory.

Liberman's results, for instance could be interpreted as follows – the pattern matching stage would have access to the whole stimulus, but the formant transition defining the plosive would be labelled as potentially a second signal based on localisation cues. Localisation cues are relatively fragile in echoic environments, so that their relative weight in an information fusion system would be low. A pattern matching system would now have to choose between a highly unlikely signal (a separate chirp and ambiguous plosive) which is corroborated by an inherently unreliable cue, or a highly likely signal that is accompanied by a potential breakdown of the localisation system in the initial part. In this light the integration of the information seems the only viable strategy. The same argument could be made for the double vowel experiments reported by Culling and Darwin [8], where synthetic vowels with different F_0 values for different formants were used. The identification rate for vowel pairs with complementary F_0 values above and below 1 kHz was found to be no worse than for pairs of vowels that use the same F_0 for all formants. In both cases performance improves if the vowel pairs differ in fundamental frequency. Again, a low-level segregation model would assign the incorrect formants to separate streams and predict poor performance while a probabilistic approach would predict that performance should be approximately the same as for non-conflicting cues.

This way of thinking may also help reconcile data that shows that formant transitions aid the segregation of simultaneous vowel-like sounds [9][2] while it is simultaneously true that the precise nature of formant transitions does not affect vowel-vowel perception [6] or the data described here. The key difference between the experiments is that the latter experiments present stimuli that could be interpreted as probable speech sounds while the former experiments either isolate [9] or excise [2] the perceptual stages.

If we postulate closely coupled processing stages that have very different underlying representations, then it is only a small step to hypothesize that the underlying representations for different aspects of speech signals also should be optimised for their specific task. A distributed representation that combines signal detectors with good temporal resolution for plosive discrimination and detectors with good spectral resolution for, for instance, vowel discrimination, is entirely plausible. This reinforces the view that when we consider the dynamics of speech perception it would be foolish to assume only one level of representation with a single set of dynamic constraints.

Acknowledgements

We are grateful to the members of the Phonetics Department at Saarbrücken and the School of Psychology at Liverpool who took part on the experiments.

References

[1]   Ainsworth, W.A. "Performance of a speech synthesis system." *Int. J. Man-Machine Studies* 6: 493-511, 1974.
[2]   Assmann, P. "The role of formant transitions in the perception of concurrent vowels." *J. Acoust. Soc. Am.* 97: 575-584, 1995.
[3]   Assmann, P. and Summerfield, Q. "The perception of speech under adverse conditions." In *Speech Processing in the Auditory System*, S. Greenberg and W.A. Ainsworth (eds.), New York: Springer Verlag, 2004.
[4]   Barker, J. and Cooke, M. "Is the sine-wave speech cocktail party worth attending?" *Speech Communication* 27(3-4): 159-174, 1999.
[5]   Bregman, A.S. *Auditory Scene Analysis: The Perceptual Organization of Sound.* Cambridge, MA: MIT Press, 1990.
[6]   Carré, R., Ainsworth, W.A., Jospa, P., Maeda, S. and Pasdeloup, V. "Perception of vowel-to-vowel transitions with different formant trajectories." *Phonetica* 58: 163-178, 2001.
[7]   Cooke, M. and Ellis, D.P.W. "The auditory organization of speech and other sources in listeners and computational models." *Speech Communication* 35: 141-177, 2001.
[8]   Culling, J.F. and Darwin, C.J. "Perceptual separation of simultaneous vowels: within and across-formant grouping by f$_0$." *J. Acoust. Soc. Am.* 93: 3454-3467, 1993.
[9]   Divenyi, P.L., Carre, R. and Algazi, A.P. "Auditory segregation of vowel-like sounds with static and dynamical spectral properties" In *Proc. IEEE Mohonk Mountain Workshop on Applications of Signal Processing to Audio and Acoustics* pp 14.1.1-4, 1995.
[10] Greenberg, S. and Ainsworth, W.A. "Speech processing in the auditory system: An overview." In *Speech Processing in the Auditory System*, S. Greenberg and W.A. Ainsworth (eds.), New York: Springer Verlag, 2004.
[11] Harding, S.M. and Meyer, G.F. "Changes in the perception of synthetic nasal consonants as a result of vowel formant manipulations." *Speech Communication* 39: 173-189, 2003.
[12] Klatt, D.H. "Software for a cascade/parallel formant synthesizer." *J. Acoust. Soc. Am.* 67: 971-995, 1980.
[13] Ladefoged, P. and Broadbent, D. "Information conveyed by vowels." *J. Acoust. Soc. Am.* 29: 98-104, 1957.
[14] Liberman, A.M. "On finding that speech is special." *American Psychologist* 37: 148-167, 1982.
[15] Liberman, A.M. and Mattingly, I.G. "The motor theory of speech perception revised." *Cognition* 21: 1-36, 1985.
[16] Lindblom, B. "Spectrographic study of vowel reduction." *J. Acoust. Soc. Am.* 35: 1773-1781, 1963.

[17] Moore, B.J.C. and Glasberg,. B.R. "Suggested formulae for calculating auditory-filter bandwidths and excitation patterns." *J. Acoust. Soc. Am.* 74: 750-753, 1983.
[18] Remez, R.E., Rubin, P.E., Berns, S.M., Pardo, J.S. and Lang, J.M. "On the perceptual organization of speech." *Psychological Review* 101: 129-156, 1994.
[19] Stevens, K.N., and House, A.S. "Perturbation of vowel articulation by consonantal context: An acoustical study." *J. Speech Hear. Res.* 6: 111-128, 1963.
[20] Repp, B.H. and Liberman, A.M. "Phonetic category boundaries are flexible." In: *Categorical Perception*, S. Harnad (ed.), Cambridge: Cambridge University Press, pp. 89-112, 1987.
[21] Warren, R.M. "Restoration of missing speech sounds." *Science*, 167, 392-393, 1970.
[22] Whalen, D.H. and Liberman, A.M. "Speech perception takes precedence over nonspeech perception." *Science* 237: 169-171, 1987.

Dynamics of Speech Production and Perception
P. Divenyi et al. (Eds.)
IOS Press, 2006

Speech Dynamics and the "Cocktail-Party" Effect

Pierre DIVENYI
Speech and Hearing Research
Veterans Affairs Medical Center
and
East Bay Institute for Research and Education
Martinez, California, USA

Abstract. To understand speech emanating from a target source, the listener in a 'cocktail-party effect' (CPE) situation must perceptually separate a dynamically changing target from a dynamically changing background. Although these dynamic changes do not occur synchronously in the target and background, investigators have resorted to presenting concurrent speech signals synchronously, except for selected keyword epochs, in order to measure speech intelligibility under speech interference (Brungart, 2001) [2]. The present study follows the rationale of that research to investigate perceptual segregation of two concurrent streams of nonspeech signals with speech-like properties: periodic harmonic sounds with the two streams differing in fundamental frequency f_0 (in all experiments), FM-like trajectory of the center frequency of a formant-like resonance (in Experiment 1), and the rhythmic AM pattern of syllabic-rate envelope fluctuations. Results show that segregation of streams with dynamic formant trajectories is easier than that of steady-state formants and that both formant trajectory pattern and rhythmic pattern discrimination is easier with larger f_0 separation between the two streams. Since elderly individuals are known to have CPE deficits, the fact that in both experiments our elderly subjects have also demonstrated consistently poorer performance than the young suggest that FM- and AM-based segregation of streams may underlie speech understanding dynamics associated with the syllable, a unit serving as the organizational interface among the various tiers of linguistic representation.

Keywords. Auditory segregation, dynamic streams, amplitude-modulation patterns, formant trajectory patterns, age-related deficits

Introduction

Speech dynamics implies constant changes over time, whether considered from the articulatory, acoustic, or perceptual points of view, or whether studied from the perspective of physics, biology, or behavioral science. As the chapters in the present book demonstrate, observing speech through the looking glass of these changes unveils a host of properties that the classic representation of speech as a sequence of static event-beads would continue to hide. In particular, Chapter 13 in the present book by Greenberg, Arai, and Grant alludes to the way dynamics may help recover a target speech source and message from the acoustic cacophony resulting from the source being located in a highly reverberant environment. For certain, reverberation will harm the intelligibility of speech [32][23] by scrambling localization cues that, under normal circumstances, help speech understanding by spatially separating multiple sources [17]. As first proposed by Cherry over 60 years ago [4], the "cocktail-party effect" (CPE) was meant to refer to the ability of listeners to use two ears instead of only one-that is, to spatially separate speech sources-in order to understand one conversation in a room full of many persons talking at once from different locations. However, multiple speech sources can also be physically co-located — for example, a single loudspeaker from which several individuals talking simultaneously — or effectively co-located due to reverberant acoustics that scramble most localization cues. When trying to understand speech by a given talker in a crowd in cases such as this in which de facto elimination of spatial cues reduces the CPE to single channel listening, one must resort to cues that are available monaurally. Thus, the CPE should be studied both as a multiple and a single spatial source phenomenon, leading to the necessity of identifying non-spatial cues that listeners use to recover the message spoken by a particular talker. The present chapter presents the argument that the dynamic nature of speech plays an important role in the separation of speech sources in a CPE situation.

That speech embodies dynamic processes strikes as a tautology. Speech has been described by Plomp [28] as "…a signal slowly varying in amplitude and frequency." Such changes in the amplitude and frequency of speech are bound to help a listener perceptually segregate it from other simultaneously present sounds, whether speech or nonspeech, if one hypothesizes that the listener can, and will, predict the direction in which amplitude and/or frequency parameters of the target speech are changing. Indeed, such predictions are regarded as indispensable for auditory scene analysis (ASA). According to Bregman [1], perceptual segregation of sources employs Gestalt principles, one of which is that of "good continuation." When in the CPE, due to a transient flare-up of noise energy, or a trough in the fluctuating speech envelope, or both, the noise interference masks the speech target, this principle will enable the listener to continue following it, even if it cannot be heard (or sufficiently heard) during that epoch. Of course, prediction based on continuation can occur on different levels: high-level linguistic analysis makes it possible to "fill in" the missed syllables or words based on sentence context [22], and a lower-level pitch analyzer tracking the smoothly changing contour of the target speaker's fundamental frequency (f_0) ensures that speech by a non-target speaker will not be mistakenly accepted as that of the target speaker. Obviously, there may be a multitude of processes operating on a number of perceptual-cognitive levels that may intervene in this game of predictions.

Estimation and recovery of "missing data" — the segment of target speech masked by noise (this latter being interpreted as any acoustic signal interfering with the target) — has been a topic much investigated by proponents of computational models of auditory scene analysis, or CASA. The starting point of these models is auditory theory: the frequency-, time-, and spatial analysis of the speech signal presented in a complex acoustic background. The acoustic scene is analyzed into a "cochleagram" (or "auditory spectrogram") that represents the scene in the time-frequency (T-F) plane at the output of monaural peripheral processing and a "periodogram" that establishes the pitch of periodic components of the scene [33]. Several of these models first establish T-F regions at which the signal-to-noise ratio is high enough that the target can be reliably identified, and regions at which it is masked (e.g., [37]). Although much of the target speech can already be recognized from these T-F masking patterns and the corresponding periodograms (such as f_0 contour, vowel quality, consonant-vowel segmentation), speech in the masked regions must be estimated.

The actual way in which this estimation takes place in a CPE situation is not known precisely, but it appears that it follows rules first proposed by Gestalt psychologists (e.g., [24]), especially as they were integrated in the coherent framework of Auditory Scene Analysis (ASA) by Bregman [1]. The rule of "good continuation," in particular, postulates that the listener will fill in the gaps of missing portions of the target speech by predictions based on intelligible portions that precede and/or follow. According to Bregman, successful segregation of auditory streams – in the present context the target speech stream and the irrelevant background – will be accomplished by processes operating on two perceptual/cognitive levels. *Primitive* segregation operates on a lower auditory sensory/cognitive level and occurs due to parametric differences between the streams that are sufficiently large so that the listener will spontaneously hear separate sources. In extreme cases, one of the sources will acquire a salience strong enough for it to "pop out" of the ensemble of sources-just as a red dot will pop out of a black-and-white image or a sudden onset of telephone ring can pop out of the cacophony of conversations at a loud gathering. While the sensory basis of primitive segregation is clear, our attention is also drawn to a segregated stream, i.e., it has definite cognitive components. In contrast, cognitive processes dominate the other, the *schema-driven* segregation, which is by definition a higher-level process. This process refers to situations such as a person recognizing his or her name spoken in a multi-speaker CPE setting, or when a listener recognizes or seeks out someone's voice or a particular topic of conversation. If this type of segregation has a sensory component, it is likely to be the result of efferent processes – i.e., cortical centers instructing the peripheral auditory system to tune to particular acoustic characteristics proper to a higher-level schema. Despite their differences, both the primitive and schema-driven segregation processes provide tools to estimate or predict data missing from the target speech: at a lower level, the dynamic changes in the speech signal occur at a slow rate (as the above quote by Plomp asserts), and therefore the missing portions may be recovered by applying the "good continuation" principle, while at a higher level, linguistic knowledge will help in finding the missing syllable, word, or phrase by selecting, among the competing ones, the alternative which forms the most phonologically, syntactically, and semantically coherent whole when taken together with the "heard" portions of the target speech. Recent results [10], consistent with this theoretical framework, showed that intelligibility of unstressed syllables and "filler words" presented at a fixed signal-to-noise ratio (SNR) is a monotonic function of the SNR of stressed "keywords." That is, the unstressed lower-SNR portions of the target speech are predicted from the inherently higher-SNR stressed syllables or words – about 85 percent of English words being monosyllabic [19].

Prediction schemes have been integral parts of CASA models and speech segregation algorithms. While detailed analysis of these models is beyond the scope of the present chapter, two "engines" in many of these models are worth pointing out. One of them is the statistical estimation of missing (or missed) T-F areas, based on T-F areas successfully "glimpsed" [5]; this estimation is solely based on acoustic properties of the target signal and the noise, thereby analogous to primitive segregation by humans. The other is the statistical estimation of speech based on higher-level (primarily learning and language) models [15], analogous to schema-driven segregation by humans. Of course, the number, the variety, and the combinations of CASA models is steadily increasing and most contemporary models, whether published or on the workbenches of investigators all over the world, incorporate to some extent both classes of missing data estimation, especially when their objective is to achieve robust automatic speech recognition (ASR, see e.g., [29]).

But how and how well do listeners achieve their predictions based on the "good continuation" Gestalt principle? It appears that they are able to follow both frequency- and amplitude-modulation (FM and AM) at the slow rates at which they occur in speech. For example, there seems to exist an inertia in the auditory system when it follows a monotonic frequency glide at an FM rate comparable to formants in diphthongs [6], suggesting that a masked portion of an FM transition can be perceptually recovered. Also, selective sensitivity to low- (syllabic-) rate AM fluctuations allows listeners to follow such fluctuations in the presence of other, even slightly different, AM fluctuations [31][34]. In the experiments described in the present chapter, we wanted to measure the ability of listeners to segregate two concurrent streams differing either in their FM trajectories or their AM patterns. In order to get a better hold on acoustic parameters, we stayed away from real speech signals; instead, our stimuli were simpler sounds that still embodied some speech properties – speech-range fundamental frequency with speech-range harmonic components, speech-range formant trajectory, and speech-range amplitude fluctuation. Throughout the study, the stimulus consisted of two concurrently presented streams, each a harmonic sinusoidal complex. The two streams were presented synchronously and with similar perceptual salience, i.e., they were identical in their total duration and average power, but they differed in their fundamental frequency and one additional feature – FM formant-glide pattern (in Experiment 1) or syllabic-rate rhythm pattern (in Experiment 2). Readers familiar with studies on informational masking in speech will recognize that the present stimuli were analogous to synchronized sentences that listeners had to segregate under the Coordinate Response Method (CRM) [2], where the sentences spoken simultaneously by two or more talkers differed in synchrony during three specific epochs at which keywords were uttered. In our experiments the different keywords in two simultaneous CRM sentences were thus replaced by either different formant trajectories or different rhythms in our two simultaneous streams. Ability to segregate in the CRM experiments was defined as the ability to associate a given talker's voice (e.g., the one who uttered the call noun "baron") with a given word (e.g., the call color "red") at a designated keyword epoch. Also similarly to the CRM, we defined ability to segregate our nonspeech streams as the ability to associate a given formant trajectory or a given rhythm pattern with the stream having either the higher or the lower fundamental frequency.

1. Experiment 1

1.1 Methods

Stimuli in Experiment 1 were two simultaneous, 400-ms streams consisting of sinusoidal harmonic complexes with different fundamental frequencies: 107 Hz in one of the streams and $107+\Delta f_0$ Hz in the other, where the frequency difference $\Delta f_0/f_0$ amounted to

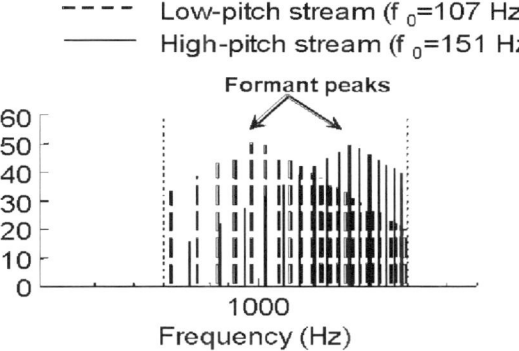

Figure 1. Line spectra of the two streams, indicating a different unique formant frequency for the low-pitch stream (dashed lines) and the high-pitch stream (solid lines). The harmonic components of both streams are kept between the same limits (500 and 3500 Hz). The frequency scale is logarithmic to show as many components as possible.

either 27 percent (close to a musical interval of Major third) or 77 percent (close to a minor seventh). As shown in Figure 1, harmonic components in both streams were limited to the range between 500 and 3500 Hz. Perceptual salience of the two streams was equalized by adjusting their output levels until their pitch strengths (i.e., the strength of the virtual pitch corresponding to the fundamental frequency according to Terhardt's model, see [35][36]) were identical. The spectrum in each of the two streams was shaped to make them acquire a resonant peak — a unique formant — by passing the harmonic complex through a four-pole Butterworth bandpass filter with a nominal bandwidth of 100 Hz. The peak frequency of this formant was modulated by first departing from, and then returning to, the same baseline frequency (1272 Hz). The formant excursion was symmetric both in frequency on a basilar membrane distance scale[1] [21] and in time: the duration of the upward and downward gliding formant transitions was identical (75, 100, or 200 ms). The transition pattern was also located in the middle of the 400-ms stimulus. That is, for transition durations shorter than 200 ms, both streams had a leading and trailing portion with a constant 1272-Hz formant frequency. The spectrum

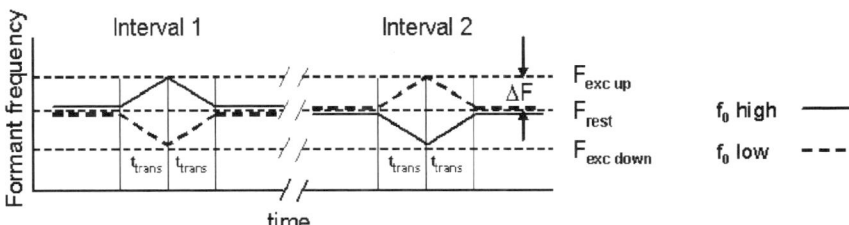

Figure 2. Schematic time-frequency diagram of a trial. The ordinate indicates peak formant frequency (i.e., the tip of the spectra in Figure 1) for the two simultaneous streams of harmonic complexes having different fundamental frequencies f_0: the higher drawn in solid, and the lower in dashed lines. The duration of the stimulus in each of the two observation intervals was 400 ms, whereas that of the formant transition t_{trans} varied from condition to condition. The transition was linear (on a basilar membrane frequency scale) between the resting frequency F_{rest} and the point of maximum excursion up or down from the resting frequency, $F_{exc\ up}$ and $F_{exc\ down}$, with ΔF designating the extent of the formant excursion..

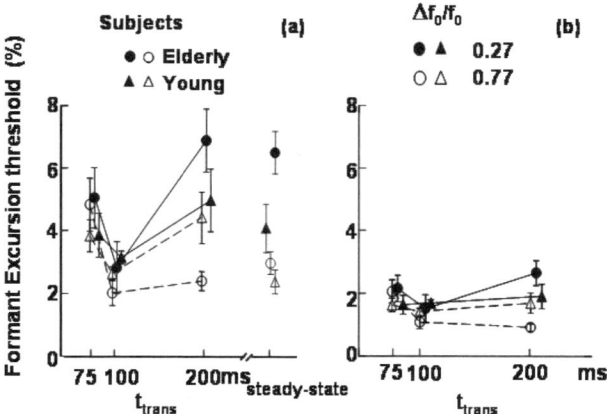

Figure 3. Formant excursion ($\Delta F/F_{rest}$) leading to segregation of the two streams at threshold performance level, as a function of the transition duration t_{trans}. Filled symbols are for the streams having f_0's different by a factor of 0.27 (~Major third), whereas the open symbols indicate an f_0 difference of 0.77 (~minor seventh). Circles indicate average data for the elderly and triangles, for the young subjects. In Panel (a), the excursion values are as observed; "steady-state" indicates the observed values for streams with fixed formant differences. In Panel (b) the data have been weighted by the extent to which the frequency excursion information is actually transmitted by a 100-ms (young subjects) and a 200-ms (elderly subjects) time window, as displayed in Table 1.

of the stimulus is illustrated in Figure 2(a).

The ability to segregate the two streams with opposite-direction formant trajectories was measured by changing the extent of formant excursions adaptively using a two-down, one-up, two-alternative, forced-choice (2AFC) procedure tracking the 70.1 percent correct performance criterion [25]. The subject was instructed to attend to the higher-f_0 stream[2] and to respond by indicating the order of the formant trajectory pattern in that stream, as shown schematically in Figure 2(b). After responding, the subject received visual feedback on the computer screen in front of him/her to indicate whether segregation of the two streams in that trial, i.e., the association of the higher f_0 and the particular formant trajectory pattern, was successful. For each subject and condition, the *auditory* extent of the formant excursion corresponding to the performance criterion was estimated as the average of the excursions in the last 10 of 12 reversals of the staircase procedure within each block of trials. The results reported represent the mean obtained in six to eight blocks. Auditory, rather than physical, formant excursion was used as the measure for the maximum frequency difference perceived because the formant frequency modulation is continuous and therefore the time spent at the peak difference is infinitesimally small. For each formant transition pattern with a given excursion, we calculated this auditory measure as the maximum formant peak frequency difference within a single auditory integration time window estimated to be 100 ms in duration. Because of the integration process under the time window, the frequency excursion available after auditory processing is less extensive than the physical.

Groups drawn from two subject populations were tested: a group of seven normal-hearing young individuals and a group of five elderly persons with minimal or no hearing loss. Pure-tone thresholds in either ear of the young subjects were 15 dB SPL or less at frequencies between 0.5 and 4 kHz, whereas those of the elderly subjects with hearing

Auditory time window (ms)	Duration of Single (up or down) Formant Transition (ms)		
	75	100	200
50	0.534	0.386	0.195
100	0.428	0.541	0.386
200	0.430	0.479	0.534

Table 1. Proportion of maximum frequency change that an auditory time window of a given duration lets through.

loss indicated a mild or moderate sloping presbycusic loss, i.e., they were at or below 25 dB SPL at 0.5 and 1 kHz, at or below 35 dB SPL at 2 kHz, and not exceeding 50 dB SPL at 4 kHz. None of the subjects had ever used, or was prescribed to use, a hearing aid. It is important to note that the stimuli were always presented at a clearly audible overall level: 86 dB SPL overall level at the envelope peaks of the stimuli.

1.2 Results

Average results of Experiment 1 by the elderly and the young subjects are illustrated in Figure 3(a) for the three transition durations (75, 100, and 200 ms) and the two f_0 separations (27 and 77 percent, approximately corresponding to a Major third and a minor seventh musical interval) used. The figure shows that segregation performance (i.e., the smallest frequency excursion at which segregation could be observed 70.1 percent of the time) by the young subjects is almost always better than that of the elderly. The results also indicate that the best performance was obtained at the 100-ms transition durations, suggesting that that particular transition duration comes close to the length of the time window used by the auditory system for gauging the extent of a slow monotonic frequency modulation. However, we also note that for the longest, 200-ms transition duration, the performance by the elderly subjects is better than that of the young, suggesting that the time window for frequency modulation is lengthened by age − a conclusion consistent with a long list of data on temporal processing by the elderly [18][16]. In fact, it can be demonstrated that a simple auditory model followed by a windowed running evaluator of frequency change shows the percentage of frequency change observable for stimuli like ours to be a joint function of the transition duration and the window size. For a comparison, formant frequency *difference thresholds* for the segregation of two streams with different f_0 and different *steady-state* formant frequency are shown as the rightmost data points on the figure. Because the frequency difference thresholds for the steady-state formants are generally lower than the frequency excursion thresholds of the dynamically changing formants, one is tempted to conclude that segregation of streams with steady-state formants is more effective than that of streams with linearly modulated formant frequencies. However, because the frequency excursion information, and thus the ability to perceive the frequency change in a transition (or glide), is limited by the auditory time window, the excursion perceived is likely to be only a fraction of the excursion in the stimulus. This fraction, in turn, is a function of the duration of the glide and the length of the window as indicated by the fractions in the rows of Table 1. The

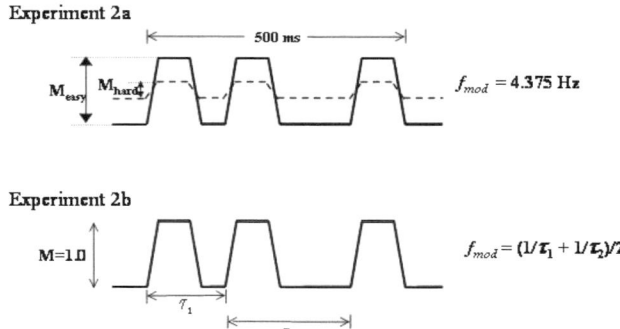

Figure 4. Schematic time envelope diagram of the stimuli in the two sub-experiments. Schematic time diagram of the amplitude-modulating (AM) waveform for one observation interval of a trial in the two sub-experiments. The ratio τ_1/τ_2 of inter-burst intervals was always kept at 0.4. In Sub-Experiment 2a, the average modulating frequency f_{mod} was held constant at 4.375 Hz, whereas the modulation index M was adaptively varied from 1.0 (solid line, M_{easy}) downward (broken line, M_{hard}). In Sub-Experiment 2b, M was held constant at 1.0 and fmod was adaptively varied from 4.0 Hz upward. The duration of a single AM burst was always 60% of τ_1, the shorter inter-burst interval, with 20-ms onset and offset ramps.

table shows that the time window transmits best frequency excursion in glides when the duration of the transition matches the length of the window. However, at best, the frequency excursion transmitted is 54%, i.e., barely more than half of the original excursion. We have reasons to believe that young listeners use a time window of about 100 ms-the "duration of a perceived event," as suggested by Efron [14]. However, the figure also shows that the elderly listeners outdid the young ones when segregating the 200-ms transitions, pointing to the likelihood that the length of the temporal window used by the elderly is about 200 ms in length. When the data in Figure 3(a) are weighted by the Table 1 efficiency fractions of the 100- (young subjects) and 200-ms (elderly subjects) windows, the resulting excursion extents at which the two streams can be segregated are decreased. These transformed data, to be interpreted as the smallest formant excursion at which the two streams can be segregated, are plotted in Figure 3(b). Comparing these excursion data with the steady-state formant difference thresholds, the conclusion is that the dynamic changes in formant frequency facilitate segregation of two streams differing in their f_0.

2.   Experiment 2

2.1 Methods

Perhaps the most important dynamic property of speech lies in the amplitude-envelope fluctuations that derive from syllabic and subsyllabic segmentation of the speech flow. In a cocktail-party situation, the envelope fluctuations of the speech by multiple talkers are superimposed on each other, leading to the question of how a listener is able to tell which segment came from which talker's speech. This question was addressed by Experiment 2, in which the two dimensions along which the streams differed from each

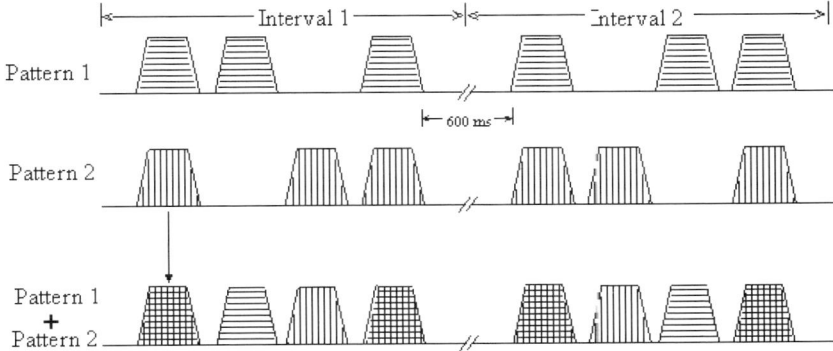

Figure 5. Schematic diagram of a trial. In each trial, Pattern 1 is randomly assigned to the higher-*f0* or lower-*f0* stream and Pattern 2 to the opposite one. The two streams were mixed and in a 2AFC paradigm. The subject's task was to identify, in the higher-*f0* stream, the pattern in the two observation intervals as either the amphibrach-dactyl Pattern 1 or the dactyl-amphibrach Pattern 2.

other were f_0, as before, and syllabic-rate rhythm. Accordingly, in this experiment, the harmonic stream carriers were amplitude-modulated by a waveform that generated three consecutive bursts separated by two unequal time intervals. In other words, the resulting rhythmic patterns were irregular: in one of the streams the first interval was longer than the second and gave way to a "0 — 0-0" *dactyl* rhythm, while in the other stream the first interval was shorter than the second, resulting in a "0-0 — 0" *amphibrach* rhythm. Holding the difference between the two intervals constant at 60%, the difficulty of discriminating, and segregating, the rhythmic patterns was controlled by varying either their perceptual salience or the rate at which they were amplitude modulated. In Sub-Experiment 2a, the perceptual salience was changed by varying the modulation index M from the easiest 1.0 (completely silent periods between the three bursts) to the most difficult 0.01 (a continuous harmonic sound with barely emerging envelope peaks during the three bursts), while holding the average modulation frequency f_{mod} constant at 4.375 Hz. In Sub-Experiment 2b, f_{mod} was changed between the easiest slow 4 Hz to the most difficult fast 20 Hz, while holding M constant at 1.0. The stimuli were presented in a two-alternative, forced-choice (2AFC) paradigm where the high-f_0 and the low-f_0 streams were paired, in succession, with the two patterns from the other dimension. Thus, in Experiment 2 a trial could consist of the high-f_0 stream having the *dactyl* rhythm presented with the low-f_0 stream having the *amphibrach* rhythm, in Interval 1, followed by the inverse pairing of f_0 and rhythm in Interval 2, or the same sounds in inverse order. Figure 4 illustrates the schematic time diagram of the stimuli in the two sub-experiments and Figure 5 the schematic diagram of a trial.

The objective of the experiment was to estimate the value of the variable affecting ease of discrimination — the modulation index M in Sub-Experiment 2a and the average modulating frequency f_{mod} in Sub-Experiment 2b — that yielded a 70.1 percent correct performance, as in Experiment 1. The results reported represent the mean obtained in six to eight blocks of trials. Forty-six elderly and nine young subjects participated.

2.2 Results

Figure 6 illustrates the results. The left panel shows the average modulation index M

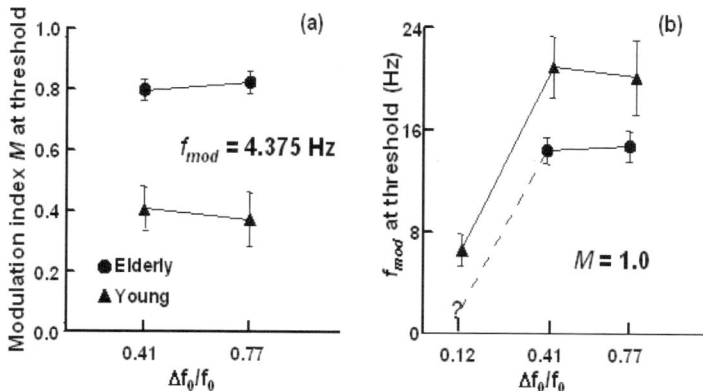

Figure 6. Panel (a) shows results of Sub-Experiment 2a: Modulation depth index M leading to threshold-level segregation of the rhythmic pattern in the two streams, as a function of the frequency ratio of the streams' fundamental frequencies $\Delta f_0/f_0$ (0.12 corresponds to a musical Major second, 0.41 to a tritone and 0.77 to about a minor seventh), obtained at the low average modulating frequency f_{mod} of 4.375 Hz. Panel (b) shows results of Sub-Experiment 2b: fmod as a function of $\Delta f_0/f_0$ obtained at full modulation depth ($M = 1.0$). Circles indicate average data for elderly subjects, while triangles indicate average data for young subjects. The question mark indicates that at a $\Delta f_0/f_0$ of 0.12 the fmod threshold for the elderly subjects could not be measured.

that yielded threshold performance, whereas the right panel shows the modulation frequency fmod at performance threshold. Both sub-experiments examined the effect of fundamental frequency difference at differences of 0.41 (half-octave or musical tritone) and 0.77(musical minor seventh). The reason for which we did not use the third-octave (0.27) f_0 difference was that many of our elderly subjects were unable to segregate the two rhythmic patterns when the fundamental frequencies were that close to each other. Since the performance appears to be quite similar at the two f_0 differences, the f_0 difference gradient is probably very steep.

The major finding in both sub-experiments is that the elderly perform significantly poorer than the young: using a low modulating frequency f_{mod} of 4.375 Hz, the young were able to segregate the two simultaneous rhythmic patterns at a modulation depth M of about 0.4, whereas the elderly needed one twice as large. We wish to point out that an average f_{mod} value of 4.375 Hz is almost exactly identical to syllabic rate amplitude fluctuations in speech and that the cadence of irregular pulses (40% difference between the long and short time intervals in the pattern) approximates rather well a long syllable-short syllable (or the inverse) succession in spoken English. Also, when using full AM depth, the young were able to segregate the streams with the different rhythmic patterns at modulating frequencies fmod of about 24 Hz at f_0 separations larger than 0.4 and about 6 Hz at the very narrow (0.12) f_0 separation, whereas at larger f_0 separations the elderly could perform the segregation task at fmod of approximately 14 Hz and were incapable of performing the task at the narrow f_0 separation. While these modulating frequencies are well above *syllabic* fluctuation rate in speech, 24 Hz is just somewhat above the range of sub-syllabic modulation frequencies necessary to resolve some phonetic features – such as the voice onset time (VOT) for voicing in stop consonant-vowel sequences – while 14 Hz is below this range, suggesting that the elderly may have to resort to acoustic cues other than VOT (such as first-formant cutback, see [26]) to understand speech.

3. Discussion

In the previous section we reported data that indicate specific limits in the human ability to perceptually segregate two streams — two sources — having different dynamic patterns. In Experiment 1, we showed the extent and the rate at which simultaneous but opposite direction formant excursions were separable and, in Experiment 2, the degree of clarity and rate needed for simultaneous but different amplitude fluctuation patterns to be segregated.

   Segregation of the two streams, in both experiments, was achieved by directing the subject to attend to one of the sources: the stream with the higher f_0 than the other stream. The fact that subjects found the task feasible is one indication that the experiments may have relied on auditory-perceptual processes similar to those needed in a CPE where the ability to separate speech sources increases as the voice pitch difference of the talkers increases [2]. For our non-speech analog of the Coordinated Response Method (CRM) stimuli, the f_0 difference appears to enable the subject to process the differences between the streams along the other dimension-dynamic patterns of formant trajectory or AM — just as the voice pitch difference enables the listener to focus on an utterance by a designated speaker. Thus, the listener in our reduced-speech experiment appears to behave similarly to one in a multiple-speaker CPE setting that focuses on the "who," the identified or designated speaker, to get to the "what," the spoken message.

   The two kinds of dynamic patterns used in the present experiment in conjunction with the f_0 dimension present an interesting extension to *grouping* — the basic paradigm thought to underlie perceptual auditory scene analysis (ASA) and implemented by the great majority of algorithms in computational auditory scene analysis (CASA). The accepted wisdom is that the auditory system and its emulated computer analog first perform a time-frequency (T-F) analysis and a subsequently intervening segregation mechanism then groups together T-F cells that are coherent either temporally or spectrally. While spectral coherence was shown to also comprise frequency components that are synchronously modulated either in amplitude or in frequency [27][38], those results were based on the behavior of sinusoidal carriers. Other studies using simultaneous synthetic vowels investigated the role of fundamental frequency modulation (f_0-FM) and found that different patterns of f_0-FM in the figure and the background do not facilitate segregation [7]. The formant modulation used in Experiment 1, an analog of diphthong patterns, is not FM *per se:* since the carrier is a complex sinusoid with unmodulated frequency components, the formant modulation is, in fact, a ripple of momentary amplitude increases propagating from one harmonic to the next like a row of dominoes. The fact that even at the rather slow rate of formant modulation used (2.5 to 6.67 Hz for the 200- to 75-ms single transition durations) the percept is close to that of a continuous frequency change, suggests that somewhere in the auditory system the perceived continuity of change is translated into something analogous to frequency modulation. We have shown [8][3] that a perceptual mechanism extending a monotonic formant modulation prolongs the modulation's extent when the trajectory is truncated before reaching its target, not unlike how a mass set in motion by some force keeps moving because of its inertia even after the force is no longer applied on it.[3] If such a velocity-sensitive mechanism is in play for the processing of the type of formant patterns used in Experiment 1, it could provide a potential explanation for why streams with modulated formant frequencies could be segregated at much smaller formant peak differences than streams with steady-state formants.

Experiment 2 provides a demonstration that grouping by synchronously amplitude-modulating harmonics of a common f_0 is possible for AM patterns presented at very slow rates for f_0 differences of half octave and larger. One notices, however, that the modulation rates used encompass the modulation frequencies dominating speech: 4 Hz indicating syllabic-rate salience and 15-to-25 Hz sub-syllabic segmentation visible mainly in the carrier frequency range above 2.5 kHz [20]. Thus, the results showing that envelope fluctuation patterns in simultaneous streams are grouped across the harmonics of a common f_0 suggest that, in speech, syllabic and sub-syllabic fluctuations up to modulation frequencies of about 25 Hz may be segregated if they are produced by speakers with voice pitch differences larger than about two semitones.

The above analysis notwithstanding, the most visibly apparent result of the two experiments is that elderly individuals with good hearing exhibited a performance generally poorer than the young in the perceptual tasks investigated. Since the same population of elderly subjects also have been found to have a poorer speech understanding in babble noise and reverberation [11], it would be tempting to conclude that the segregation tasks in our two experiments underlie robust speech intelligibility. While this may be the case, it is also well known that, unfortunately, all kinds of auditory abilities, especially those requiring temporal processing, diminish with aging [18][12][9] and, therefore, age-related deficits in the two tasks examined here only fit a generalized geriatric decline. To show that these tasks embody speech processing better than others, we would have to conduct a large-scale investigation and perform robust statistical analyses. To date, we have conducted only one such study [13], which indicated a significantly high correlation between speech understanding in babble noise and segregation of syllabic-range AM patterns. Without further statistical evidence we can only state that the present experimental results are not inconsistent with the general view of temporal processing dysfunction in elderly individuals, possibly due to an overall slowing-down of central nervous activity [30].

We would like to conclude that the stimuli in the present experiments were modeled after variations in speech − i.e., they signify two instances of the dynamic processes comprising speech. Future theoretical work, which would quantitatively characterize speech as an ensemble of dynamic functions, as opposed to the classic beads-on-a-string representation, would be able to account for the phenomena described by most chapters in the present volume and would become the ultimate tribute to L. A. Chistovich and her colleagues who laid the foundations for it.

Acknowledgments

The author wishes to thank Kara Haupt, Alex Brandmeyer, and JC Sander for their help in collecting and analyzing data, and Steve Greenberg for his helpful comments on an earlier version of the manuscript. The research was supported by grant AG07998 from the National Institute on Aging and the Veterans Affairs Medical Research.

Endnotes

1. This scale is equivalent to the equal-rectangular-bandwidth, or ERB, scale.
2. In pilot experiments we noted that the stream with the higher pitch (f_0 high) was somewhat more salient perceptually than the stream with the lower pitch, consistent with centuries' worth of musical writing and practice putting the melody intended to be heard into the treble.
3. A similar finding has been reported showing that a tone sweep preceding the noise masker decreases the forward-masked threshold of a tone the frequency of which is on the trajectory of the sweep interrupted by the noise [6].

References

[1] Bregman, A.S. *Auditory Scene Analysis: The Perceptual Organization of Sound.* Cambridge, MA: MIT Press, 1990.
[2] Brungart, D.S. "Informational and energetic masking effects in the perception of two simultaneous talkers." *J. Acoust. Soc. Am.* 109: 1101-1109, 2001.
[3] Carré, R. and Divenyi, P.L. "Modeling and perception of 'gesture' reductions." *Phonetica*, 57:, 152-169, 2000.
[4] Cherry, C. "Some experiments on the recognition of speech with one and with two ears." *J. Acoust. Soc. Am.* 26: 975-979, 1953.
[5] Cooke, M.P., Green, P., Josifovski, L. and Vizinho, A. "Robust automatic speech recognition with missing and unreliable acoustic data." *Speech Communication* 34: 267-285, 2001.
[6] Crum, P.A. *Effects of Frequency Velocity on the Predicted Path of a Dynamic Sound.* Unpublished Doctoral Dissertation. Deparment of Psychology, Universeity of California, Berkeley, 2005.
[7] Culling, J.F. and Summerfield, Q. The role of frequency modulation in the perceptual segregation of concurrent vowels, *J. Acoust. Soc. Am.* 98: 837-846, 1995.
[8] Divenyi, P., Lindblom, B., and Carré, R. "The role of transition velocity in the perception of V1V2 complexes." *Proc. XIIIth International Congress of Phonetic Sciences*, pp. 258-261, 1995.
[9] Divenyi, P. "Masking the feature-information in multi-stream speech-analogue displays." In *Speech Separation by Humans and Machines*, P. Divenyi (ed.), New York: Kluwer, pp. 269-281, 2005.
[10] Divenyi, P. "Humans glimpse, too, not only machines (hommage à Martin Cooke)." *Forum Acusticum*, 2005.
[11] Divenyi, P.L. and Haupt, K.M.. "Audiological correlates of speech understanding deficits in elderly listeners with mild-to-moderate hearing loss. I. Age and laterality effects." *Ear and Hearing* 18: 42-61, 1997.
[12] Divenyi, P.L. "Beyond presbyacusis: Non-hearing loss-related temporal processing deficits in the elderly." *J. Acoust. Soc. Am.* 107: 2796-2797, 2000.
[13] Divenyi, P.L. and Haupt, K.M. "Auditory segregation of syllable-length low-frequency amplitude-modulated sinusoidal patterns by elderly listeners." *Abstracts of the Twenty-third Midwinter Research Meeting, Association for Research in Otolaryngology*, 2000.
[14] Efron, R. "Conservation of temporal information by perceptual systems." *Percept. Pyschophys.* 14: 518-530, 1973.
[15] Ellis, D.P.W. "Using knowledge to organize sound: The prediction-driven approach to computational auditory scene analysis, and its application to speech/nonspeech mixtures." *Speech Communication* 27: 281-298, 1999.
[16] Fitzgibbons, P.J. and Gordon-Salant, S. "Age effects on discrimination of timing in auditory sequences." *J. Acoust. Soc. Am.* 116: 1126-1134, 2004.
[17] Freyman, R.L., Helfer, K.S., McCall, D.D. and Clifton, R.K. "The role of perceived spatial separation in the unmasking of speech." *J. Acoust. Soc. Am.* 106: 3578-3588, 1999.
[18] Gordon-Salant, S. and Fitzgibbons, P.J. "Profile of auditory temporal processing in older listeners." *J. Speech Lang. Hear. Res.* 42: 300-311, 1999.

[19] Greenberg, S., Carvey, H.M., Hitchcock, L. and Chang, S. "Beyond the phoneme A juncture-accent model for spoken language." *Proc. Second International Conference Human Language Technology Research*, pp. 36-43, 2002.

[20] Greenberg, S. and Arai, T. "What are the essential cues for understanding spoken language?" *IEICE Trans. Inf. & Syst.* E87: 1059-1070, 2004.

[21] Greenwood, D.D. "Auditory masking and the combination band."*J. Acoust. Soc. Am*. 33: 484-502, 1961.

[22] Kalikow, D.N., Stevens, K.N., and Elliott, L.L. Development of a test of speech intelligibility in noise using sentence materials with controlled word predictability, *J. Acoust. Soc. Am*. 61: 1337-1351, 1977.

[23] Kidd, G., Jr., Mason, C.R., Brughera, A., and Hartmann, W.M. "The role of reverberation in release from masking due to spatial separation of sources for speech identification" *Acta Acustica*, 2005.

[24] Koffka, K. *Principles of Gestalt psychology*. New York: Harcourt Brace Jovanovich, 1935.

[25] Levitt, H. "Transformed up-down methods in psychoacoustics." *J. Acoust. Soc. Am*. 49: 467-477, 1971.

[26] Lisker, L. "Is it VOT or first-formant detector?" *J. Acoust. Soc. Am*. 57: 1547-1551, 1975.

[27] Moore, B.C.J. and Shailer, M.J. "Modulation discrimination interference and auditory grouping." *Phil. Trans/ Royal Soc. Lond. B (Biol. Sci.)* 336: 339-346, 1992.

[28] Plomp, R. "Perception of speech as a modulated signal." *Proc. Tenth International Congress Phonetic Sciences*, pp. 29-40, 1983.

[29] Raj, B., Seltzer, M. and Stern, R.M. "Reconstruction of missing features for robust speech recognition." *Speech Communication* 43: 275-296, 2005.

[30] Salthouse, T.A. *Theoretical Perspectives on Cognitive Aging*. Hillsdale, N.J.: Erlbaum, 1991.

[31] Shailer, M.J. and Moore, B.C.J. "Effects of modulation rate and rate of envelope change on modulation discrimination interference." *J. Acoust. Soc. Am*. 94: 3138-3143, 1993.

[32] Shinn-Cunningham, B. "Speech intelligibility, spatial unmasking, and realism in reverberant spatial auditory displays." *Proc. ICAD*, Kyoto, 2002.

[33] Slaney, M. *Lyon's Cochlear Model*. Cupertino, CA: Apple Computer Technical Report, 1988.

[34] Takeuchi, A.H. and Braida, L.D. "Recognition of amplitude-modulation patterns in the presence of a distractor. II. Effects of dichotic presentation and unmodulated distractors." *J. Acoust. Soc. Am*. 98: 142-147, 1995.

[35] Terhardt, E., Stoll, G., and Seewann, M. "Algorithm for extraction of pitch and pitch salience from complex tonal signals." *J. Acoust. Soc. Am*. 71: 679-688, 1982.

[36] Terhardt, E., Stoll, G. and Seewann, M. Pitch of complex signals according to virtual-pitch theory: Tests, examples, and predictions, *J. Acoust. Soc. Am*. 71: 671-678, 1982.

[37] Wang, D.L. "On Ideal Binary Mask as the computational goal of auditory scene analysis." In Speech Separation by Humans and Machines, P. Divenyi (ed.), New York: Kluwer, pp. 179-196, 2004.

[38] Yost, W.A. and Sheft, S. "Modulation detection interference: across-frequency processing and auditory grouping." *Hear. Res*. 79: 48-58, 1994.

Dynamics of Speech Production and Perception
P. Divenyi et al. (Eds.)
IOS Press, 2006

Fluctuations in Amplitude and Frequency Enable Interaural Delays to Foster the Identification of Speech-Like Stimuli

Richard M. STERN[1], Constantine TRAHIOTIS[2] and Angelo M. RIPEPI[1]
*[1]Department of Electrical and Computer Engineering
and Biomedical Engineering Program,
Carnegie Mellon University, Pittsburgh, Pennsylvania, USA*
*[2]Department of Neuroscience and Department of Surgery (Otolaryngology)
University of Connecticut Health Center, Farmington, Connecticutt, USA*

Abstract. In this study, we describe the results of two experiments that help clarify the conditions under which interaural time delays can facilitate the identification of simultaneously-presented vowel sounds. In one experiment we measured the intelligibility of simultaneously-presented natural speech and speech that had been degraded in a manner that precluded the use of pitch information. In a second experiment we measured the identification accuracy gained by adding pitch and amplitude information to whispered vowel-like sounds. The major results of these experiments are twofold. First, interaural time delays can indeed facilitate the identification of simultaneously-presented speech-like sounds, even when cues based on common fundamental frequency are not available. Second, the ease with which the very potent contribution of interaural timing information can be exploited is strongly facilitated in turn by the presence of dynamic variations in the stimuli (such as the monaural amplitude and frequency fluctuations that are characteristic of natural speech sounds).

Keywords. Phonetic identification, interaural delays, amplitude modulation, frequency modulation, coincidence detection

Introduction

This presentation and paper are concerned with the ways in which the use of cues based on interaural time delay (ITD) can foster the separation and identification of multiple simultaneously-presented speech-like stimuli. We begin with a review of some of the major trends of research in binaural modeling, particularly with regard to models based on the interaural cross-correlation of the auditory-nerve response to the stimuli. We then present and discuss the results of two experiments that serve to clarify the extent to which differences in ITD can facilitate the separate perception of competing streams of natural speech, and the important role that is played by the presence of dynamic variations in these stimuli.

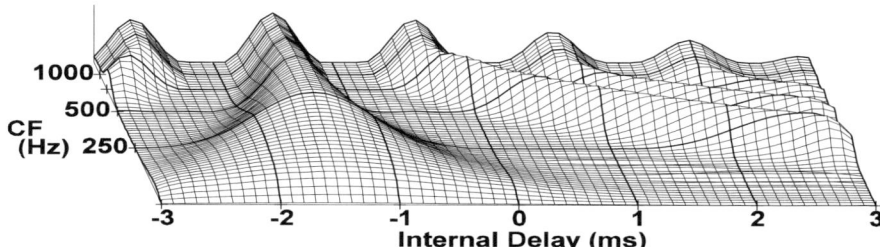

Figure 1. The average value of the instantaneous number of coincidences as a simultaneous function of characteristic frequency and internal delay. The stimulus is a low-frequency bandpass noise with a center
frequency of 500 Hz and an ITD of –1.5 ms.

The "modern era" of binaural modeling can be said to have begun with Jeffress's
prescient paper (Jeffress, 1948) suggesting that a neural coincidence mechanism could
underlie human ability to process small interaural time differences in impinging stimuli.
Jeffress suggested that central units could internally code external interaural delays that
record coincidences of neural impulses from pairs of more peripheral nerve fibers tuned
monaural to the same center frequency. Since then, numerous behavioral and physiological investigations have confirmed the utility and general validity of his observation.
Current models include Jeffress's coincidence mechanism after peripheral processing of
the signals that includes bandpass filtering, nonlinear rectification, and compression.

An intuitive understanding of how such cross-correlation-based models can be used
to understand the binaural representation of signals presented with external delays can
be obtained by considering a three-dimensional "cross-correlation surface." Figure 1 is a
representation of the relative response of an array of coincidence counting units plotted
when the signal is a bandpass noise having a center frequency of 500 Hz, a bandwidth of
800 Hz, and presented with an external interaural delay of –1.5 ms. The responses are
plotted as a simultaneous function of internal interaural delay (along the horizontal axis)
and center frequency of the peripheral input fibers (along the oblique axis). As can be
seen, the value of the external delay, –1.5 ms, can be inferred from the "straight" or vertical ridge of the pattern of cross-correlation observed at that internal delay. The remaining, curved, ridges are observed because the cross-correlation functions of the
narrowband outputs resulting from peripheral filtering have repetitive peaks of activity
that are spaced at intervals of internal delay equal to the reciprocal of the center frequency of the peripheral bandpass filters. Similarly, speech or speech-like information
stemming from an external source of sound would be expected to result in a straight
ridge of activity corresponding to the internal delay associated with the external delay
with which the signal arrives at the two ears. Within this framework the ability to "separate" or understand two sources of auditory information presented simultaneously can
be thought about as the ability to parse and/or track the information that corresponds to
the respective ridges in the cross-correlation produced by the sources.

Consistent with this view, it is widely accepted that the ability to understand speech
in the presence of competing sounds improves when the speech and competing sounds
are spatially separated. Such an outcome has been observed in experiments using natural free-field stimuli (*e.g.* [2][16]) and in experiments utilizing stimuli presented via earphones (*e.g.* [3][10][9][16][12][7]).

These observations notwithstanding, the results of several experiments using earphones indicate that listeners are unable to achieve separate identification of simultaneously-presented vowel-like sounds solely on the basis of their ITDs (*e.g.* [4][8][6]). Nevertheless, and important for our purposes, Darwin and Hukin did note that the presence of an ITD can enhance the identification of vowel-like sounds when there is plausible independent evidence of an additional sound source. Taken at face value, the inability to identify artificially-generated vowels on the basis of ITD appears to be inconsistent with the ease with which one can simultaneously perceive naturally-occurring speech emanating from spatially-separated sources.

This investigation is an attempt to understand the factor(s) underlying the differences between these two types of outcomes. Toward that end we conducted two separate, but related, experiments. In the first experiment we attempted to reduce or eliminate pitch-based cues which are inherent in natural speech sounds. This tested the hypothesis that pitch cues could be highly salient, if not necessary, for the identification for the identification of sources of sounds having differing ITDs. In the second experiment we attempted to assess the extent to which the addition of amplitude and/or frequency modulation could combine with ITD to enhance the identification of bandpass-filtered vowel sounds, using stimuli similar to those employed by Culling and Summerfield. It is well known that (monaural) pitch and amplitude cues foster the perceptual segregation of independent sources of sound (*e.g.* [1][15][5]), and it seemed reasonable to expect that the separate perception of simultaneously-presented sources of sounds based on ITD could be facilitated by the presence of monaural modulations in amplitude and/or frequency.

The results of Experiment 1 indicate that the identification of simultaneously-presented natural speech sounds is improved when the ITDs with which they are presented are different, even when pitch information is not available as a cue. The results of Experiment 2 indicate that the addition of speech-like variations in amplitude and frequency can improve the ability to use ITDs in order to identify vowel-like sounds similar to those employed by Culling and Summerfield. This latter finding is consistent with some of the observations of [6].

1. Experiment 1: Intelligibility of Interaurally-delayed Natural Speech Sounds Devoid of Pitch Information

In this experiment we measured the extent to which pitch information plays a role in the perceptual segregation of interaurally-delayed natural speech. Said differently, we measured intelligibility of speech after removing potentially useful information concerning pitch and harmonicity.

1.1 Stimuli and experimental procedure

The stimuli were taken from the SATASK database recorded by the US Army Research Laboratory [9]. This database consisted of recorded sentences of speech of the form "(NAME) write the number (NUMBER) on the (COLOR) (OBJECT)". Four names, eight numbers, eight colors, and nine object names were used, all of which were monosyllabic. The sentences were spoken by four males and digitally recorded with a sampling rate of 11,025 Hz under carefully controlled conditions. Efforts were made to ensure that all sentences were spoken at the same rate so that the major content words would occur at coincident times if the signals were combined.

Pairs of sentences selected randomly from the possible combinations of four names, eight numbers, eight colors, and nine object names were combined digitally and presented binaurally. One of the two sentences always began with the NAME "Troy" and will be referred to as the target sentence. The other sentence will be referred to as the masker sentence. An example of a target sentence could be "Troy, write the number 4 on the green fork". A corresponding masker sentence could be "Ron, write the number 2 on the black kite". The two sentences were combined with a target-to-masker ratio of 0 dB. In some blocks of trials both sentences were presented with zero ITD, causing both sentences to be perceived in the center of the head when the stimuli were presented diotically over headphones. In other blocks of trials one of the two sentences would be presented with zero ITD while the other would be presented with a 363-μs ITD, causing the dichotically-presented sentence to be perceived toward the leading (right) ear. (With a sampling rate of 11,025 Hz, 363 ms is the closet integer sample delay to the ITD of 400 ms that had been used in the experiments of Culling and Summerfield.)

The pairs of sentences were presented in blocks of 25 trials. They were always composed of speech from two different talkers, and the particular combination of NAME, NUMBER, COLOR, and OBJECT used within each target-masker set was unique. Using a computer terminal with a graphical user interface, the listener's task was to choose the NUMBER, COLOR, and OBJECT that corresponded to the sentence that started with the name TROY. The listeners were required to respond on each trial before the next trial could begin. One hundred sentences from each condition were presented to each of two listeners.

The sentences were presented in five different fashions: natural, vocoded with natural pitch contours, vocoded in monotone style with the target and masker presented at two fixed fundamental frequencies (90 and 100 Hz, respectively), vocoded in monotone style with both target and masker presented with the same fundamental frequency (100 Hz), and whispered. The term "natural" refers to the original speech as recorded in the SATASK database. The various "vocoded" and "whispered" conditions were obtained using LPC waveform coding methods. The incoming speech was windowed using a series of 20-ms Hamming windows which overlapped by 10 ms. Fourteen LPC coefficients were obtained for each windowed segment using the Levinson-Durbin method (e.g. [13]). These coefficients characterize the time-varying spectral profile of the incoming speech, but do not contain detailed information about the excitation signal. The monotone speech signals were obtained by exciting the linear filter specified by the (time-varying) LPC coefficients with a periodic impulse train. The vocoded speech with natural pitch contours was also obtained by exciting the LPC-derived filter with an impulse train, but with an instantaneous frequency that equaled the fundamental frequency of the voiced segments of the original signal. Pitch was estimated using the pitch-extraction algorithm of the commercially-available Entropic Signal Processing System [14]. The "whispered" speech was obtained by exciting the filter specified by the LPC coefficients with white noise. The use of the monotone and whispered speech conditions enabled us to present speech-like stimuli for which grouping cues associated with fundamental frequency were either difficult to separate (as in the case of two sentences of monotone speech presented simultaneously with precisely the same funda-

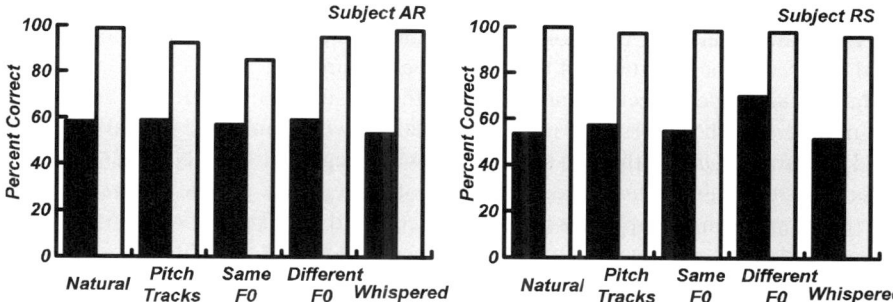

Figure 2. Percent correct identification of the content words in the sentences of Experiment 1. Conditions from left to right are natural speech, vocoded speech with natural pitch tracks, vocoded monotone speech with the same fundamental frequency (F0), vocoded monotone speech with different fundamental frequencies, and vocoded whispered speech. The darker bars represent results obtained with target ITD of zero μs while the lighter bars represent data obtained with target ITD of 363 μs. Masker ITD was zero ms in all cases.

mental frequency), or non-existent (as in the case of simultaneously-presented whispered speech).

1.2 Results and discussion

Figure 2 displays the percentage of words correctly identified for each of the five experimental conditions, presented separately for two listeners, the first and third authors. The reader is reminded that the masker sentence was always presented with zero ITD. The darker and lighter bars represent data obtained when the target ITD was 0 ms or 363 ms, respectively. Because there were 8 numbers, 8 colors, and 9 objects to identify, chance performance for this task is about 12 percent correct.

For our purposes the most important feature of the data is that identification accuracy was consistently better for target stimuli presented with the ITD of 363 ms. This verifies that ITDs per se can, under appropriate circumstances, facilitate the intelligibility of competing speech-like stimuli. In addition, performance did not vary greatly over the five different types of stimuli. Note that, in particular, a binaural advantage was observed even for conditions in which the fundamental frequencies were the same (the "Same F0" condition) or nonexistent (the "Whispered" condition). We interpret this outcome to mean that ITDs can aid speech intelligibility even when the sources of speech cannot be segregated on the basis of information stemming from variations of pitch. It is interesting listeners were able to perform much better than chance (12 percent) when both targets and maskers were presented with zero ITD. We believe that this is a consequence of the limited masking effects that result when the targets and maskers are presented at an energy ratio of 0 dB.

2. Experiment 2: Identification of Simultaneously-presented "Whispered" Vowels Having Speech-like Contours of Pitch and Amplitude

2.1 Stimuli and experimental procedure

The purpose of this experiment was to evaluate the extent to which modulations in amplitude and/or frequency can facilitate the identification of speech-like sounds based on ITD. As in the previous experiment, we employed stimuli that were "intermediate" between natural speech and the whispered vowels used by Culling and Summerfield [4]. Data were also obtained with such modulations absent.

The stimuli included whispered vowels similar to those generated by Culling and Summerfield as well as versions of such signals that were modulated by the amplitude and/or frequency contours of natural speech. Each of four whispered vowels (which were labeled "AR", "EE", "OO", and "ER") were constructed by passing white noise through time-invariant filters each of which had two narrow rectangular passbands. Four finite-impulse-response equiripple filters were employed that were obtained using the Parks-McClellan algorithm (e.g. [11]). The center frequencies of the passbands were the four center frequencies used by Culling and Summerfield: 225, 625, 975, and 1925 Hz. The filters had transitional bandwidths of 50 Hz and a length of 512 samples. The sample rate was 11,025 Hz, as in Experiment 1. For each trial, independent tokens of each type of stimulus were generated by exciting the appropriate filter with a statistically-independent white noise excitation function.

Contours of amplitude modulation of speech were obtained by measuring the short-term energy of speech waveforms from the Koehnke and Besing SATASK database. Sentences were selected from that database in the same manner as described in the previous experiment. Contours of frequency modulation were obtained by estimating the pitch of the SATASK sentences, again using the pitch-extraction algorithm in the ESPS package of Entropic Research Laboratory. The duration of the sentences was approximately three seconds.

Data were collected using unmodulated whispered vowels, whispered vowels with natural amplitude-modulation contours, whispered vowels with natural frequency-modulation contours, and whispered vowels presented with both natural amplitude and frequency modulation contours. Gaussian noise presented at −30-dB re the level of the vowel sounds was added in order to mask low-level off-frequency sideband information resulting from the modulation of the signals. The unmodulated whispered vowel sounds were similar to the stimuli used by Culling and Summerfield, but approximately three seconds in duration.

For each block of trials, two equal-level vowel waveforms, either an "AR" and an "EE" or an "OO" and an "ER" were combined digitally. One of the two vowels was presented with zero ITD and would be perceived, in isolation, in the center of the head. The other vowel was presented with a 363-μs ITD, and would be perceived, in isolation, toward the right ear. The task was to identify which of the four types of vowels, "AR", "EE", "ER", or "OO", was perceptually toward the right side of midline. As authors and experimenters, the listeners knew that only four combinations of vowel identity and intracranial position were possible, and this information could sometimes be used to improve identification accuracy. This limitation of stimulus conditions was necessary to avoid the presentation of pairs of vowels having overlapping spectral components.

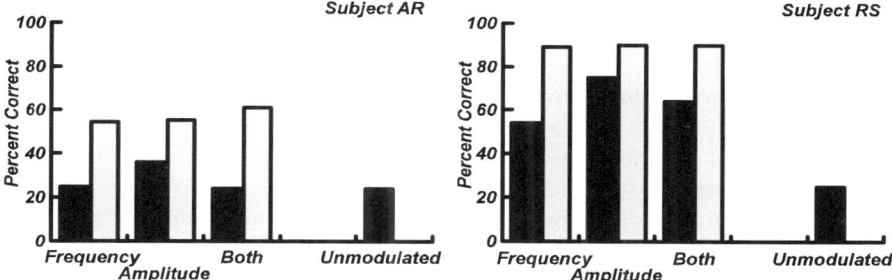

Figure 3. Results of Experiment 2 whispered vowels presented with frequency modulation, amplitude modulation, both frequency and amplitude modulation, and no modulation were identified. The lighter bars indicate data obtained when the modulation contours for the two vowels were drawn from the different utterances and the darker bars indicate data obtained when the modulation contours of the two whispered vowels were identical.

Data were collected in four blocks of 25 trials for each stimulus condition. Identification accuracy was obtained for conditions in which the two simultaneously-presented stimuli had different amplitude- and/or frequency-modulation contours (extracted from two different SATASK sentences) and for conditions in which the two simultaneously-presented stimuli had identical amplitude- and/or frequency-modulation contours (extracted from a single SATASK sentences). Finally, control data were obtained with the stimuli unmodulated by either amplitude or frequency. These unmodulated stimuli were very similar to the stimuli used by Culling and Summerfield, except that they were of much longer duration.

2.2 Results and discussion

Figure 3 summarizes the results for the two listeners, plotted separately. Percentage of correct identifications is plotted for each of the four types of stimulus conditions. The lighter bars indicate data obtained when the modulation contours for the two vowels were drawn from different utterances and the darker bars indicate data obtained when the modulation contours of the two whispered vowels were identical.

Because there were only four possible responses, chance performance is nominally 25 percent correct. The fact that the no-modulation condition results in performance near chance confirms the major results of Culling and Summerfield [4] experiment. That is, when there was no modulation of the stimuli, the listeners were unable to use the ITD of 363 μs in order to perceptually segregate and identify the target vowel.

Performance improved substantially when the vowel sounds were modulated by two different frequency and/or amplitude contours, an outcome that is consistent with the results of Experiment 1. For those conditions, identification accuracy was between 54 and 61 percent correct for Subject AR and between 89 and 90 percent for Subject RS. (These differences in performance are likely to be a consequence of RS's having had vast experience as a subject in binaural hearing experiments.) As indicated by the solid bars, Subject RS was also able to perform the discriminations at a level of between 54 and 75 percent correct when the two vowel sounds were modulated by the same pitch and/or amplitude contours, although the identification task was considerably more difficult than it was when the modulating waveforms were different for the two vowels. RS's data are well above chance for all conditions, even assuming that he is able to make use of all available monaural information. Subject AR obtained relatively little improvement in performance over chance when the two vowels were modulated identically, although amplitude modulation provided a small benefit.

3. General Conclusions

We conclude from the results of the two experiments that ITD per se can indeed be an extremely useful cue for fostering the identification of simultaneously-presented speech-like sounds. The results of Experiment 1, particularly with whispered speech, indicate that ITDs can facilitate speech intelligibility even when "grouping" cues based on common fundamental frequency are not available. The results of Experiment 2 indicate that listeners are able to use ITDs to foster the separation and identification of speech-like sounds and whispered vowels when the stimuli contain naturally-occurring amplitude and frequency modulations. We note that the information derived from modulating the stimuli is, in principle, monaural in nature and appears to be necessary for the binaural cues based on ITD to become effective in increasing the intelligibility of competing sources of speech. Based on these results, it appears that Culling and Summerfield's [4] findings were at least in part a consequence of the absence of dynamic variations in their stimuli.

Acknowledgments

This research was partially supported by a graduate research assistantship to Angelo Ripepi from the Carnegie Mellon University Biomedical Engineering Program. C. Trahiotis was supported by Research Grant No. NIH DC-00234 from the National Institute on Deafness and Other Communication Disorders, National Institutes of Health. The experimental data reported here were obtained by Angelo Ripepi in partial fulfillment of the requirements for the degree of Master of Science at Carnegie Mellon University.

References

[1] Bregman, A.S. *Auditory Scene Analysis: The Perceptual Organization of Sound*, MIT Press, Cambridge, MA, 1990.
[2] Bronkhorst, A.W. and Plomp, R. "A clinical test for the assessment of binaural speech perception in noise," *Audiology* 29, 275–285, 1990.
[3] Bronkhorst, A.W. and Plomp, R. "Effect of multiple speech-like maskers on binaural speech recognition in normal and impaired hearing," *J. Acoust. Soc. Am.* 92, 3132-3139, 1992.
[4] Culling, J.F. and Summerfield, Q. "Perceptual separation of concurrent speech sounds: Absence of across-frequency grouping by common interaural delay," *J. Acoust. Soc. Am.*, 98, 785-797, 1995.
[5] Darwin, C.J. and Carlyon, R.P. "Auditory Grouping," in *Handbook of Perception and Cognition, Volume 6: Hearing*, B.C.J. Moore, ed., New York: Academic Press, 1995.
[6] Darwin, C.J. and Hukin, R.W. "Perceptual segregation of a harmonic from a vowel by interaural time difference and frequency proximity," *J. Acoust. Soc. Am.* 102, 2316–2324, 1997.
[7] Hawley, M.L., Litovsky, R.Y., and Colburn, H.S. "Speech intelligibility and localization in a multi-source environment," *J. Acoust. Soc. Am.* 105, 3436-3448, 1999.
[8] Hukin, R.W. and Darwin, C.J. "Effects of contralateral presentation and of interaural time differences in segregating a harmonic from a vowel," *J. Acoust. Soc. Am.* 98, 1380–1387, 1995.
[9] Koehnke, J. and Besing, J.M. "A Procedure for Testing Speech Intelligibility in a Virtual Listening Environment," *Ear & Hearing*, 17, 211-217, 1996.

[10] Nilsson, M.J. and Soli, S.D. "Norms for a headphone simulation of the hearing in noise test: comparison of physical and simulated spatial separation of sound sources," *J. Acoust. Soc. Am.* 95, 2994, 1994.

[11] Oppenheim, A.V., Schafer, R.W., and Buck, J.R. *Discrete-Time Signal Processing (Second Edition)*, Upper Saddle River, NJ: Pearson Education Publishers, 1999.

[12] Peissig, J. and Kollmeier, B. "Directivity of binaural noise reduction in spatial multiple noise-source arrangements for normal and impaired listeners," *J. Acoust. Soc. Am.* 101, 1660–1670, 1997.

[13] Rabiner, L.R. and Schafer, R.W. *Digital Processing of Speech Signals*, Prentice-Hall, Englewood Cliffs NJ, 1978.

[14] Talkin, D. "A Robust Algorithm for Pitch Tracking (RAPT)", in *Speech Coding and Synthesis*, W.B. Kleijn and K.K. Paliwal, eds., Amsterdam, NL: Elsevier Science, pp. 495-518, 1995.

[15] Yost, W.A. "Auditory Image Perception and Analysis," *Hearing Res.* 56, 8-19, 1992.

[16] Yost, W.A., Dye, R.H. Jr., and Sheft, S. "A Simulated "Cocktail" Party" with Up to Three Sound Sources," *Percept. Psychophys.* 58, 1026–1036, 1996.

Dynamics of Speech Production and Perception
P. Divenyi et al. (Eds.)
IOS Press, 2006

Vowel Normalisation: Time-domain Processing of the Internal Dynamics of Speech

Richard E. TURNER[1], Marc A. AL-HAMES[1], David R. R. SMITH[1], Hideki
KAWAHARA[2], Toshio IRINO[2] and Roy D. PATTERSON[1]
[1] *Centre for the Neural Basis of Hearing*
Dept. of Physiology, Development and Neuroscience, University of Cambridge, UK
[2] *Faculty of Systems Engineering, Wakayama University, Wakayama, Japan*

Abstract. Human listeners can identify vowels regardless of speaker size, although
the sound waves for an adult and a child speaking the 'same' vowel would differ enor-
mously. The differences are mainly due to differences in vocal tract length (VTL) and
glottal pulse rate (GPR) which are both related to body size. ASR machines are notoriously bad at understanding children if they have been trained on the speech of an
adult. In this paper, we propose that the auditory system adapts its analysis of speech
sounds, dynamically and automatically to the GPR and VTL of the speaker on a sylla-
ble-to-syllable basis. In this paper, we illustrate how this rapid adaptation might be
performed with the aid of a computational version of the auditory image model, and
we propose that an auditory preprocessor of this form would improve the robustness
of speech recognizers.

Keywords. Vowel normalisation, pitch synchronous analysis, auditory preprocessing

Introduction

Human listeners can identify specific vowels regardless of the speaker and they also
know whether the speaker is a man, woman or child. This is possible even though the
sound waves for a particular vowel are very different when spoken by men, women and
children. For example, if we compare the vowel /a/ spoken by a man and a child, the
most prominent spectral peaks (the formants) and the repetition rate (glottal pulse rate)
will both be greater in the case of the child. The formant frequency differences are due
largely to changes in vocal tract length (VTL), which varies with age and sex
[25][11][7]. The glottal pulse rate (GPR), or voice-pitch, differences are due to variation
in vocal cord size, mass and tension [24]. Somehow, the auditory system automatically
extracts from the sound both the specific vowel spoken (VT shape information) and the
size of the speaker (man, woman or child). How is this done?

There are currently two candidate theories. One argues that the auditory system includes an active re-scaling process [13] that is applied to all sounds at an early point in the auditory system. This Mellin Transform (MT) [6] maps all input sounds to a nominal scale [14], thereby reducing variability in the shape information whilst segregating the size information. In the process, the MT normalises vowels for VTL. The other theory posits that the speech centre in the brain learns the statistics of variation in GPR and formant frequency while learning speech as a child [1][2]. The vowel /a/, as spoken by a child and an adult, are heard as the same vowel because the auditory system has learnt that a high GPR is correlated with high formant frequencies and *vice versa*.

In this chapter we review the MT and show how a time-domain model of auditory perception, the Auditory Image Model (AIM), can be modified to include the MT. We show that the resulting Mellin Images (MI) provide information about both the shape and length of the vocal tract, and that a simple mixture-of-Gaussians classifier can be used to categorise the MIs of different vowels. We show how a range of vowels, scaled in GPR and VTL to represent different size speakers, can be reliably classified from the MIs of the vowels. With regard to theories of human vowel normalisation, if vowel perception is based on learnt statistical variation, then categorisation should break down when the scaling of VTL and GPR exceeds the normal human range. An active re-scaling process, used to transform all sounds, might be expected to work across a much wider region of changes in GPR and VTL. We report categorisation tests which showed that AIM with the MI extension was able to recognise vowels scaled well beyond the normal speech range. We also measured vowel recognition psychophysically and showed that performance is excellent over a region considerably greater than that of normal speech. Finally, we measured discrimination performance (resolution) along the GPR and VTL dimensions and showed that speaker size remains a useful cue well beyond the range of normal experience.

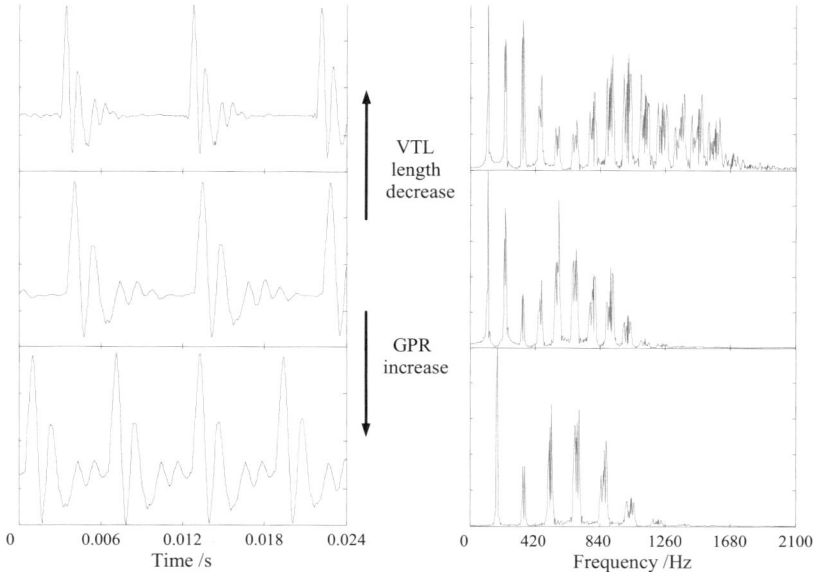

Figure 1. Waveforms (left) and spectra (right) of the vowel /a/ illustrating the effect of scale changes of VTL and GPR. Decreasing VTL causes an expansion of the spectral envelope which leads to higher formant frequencies. Increasing GPR causes the spacing of the harmonics to expand under the spectral envelope.

1. Theoretical Background

In this section we explain the motivation for including the Mellin Transform in models of auditory processing. We then go on to describe the extension of the Auditory Image Model to include the MT, and discuss the structure of the resultant Mellin Images.

1.1 Scaling Vowels in GPR and VTL

Vowels are complex tonal sounds largely characterised by their pitch and formant frequencies. The pitch is determined by the rate at which the larynx produces glottal pulses (GPR). The vowel type is determined by the placement of the tongue which largely controls the shape of the oral cavities and, thereby, the formant frequencies. For a given vowel, the size of the speaker (or more accurately, the VTL) affects the absolute frequencies of the formants – a large male has a longer vocal tract and, consequently, lower formant frequencies than a small child. It is the case, however, that the ratio of the formant frequencies is similar [8], and it is this which is thought to characterise the vowel type. Figure 1 presents the waves and Fourier spectra of three versions of the vowel /a/ to illustrate the effects of scaling VTL and GPR. A 'standard' version of the vowel appears in the middle row. The upper row shows what happens when the vocal tract is reduced in length; the glottal pulses occur at the same rate and so the GPR is unchanged, but the duration of the resonance within the glottal period decreases, and as a result, the spectrum expands. The lower row shows what happens when the glottal period is reduced; the duration of the resonance within the glottal period is largely unaffected and the *envelope* of the spectrum is largely unaffected, but the spacing of the harmonics

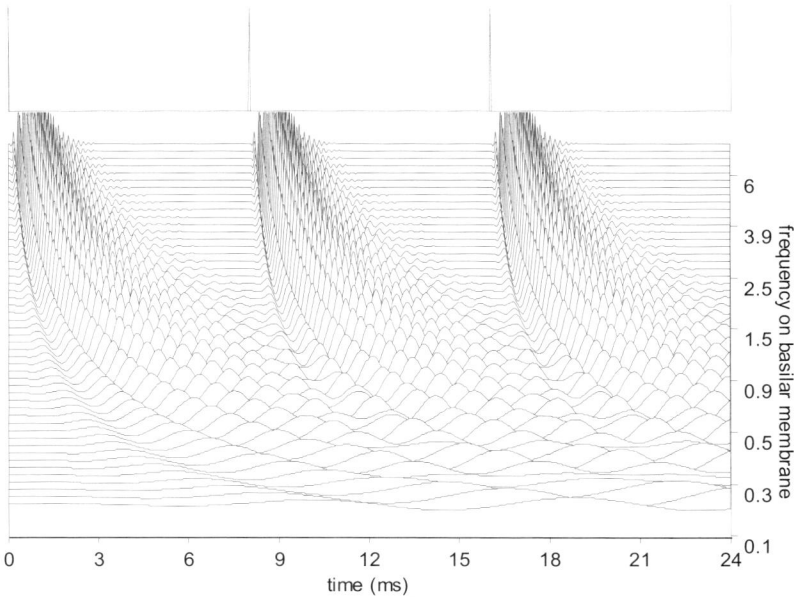

Figure 2. Simulation of basilar membrane motion in response to a click-train with an 8-ms period using a gammatone auditory filterbank. In the high frequency channels the filter response dies away before the next click. In the low frequency channels the cycles of the impulse response interact.

under the envelope expands as the GPR rises. The figure shows that the effects of scaling VTL and GPR can be largely independent.

The MT segregates dilation information from shape and structure information, and it can transform the two resonances in the middle and upper rows of Figure 1 into an invariant form that reveals that they came from vocal tracts with the same shape. However, the MT is not shift invariant and so the representation of the resonance has to be transformed, prior to the application of the MT, into a form where the zero of the MT occurs at the start of the resonance. In other words, the MT analysis has to be pitch synchronous. This property is very difficult to achieve in spectral models of auditory processing. It arises naturally, however, in time-domain models of auditory processing that focus on the time-interval information produced by the cochlea in the auditory nerve. In the next subsection, we describe how the Auditory Image Model of perception performs the preprocessing required by the MT, and then we explain how the MT can normalise vowels as they appear in the auditory image.

1.2 Auditory Images

The Auditory Image Model was developed to explain auditory perception in terms of the neural patterns produced by sounds in the cochlea [20][21][1], and to illustrate the dynamic response to sounds in high-resolution video format. Recently, a modular Matlab version of AIM has been created to facilitate further development of time-domain auditory models [3]. It is referred to as AIM-mat and we have extended AIM-mat to incorporate a module that transforms auditory images into Mellin Images (MIs). This section outlines the construction of auditory images using a click-train to emphasise the form of the impulse response of the auditory system.

1.2.1 Basilar Membrane Motion

In AIM-mat, the motion of the basilar membrane is simulated by a bank of bandpass filters whose centre frequencies are evenly distributed along a quasi-logarithmic scale referred to as an ERB scale [10]. The impulse response of the filter is well described by the gammatone function [4][5] or, more generally, by the gammachirp function [12]. The centre frequency of a filter is the carrier of the impulse response and the damping exponential tail of the impulse response determines the filter bandwidth, which is about 10% of the centre frequency. AIM-mat's simulation of the basilar membrane motion (BMM) in response to a click-train is shown in Figure 2. Figure 3A provides a simplified schematic explanation. Repeated ridges of BM displacement are observed (Figure 2), and they can be labelled by their integer ridge value, h (Figure 3A). The BM performs a spectral analysis of the sound in the form of a wavelet transform. This transform preserves scale information [12][14] and enables the auditory system to exploit the advantages of spectral analysis and scale analysis within a single system.

1.2.2 Neural Activity Pattern

The inner hair cells along the basilar membrane convert BMM into a neural activity pattern (NAP). AIM simulates the process with half-wave rectification, compression and low-pass filtering to limit phase locking and then the local contrast is enhanced with 2-dimensional, adaptive thresholding (2D-AT).

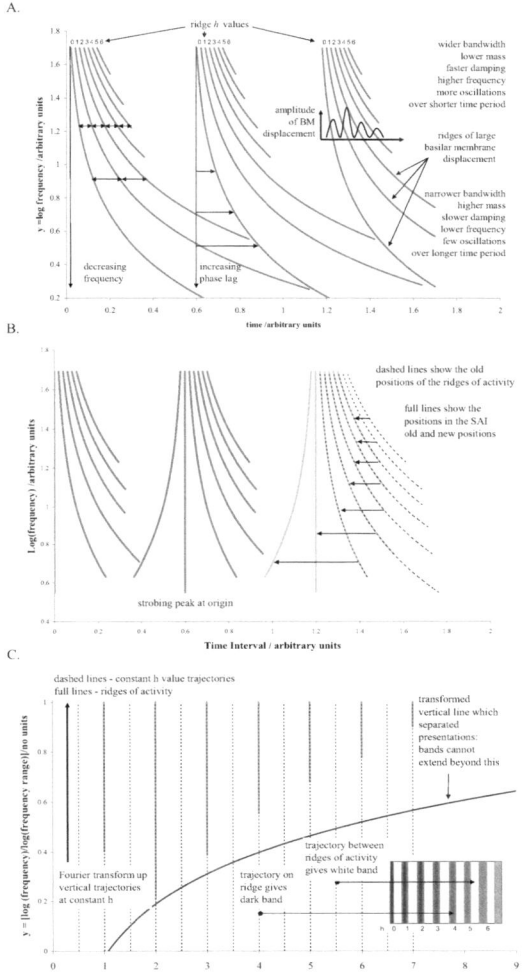

Figure 3. A. Schematic of basilar membrane motion. Each click produces an impulse response in all the filters. The lower frequency filters have greater phase lags, they oscillate for a longer time, but for fewer oscillations. Height out of the plane represents BM displacement. The ridges of activity have well defined trajectories described by maxima in the cosine function of the impulse response. We label them with integer values, h. B. Schematic showing strobing in the NAP. The second peak is typically the largest and is used at the strobe point that defines the zero of the time-interval dimension of the auditory image. C. Size Shape Image for the click-train: The upper channels are expanded by transformation to log time-interval, and aligned vertically in accordance with their *h* value (that is, the cycle of the impulse response). The MT is completed by calculating the spatial frequencies for each value of *h* using a Fourier Transform.

1.2.3 Strobed Temporal Integration and the Stabilized Auditory Image

If the intensity of a pure sinusoid is modulated in time, then as the modulation rate increases from 1-100 Hz, the perception of level fluctuation fades away (around 30 Hz)

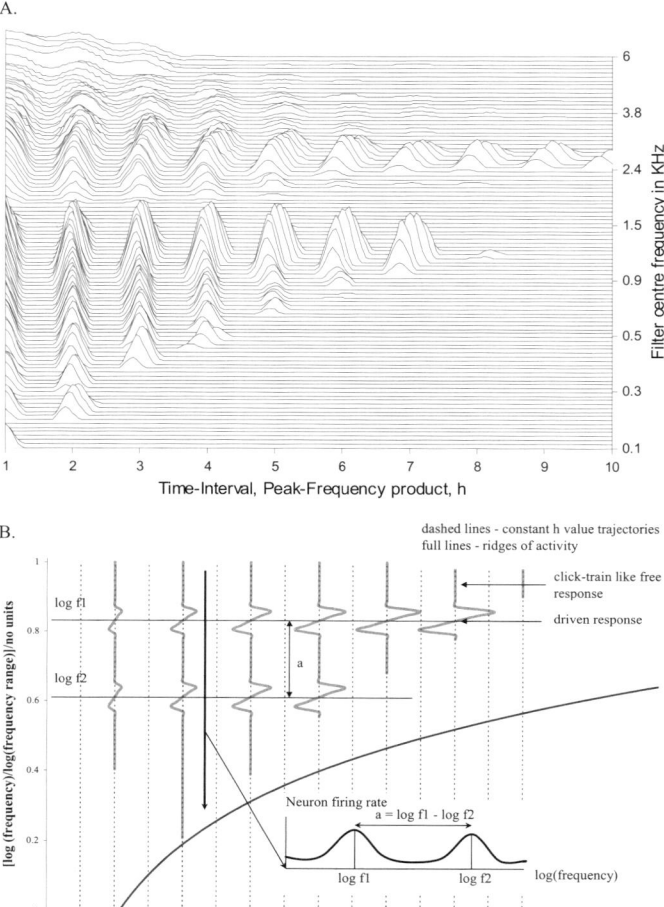

Figure 4. A. The SSI for a double damped sinusoid generated by AIM-mat: Two high activity peaks are present at the formant frequencies. B. Predicted SSI for the double damped sinusoid: High activity peaks at the formant frequencies are seen superimposed on the click response. '*a*' is defined as the separation of two formants in log-frequency space.

and is replaced by the perception of periodicity pitch [23]. This implies that some type of temporal integration occurs in the auditory system. It is important to note, however, that we hear detailed timbre information in music and speech which indicates that the auditory system has a special form of integration that preserves the fine structure of sounds.

Strobed Temporal Integration (STI) is one candidate for this special integration process. Successive copies of the repeating neural pattern produced by the vowel are mapped onto one, stabilised copy of the pattern. The result is referred to as a Stabilised

Auditory Image (SAI). To achieve this, the start of each glottal cycle needs to be mapped to zero on the time interval axis, in each channel. The ridge with the greatest activity can be used to coordinate the mapping [19]. Periodic sounds build up a stationary image over time in a stroboscopic fashion (see Figure 3B). By stabilising the neural representation of the impulse response of the vocal tract, STI bridges the gap between the wavelet transform and the MT.

1.3 The Size Shape Image and the Mellin Image

A click train is like a stream of glottal pulses measured at the larynx before they pass through the vocal tract. The SAI of the click train is the multi-channel impulse response of the auditory system. The vocal tract resonates at formant frequencies and imposes a structure on the auditory impulse response. As the vocal tract becomes shorter, the formants move up along the ridges of the impulse response, contracting in time as they go. The problem is how to normalise for the frequency shifting and time-interval compression to produce a size invariant representation of the resonance information.

The ridges of activity in the multi-channel impulse response are lines along which the product of time interval and filter centre-frequency are constant, and this product variable is h, the abscissa of the Mellin transform. Along the peak of each ridge of the impulse response, the value of h is an integer. If we take the spectra as they exist along the ridges (and the valleys) and plot them as a function of h (Figure 4A), the result is what Irino and Patterson [13] refer to as a Size Shape Image (SSI). The ordinate in the SSI remains log frequency. Mellin Images are then produced from the SSI by performing a Fourier transform (FT) of the activity on lines of constant h. These Mellin coefficients indicate the strength of spatial frequency components in the SSI. The resulting Mellin Image is a two dimensional plot with h value along the abscissa and spatial frequency along the ordinate [14]. The MI of a click-train is shown in Figure 5A. It contains vertical banding, a feature present in the MIs of all periodic sounds. This MI is essentially what a stream of glottal pulses would produce in the absence of the vocal tract. The activity is restricted to low spatial frequencies since clicks produce essentially flat spectra along the ridges of the multi-channel impulse response, and the activity occurs at integer values of h since it is restricted to the impulse response ridges. The phases of the spatial frequency coefficients encode the size information separately from the vowel information.

1.4 Summary of MI construction

The MI is constructed in three stages: A scale preserving wavelet analysis simulates the spectral analysis of the cochlea. The repeating neural patterns produced by periodic sounds are stabilised and anchored on zero by strobed temporal integration, to produce an Auditory Image. Finally, a spatial Fourier analysis is performed down the ridges of the auditory impulse response and the frames of spatial frequency coefficients are plotted as a function of ridge number, h, to produce the Mellin Image.

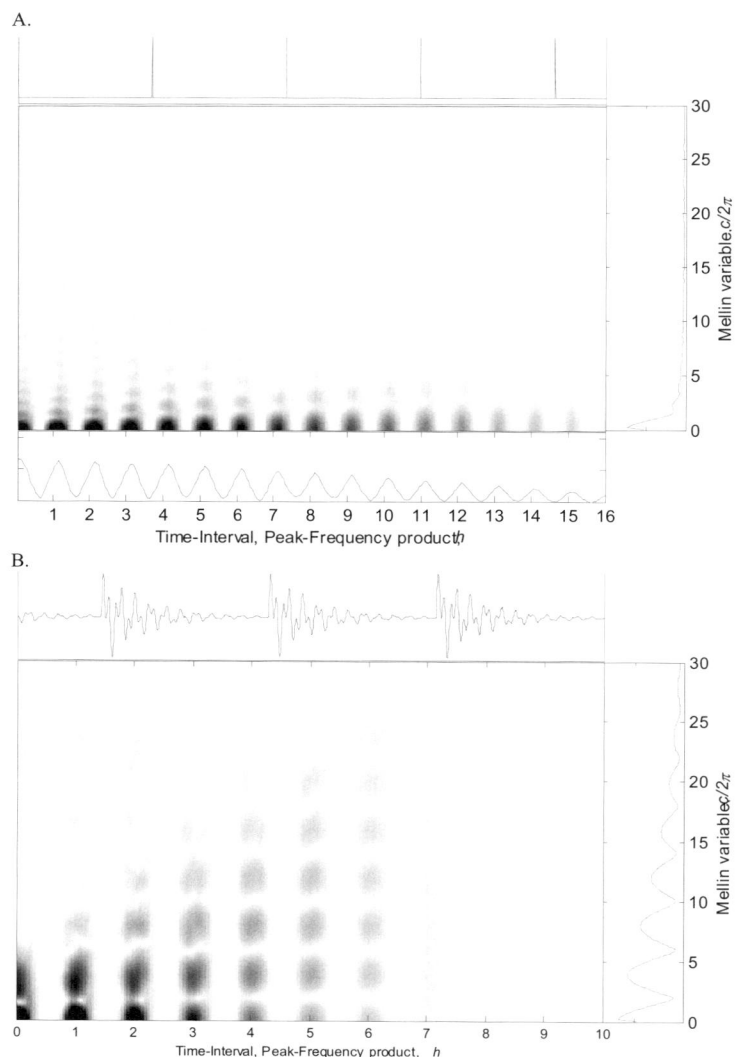

Figure 5. A. Mellin Image of click-train: Characteristic vertical banding is observed together with large contributions from the low frequency Mellin coefficients. The right-hand panel shows horizontal summation of Mellin coefficient intensities across the entire Mellin Image. The lower panel shows vertical summation.B. The Mellin Image for a double damped sinusoid with carrier frequencies of 2600 Hz and 1100 Hz and a repetition rate of 100 Hz.

2. Mellin Images of Vowel Sounds

This section describes the form of vowel information in the MI.

2.1 The Double-Damped Sinusoid: a simple model of the vowel

The majority of the information in a vowel is concentrated in the first two formants, and the ringing response of the formants as they are struck by a stream of glottal pulses can be simulated by a 'double damped sinusoid'. A single damped sinusoid has an envelope which has an abrupt onset and an exponential, or 'damped', decay. The double damped sinusoid is simply the linear addition of two sinusoids with the same envelope. The SSI produced by AIM-mat in response to the double damped sinusoid is presented in Figure 4A. A schematic of the SSI is presented in Figure 4B to illustrate the important features. For *h* values of 0 and 1, there is a broad frequency response due to the abrupt onset of each cycle. Thereafter, two horizontal ridges of activity develop in the SSI centred on the two formant frequencies, f1 and f2. When the FT is applied to ridges with *h* values greater than about two, it fits the ridges with a sum of sinusoids which have maxima that are coincident with the peaks of the two ridges. This constrains the wavelengths of the spatial frequency components to be multiples of a constant, *a*.

The Mellin Image of the double damped sinusoid is shown in Figure 5B and it shows that a set of horizontal bands develops for *h* values greater than two at harmonics of a fixed value, which in this case is about four. In Fourier terms, the banding occurs at spatial frequency values of:

$$\omega = \frac{n\pi}{a}$$

where *n* is an integer and *a* is the separation of horizontal ridges in the SSI. These are the main features of a pair of formants as they appear in the SSI and MI. Vowel sounds similarly produce Mellin Images with horizontal banding that reflects the formant spacing, and contrast that reflects the regularity, or degree of voicing.

2.2 The role of logarithmic frequency in the scale transform.

The tonotopic axis of the cochlea is a quasi-logarithmic frequency axis which is very different from the linear frequency scale of the standard spectrogram. In the linear frequency domain, a reduction in VTL not only causes an increase in the formant frequencies, it also causes the spacing between the formants to increase. On a logarithmic frequency axis, the formants still shift up but the distance between them remains fixed. The spatial FT in the MT codes the spacing between the formants in the magnitude of the coefficients, and separately, it codes the shift produced by the reduction in VTL in the phase of the coefficients. In this way the auditory system can perform a frequency analysis and then segregate information about the shape and size of the vocal tract of the speaker.

2.3 Vowel images

There is a high-fidelity vocoder, referred to as STRAIGHT [15], which is a sophisticated speech processing package that dissects and analyses an utterance at the level of individual glottal cycles. It segregates the GPR and VTL information and stores them separately, so that the utterance can be resynthesized later with arbitrary shifts in GPR and VTL. Utterances recorded from a man can be transformed to sound like women and children.[2] The advantage of STRAIGHT is that the spectral envelope of the speech that carries the vocal tract information is transformed, as it is extracted, to remove the har-

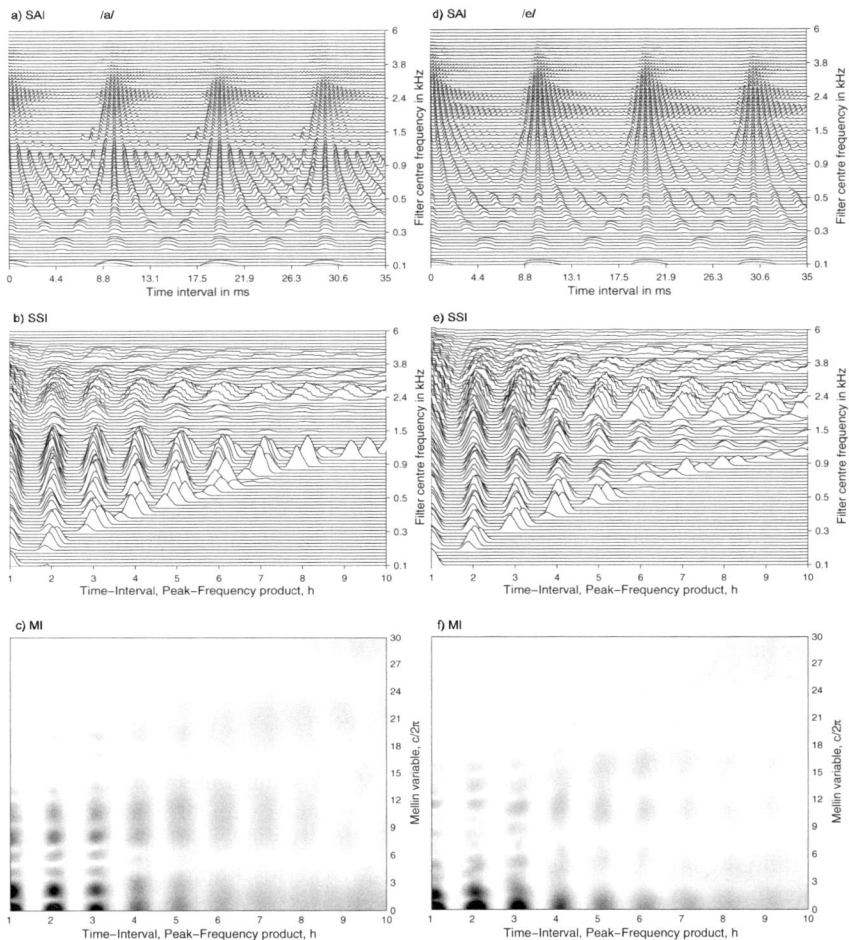

Figure 6. Auditory Images of the vowels /a/ (left) and /e/ (right): Stabilised Auditory Images (SAIs) (a,d), Size-Shape Images (SSIs) (b,e) and Mellin Images (MIs) (c,f). The vowels had a GPR of 100Hz and the VTL was about 17 cm.

monic structure associated with the original glottal pulse rate (GPR), and the harmonic structure associated with the frame rate of the analysis window. As a result, the resynthesized utterances are of extremely high quality even when the speech is resynthesized with GPR and VTL values well beyond the normal range of human speech. We characterise the change in VTL by the Spectral Envelope Ratio (SER), that is, the VTL of the input speech over the VTL of the resynthesised speech. Small values of SER indicate expansion of the vocal tract to simulate large adult males and large values of SER indicate compression of the vocal tract to simulate children.

We collected examples of the canonical English vowels (/a/, /e/, /i/, /o/, /u/), as spoken by an adult male using a high quality microphone (SM58-LCE, Shure). The vowels were spoken in /hVd/ format in one relatively natural sequence which sounded like *'haard, hayed, heed, hoed, who'd'*. The sounds were digitised into 'wav' files with 16-bit resolution and a sampling rate of 44.1 kHz. The vowels were excised out of the /hVd/ sequences, preserving the initial onset of the vowel whilst avoiding the preceding aspiration associated with the   /h/. A cosine-squared amplitude function (5 ms onset, 30 ms offset, 215 ms plateau) was used to gate the vowels, and they were normalised to a fixed RMS value (0.1, relative to the maximum $d\pm1$) and to a fixed GPR (100 Hz) corresponding to a large male speaker. STRAIGHT was then used to produce a library of vowels with one of twenty six glottal pulse rates (from 50 Hz to 300Hz in 10Hz steps) combined with one of twenty six VTL scalings (SERs from 0.5 to 3.0 in steps of 0.1). These 676 combinations span a range greater than that which occurs naturally in the population [22][7][11] with the emphasis on lower glottal pulse rates than in Assmann *et al.* [1].

2.4 Characteristics of vowels in the Mellin Image

The SAI, SSI and MI of an /a/ and an /e/ are shown in Figure 6. The MI of the /a/ is characterised by a horizontal band between spatial frequency values of 8 and 13, and another, higher, band between values of 17 and 23. In contrast, The MI of the /e/ has a narrow band at low spatial frequencies between 3 and 6, and a broad middle band between 9 and 18 which divides into two narrow bands as *h* grows above 5. There is a wealth of information encoded in the details of these MI and those of the other vowels. At this point, we proceed to demonstrate how it is used in VTL normalisation.

3.   Recognition of Vowels Using the Mellin Image

We evaluated the normalisation properties of the MI by simulating the process of vowel recognition. A library of Mellin Image templates for vowels with different combinations of GPR and SER was generated from the canonical five vowels, and then MIs from test vowels were classified by comparison with the MIs in this library. The classification was performed with a 'Mixture of Gaussians' model and a Euclidean distance measure [18]. Briefly, the classification process is as follows: The MI of a test vowel is compared with the MIs in the library and the classifier generates the probability that the MI originates from each of the five vowel classes. The test MI is then attributed to the vowel class corresponding to the highest probability. These probabilities are also used to construct a confusion matrix that can be used to derive confidence limits for the classification. From the probabilities, it is possible to summarise the performance of the recognition process using a log-pseudo-likelihood quantity. This simple discrimination tool will reveal whether the MI is successful in normalising vowels with a range of GPR and VTLs. If it proves successful, more advanced feature extraction techniques can be developed later.

   Initially, the confusion matrix was generated for a library with templates of all 3380 vowels to show that all of them could be correctly identified. Then the size of the library was reduced in stages as performance was monitored. The analysis showed that the library could be reduced to one template for each vowel type. As a test of the generalisation, we created three sets of five templates to represent the vowels of a man, a woman and a child, and tested them with the entire vowel set. Figure 7 presents the recognition performance for the three recognisers, and it shows that performance is good throughout

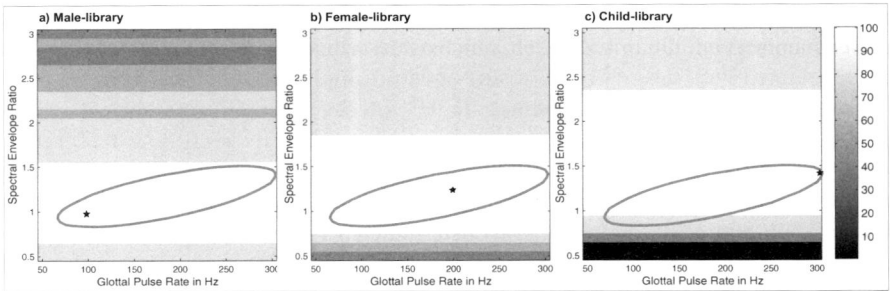

Figure 7. Vowel recognition results with templates representing a typical male (a), female (b), and child (c). The star indicates the GPR and the scale of the template. The grey ellipses mark the region of natural human speech. The results are the average recognition rates for all five vowels. Chance-probability is 20%. White areas show correct classification of all five vowels.

most of the GPR-SER domain, for all three recognisers. The best overall performance was 86.2% for the library of templates associated with the woman, followed by the libraries of the child (83.1%) and then the man (78.5%). Comparison of the three panels in Figure 7 reveals that the area of perfect performance moves up in the SER dimension as the library proceeds from the man to the child. This indicates that the range of successful normalisation is limited; however, the area is much larger than the range of natural human speech (shown by the oval).

3.1 Summary

The Matlab version of AIM has been extended to include a module that normalises the auditory image for changes in VTL and converts the auditory image into a Mellin Image. A set of test vowels was constructed using STRAIGHT; there were 3380 vowel sounds with GPR and VTLs that span an area of the GPR-VTL space five times larger than the region of natural variation. A simple classifier, based on a Euclidean Distance measure, was developed and a sequence of tests revealed that excellent categorisation of the entire set of 3380 vowels could be achieved when the classifier was limited to a set of only five templates, one for each vowel type. The recognition performance is excellent throughout the range of GPR-VTL values encountered in normal speech and well beyond, indicating the value of vowel normalisation by AIM with the Mellin transform.

4.   Comparison with Human Vowel Normalisation

4.1 Motivation

Assmann *et al.* [1][2] have suggested that vowel normalisation is based on learnt statistical correlation; that is, one learns that a child's /a/ has the same meaning as an adult's /a/ through experience, despite the differences in GPR and formant frequencies. They used STRAIGHT to produce a set of vowels with GPR and VTL values covering the range in normal human speech and showed that a neural net could learn the variability and eventually categorise the vowels correctly. If the auditory system performs vowel normalisation with a transform rather than statistical learning, then we might expect that humans can recognise vowels across a range of GPRs and VTLs far greater than that normally encountered in human speech, much as described for AIM with the MI above.

4.2 Vowel Discrimination Experiment

This section presents a pilot study designed to delimit the range of the GPR-VTL space over which vowel recognition is possible. We also measured the sensitivity to change along the VTL and GPR dimensions, to determine the resolution (granularity) of the space.

4.2.1 Methods

STRAIGHT was used to produce vowels with pitches from 12.5 to 750 Hz and SERs from 0.1 to 3.5; these limits are well beyond the human range. The vowel identification experiment employed a single interval five-alternative, forced-choice paradigm in which the listener heard a scaled version of one of five stationary English vowels and had to identify the vowel spoken, by selecting the appropriate letter-key on the keyboard. There was no feedback. There were 50 different combinations of GPR and SER for each vowel, and they were presented in a pseudo-random order. Data were collected over ten sessions giving five repetitions at each combination of GPR and SER. The points were chosen to sample the normal range of GPR and VTL densely [22][7][11], as well as exploring the extreme ranges more sparsely where performance breaks down. The sounds were played from the 16-bit sound card of a Dell desktop PC via Sennheiser HD437 headphones.

4.2.2 Results and Discussion

Figure 8 shows vowel identification, as a function of GPR and SER averaged over three listeners, using a 2D surface plot in which grey tone shows percent correct. The sample points are shown as circles with interpolation between the data points. The heavy black line marks the 50% identification contour (d'=1.0 in a 5AFC paradigm), defined as the threshold for vowel identification. The results show that identification performance is above threshold for GPR and SER values well beyond the natural range, with no feedback and essentially no training. The area of good recognition performance is approximately 15 times the range encountered in normal speech. Neural nets do not generalise well beyond the data they are trained on [17], and it seems unlikely that a model that has lent the statistical correlations of the normal range would be able to recognise vowels over a much wider range. The range of the human performance is, however, consistent with the range achieved with AIM and the MI, which supports the hypothesis that the auditory system has an active normalisation mechanism and this is the basis of vowel normalisation in humans.

4.3 Discrimination of Glottal Pulse Rate and VTL (SER)

Having mapped vowel identification in the space of GPR and VTL, we then investigated the sensitivity to change along the two dimensions, measuring the Just Noticeable Differences (JNDs) for glottal pulse rate and VTL. The perceptual cue to a change in SER is a change in speaker size. We measure the SER JND both within and beyond the normal speech range.

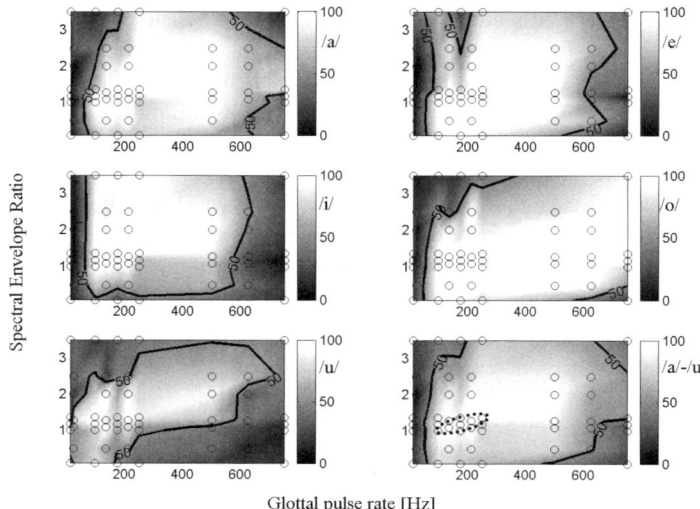

Glottal pulse rate [Hz]

Figure 8. Vowel identification as a function of glottal pulse rate (Hz) and Spectral Envelope Ratio (SER). The unit of the ordinate is in multiples of the VTL of the original speaker (RP, male, VTL ~ 17 cm). The GPR values were 12.5, 25, 100, 137.5, 175, 212.5, 250, 500, 625 and 750 Hz. The SER values were 0.1, 0.5, 1, 1.09, 1.18, 1.27, 1.36, 2.0, 2.5 and 3.5. The data are presented as a 2D surface plot with grey tone showing percent correct. Sample points are shown as circles, with cubic interpolation between data points. Each data point is based on 15 repetitions, five from each of three listeners. The average for all five vowels is shown on the bottom right (in this case each data point is based on 75 repetitions). The thick black contour line marks the identification threshold (50%, d'=1.0) in our 5AFC experiment. The ellipse (bottom-right panel) shows the range of GPR and SER in the normal population (e.g. [22]).

4.3.1 Methods

We used a two interval two-alternative forced-choice paradigm with the method of constant stimuli. The same vowels were used as in the vowel identification experiment. Each trial consisted of two intervals, one containing the standard stimulus and the other containing the test stimulus. The interval containing the standard stimulus was determined pseudo-randomly. The listener had to choose the interval containing the vowel spoken by the smaller speaker (discrimination of speaker size) or the interval containing the higher GPR (discrimination of glottal pulse rate). No feedback was given. Six-point psychometric functions were measured with at least 20 trials per point. Each experimental session consisted of the five standard stimuli with their associated six test stimuli. There were ten experimental blocks per experimental session where the thirty test stimuli were presented in pseudo-random order. Data were collected for three listeners over two or three experimental sessions for each set of psychometric functions.

4.3.2 Results and Discussion

Speaker size discrimination: We began by measuring the JND[3] for speaker size at the centre of the normal range for humans. The standard stimuli were the five English vowels each with a GPR of 175 Hz and a SER of 1.18. The six test stimuli for each standard had the same GPR (175 Hz) as the standard but a range of SERs bracketing 1.18. The psychometric functions for speaker size discrimination were generated separately for the five English vowels tested. The percentage of trials on which the test stimulus was judged to be spoken by the smaller speaker was plotted as a function of the SER of the test stimulus. A best-fitting cumulative Gaussian curve [9] was fitted through the data points. The cue for the listener was the perceived size of the speaker and using the cue seemed entirely natural. The point of subjective equality was typically within 2% of the standard SER indicating accurate perception of speaker size.

We then measured speaker size discrimination where performance has begun to drop (SER of 2.36), reasoning that discrimination might be expected to deteriorate at this point. At more extreme values, the scaled vowels were not intelligible, and much beyond a scale factor of 2.36 it was difficult to discern speaker characteristics. The standard stimuli were the five English vowels (GPR of 175 Hz, SER of 2.36); the six test stimuli for each standard had the same GPR (175 Hz) and a range of SERs bracketing 2.36. The JND for speaker size is worse for higher SERs (smaller VTLs): 11.52% ±0.98% across the three listeners for a SER of 2.36 compared to 8.83% ±0.78% for a SER of 1.18. We would expect deterioration in the JND given that vowel identification has begun to deteriorate and speaker characteristics are difficult to discern.

Glottal pulse rate discrimination: We also measured the JND for glottal pulse rates at the centre of the normal range for humans with the same vowels (GPR of 175 Hz, SER of 1.18) and their six test stimuli (SER of 1.18 with glottal pulse rates bracketing 175 Hz). The JND for vowel GPR was 4.09% ± 1.05%.

4.4 Summary of human vowel normalisation

We have mapped the region of GPR and SER where vowel identification is essentially errorless (Figure 8) and showed that excellent performance is maintained over a region considerably greater than that of normal speech. This supports the hypothesis that the auditory system includes a scale transform of some sort. Whilst Assmann *et al.* [1][2] emphasise that the performance outside the normal range eventually falls, we emphasise that the region of errorless performance is larger than the range normally encountered. We also measured sensitivity to changes in SER and GPR. Our principal finding is that listeners hear speaker size in scaled vowels even when they are beyond the normal range. The full extent of the range has been recently measured by Smith *et al.* [24].

5.   Conclusion

The chapter began with a description of a Matlab version of the auditory image model (AIM) and a review of the mathematical framework of the Mellin transform. A Matlab module was then introduced to convert the auditory image into a Mellin Image which normalises the auditory images for size. The structure of the Mellin Image was illustrated with a simulated, two-formant vowel and two natural vowels. A larger set of scaled vowels was produced with the vocoder, STRAIGHT, and a simple classifier was used to demonstrate the value of the Mellin Transform as a tool for the normalisation of vocal tract length. Excellent vowel recognition was observed over a GPR-VTL space five times larger than that naturally encountered in speech. Human recognition performance was measured for scaled vowels and the region of good performance was found to be approximately 15 times larger than that encountered in normal speech. This supports the hypothesis that the auditory system includes an active normalisation process something like the Mellin transform.

Glossary of Terms

2D-AT	Two dimensional adaptive thresholding - cross channel sharpening of neural activity pattern
5-AFC	Five alternative forced choice - experimental paradigm where the subject is forced to choose one of five choices on each trial of an experiment
AI	Auditory Image - a representation of stimulus information in sounds to which we have perceptual access
AIM-mat	The auditory image model in Matlab - a computer simulation of the auditory processing required to produce the initial perception produced by a sound
BM	Basilar membrane - a membrane in the inner ear that transduces a sound wave into mechanical motion
BMM	Basilar membrane motion
GPR	Glottal Pulse Rate - the rate at which the vocal folds open and shut, alternatively called the voice-pitch
JND	Just noticeable difference - measure of the slope of the psychometric function
MI	Mellin image - the three dimensional, scale invariant image produced in the auditory model
MT	Mellin transform - an integral transform that is scale invariant but not shift invariant. The opposite is true of the Fourier Transform.
NAP	Neural activity pattern - the pattern of neural activity produced by a sound in the auditory nerve
SAI	Stabilised auditory image - the static perception produced by a periodic sound. The process is simulated by Strobed Temporal Integration.
SER	Spectral envelope ratio - frequency dimension scaling factor; the reciprocal of the VTL scaling factor
SSI	Size shape image - an intermediate stage in the conversion of an Auditory Image into a Mellin Image
STI	Strobed temporal integration - an integration process that stabilises the repeating neural representation produced by a periodic sound whilst preserving the phase-locking information
VT	Vocal tract
VTL	Vocal tract length - length of the supra-laryngeal vocal tract measured from the glottis to the lips

Endnotes

1. The AIM-mat software can be downloaded from http://www.pdn.cam.ac.uk/cnbh/aimmanual/index.html.

2. Examples of scaled vowels can be found at:
http://www.pdn.cam.ac.uk/cnbh/web2002/bodyframes/sounds_movies/scaled_vowels.htm

3. We define the JND as $[(76\%-50\%)/50\%]*100\%$. The point of subjective equality (50% correct) represents the matching point (chance performance of d'=0.0 in our 2AFC experiment). The 76% correct point is the traditional discrimination criterion value (d'=1.0 in our 2AFC experiment). The values were read off the best-fitting cumulative Gaussian.

References

[1] Assmann, P.F., Nearey, T.M. and Scott, J.M. "Modelling the perception of frequency-shifted vowels." *Proc. 7th Int. Conf. Spoken Lang. Proc.*, 2002.

[2] Assmann, P.F. and Nearey, T.M., "Frequency shifts and vowel identification." *Proc. 15th Int. Cong. Phon. Sci.*, 2003.

[3] Bleeck, S., Ives, T. and Patterson, R.D. "Aim-mat: The auditory image model in MATLAB." *Acta Acoustica* 90: 781-788, 2004

[4] Boer, E. de "Synthetic whole nerve action potentials for the cat." *J. Acoust. Soc. Am.* 58: 1030-1045, 1975.

[5] Carney, L. and Yin, C. "Temporal coding of resonances by low frequency auditory nerve fibres: single fibre responses and a population model." *J. Neurophysiol.* 60: 1653-1677, 1988.

[6] Cohen, L. "The scale transform." *IEEE Trans. Acoust. Speech Sig. Proc.* 41: 3275-3292, 1993.

[7] Fitch, W.T. and Giedd, J. "Morphology and development of the human vocal tract: A study using magnetic resonance imaging." *J. Acoust. Soc. Am.* 106: 1511-1522, 1999.

[8] Flanagan, J. *Speech Analysis, Synthesis and Perception* (2nd ed.). New York: Springer Verlag, 1972.

[9] Foster, D.H. and Bischof, W.F. "Bootstrap estimates of the statistical accuracy of thresholds obtained from psychometric functions." *Spatial Vision*, 11: 135-139, 1997.

[10] Glasberg, B.R. and Moore, B.C.J. "Derivation of auditory filter shapes from notched-noise data." *Hear. Res.* 47: 103-138, 1990.

[11] Huber, J.E., Stathopoulos, E.T., Curione, G.M., Ash, T.A. and Johnson, K. "Formants of children, women and men: The effects of vocal intensity variation." *J. Acoust. Soc. Am.* 106: 1532-1542, 1999.

[12] Irino, T. and Patterson, R. "A time-domain, level dependent auditory filter: The gammachirp." *J. Acoust. Soc. Am.* 101: 412-419, 1997.

[13] Irino, T. and Patterson, R.D. "Stabilised wavelet Mellin transform: An auditory strategy for normalising sound-source size." *Proc. Eurospeech, pp.* 1899-1902, 1999.

[14] Irino, T. and Patterson, R. "Segregating information about the size and shape of the vocal tract using a time-domain auditory model: The stabilised wavelet Mellin transform." *Speech Comm.* 36(3-4): 181-203, 2002.

[15] Kawahara, H. and Irino, T. "Underlying principles of a high-quality speech manipulation system STRAIGHT and its application to speech segregation." In *Speech Separation by Humans and Machines*, P. Divenyi (ed.), Norwell, MA: Kluwer, pp. 167-180, 2005.

[16] Kawahara, H., Masuda-Kasuse, I.. and de Cheveigne, A. "Restructuring speech representations using pitch-adaptive time-frequency smoothing and instantaneous-frequency-based F0 extraction: Possible role of repetitive structure in sounds." *Speech Communication*, 27(3-4): 187-207, 1999.

[17] LeCun, Y. and Bengio, Y. "Convolutional networks for images, speech, and time-series." In *The Handbook of Brain Theory and Neural Networks*, Cambridge, MA: MIT Press, 1995.

[18] Mackay, D.J. *Information Theory, Inference and Learning Algorithms*. Cambridge: Cambridge University Press, 2003.

[19] Patterson, R.D. "The sound of a sinusoid: Time-interval models." *J. Acoust. Soc. Am.* 96: 1419-1428, 1994.
[20] Patterson, R., Allerhand, M. and Giguère, C "Time domain modelling of peripheral auditory processing: A modular architecture and a software platform." *J. Acoust. Soc. Am.* 98: 1890-1894, 1995.
[21] Patterson, R.D. "Auditory images: How complex sounds are represented in the auditory system." *J. Acoust. Soc. Am.* 21: 183-190, 2000.
[22] Peterson, G.E. and Barney, H.I. "Control methods used in the study of vowels." *J. Acoust. Soc. Am.* 24: 75-184, 1952.
[23] Pressnitzer, D., Patterson, P. and Krumholz, K. "The lower limit of pitch." *J. Acoust. Soc. Am.* 24: 75-184, 2001.
[24] Smith, D.D.R., Patterson, R.D., Turner, R., Kawahara, H., and Irino, T. "The processing and perception of size information in speech sounds." *J. Acoust. Soc. Am.* 117: 305-318, 2005.
[25] Titze, I.R. "Physiologic and acoustic differences between male and female voices." *J. Acoust. Soc. Am.* 85: 1699-1707, 1989.
[26] Yang, C. and Kasuya, H. "Dimension differences in the vocal tract shape measured from MR images across boy, female and male subjects." *J. Acoust. Soc. Jap.* 16: 41-44, 1995.

Dynamics of Speech Production and Perception
P. Divenyi et al. (Eds.)
IOS Press, 2006

The Role of Temporal Dynamics in Understanding Spoken Language

Steven GREENBERG[1], Takayuki ARAI[2] and Ken W. GRANT[3]
[1]Silicon Speech, Santa Venetia, California, USA
[2]Sophia University, Tokyo, Japan
[3]Walter Reed Army Medical Center, Washington, D.C, USA

Abstract. Classical models of speech recognition assume that a detailed, short-term analysis of the acoustic signal is essential for accurately decoding the speech signal and that this decoding process is rooted in the phonetic segment. This chapter presents an alternative view, one in which the time scales required to accurately describe and model spoken language are both shorter and longer than the phonetic segment, and are inherently wedded to the syllable. The syllable reflects a singular property of the acoustic signal - the modulation spectrum - which provides a principled, quantitative framework to describe the process by which the listener proceeds from sound to meaning. The ability to understand spoken language (i.e., intelligibility) vitally depends on the integrity of the modulation spectrum within the core range of the syllable (3-10 Hz) and reflects the variation in syllable emphasis associated with the concept of prosodic prominence ("accent"). A model of spoken language is described in which the prosodic properties of the speech signal are embedded in the temporal dynamics associated with the syllable, a unit serving as the organizational interface among the various tiers of linguistic representation.

Keywords. Modulation spectrum, speech perception, intelligibility, syllables

Introduction

Models of spoken language have traditionally focused on two disparate aspects of speech recognition—the acoustic–phonetic properties of the speech signal [22] and the psychological processes associated with lexical access [19]. Such traditional models assume that speech can be characterized simply as a sequence of words containing strings of phonemic constituents. Within this traditional "beads–on–a–string" framework the process of lexical recognition is primarily one of decoding the phonemes associated with the speech signal, attempting to deduce the sequence of words uttered by the speaker via a process of phonetic characterization. Such phonetic–segment models possess a beguiling simplicity and directness—word recognition is simply a matter of decoding the sequence of phones uttered and then proceeding to "look up" the word in a mental lexicon, akin to the process by which a reader retrieves an entry in a dictionary [11].

However attractive such sequential models may be in the abstract, they fail to account for many properties of spoken language such as (1) the ability of listeners to

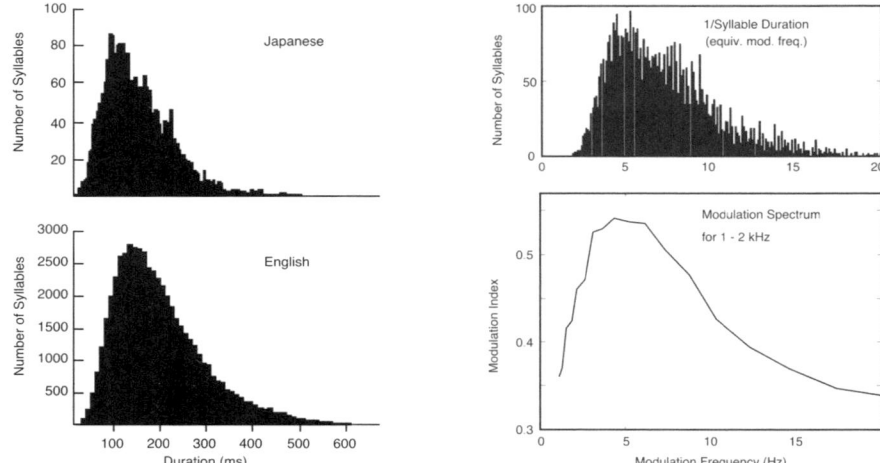

Figure 1. (a) Statistical distribution of syllable duration for spontaneous material in Japanese and American English. (b) The relation between the distribution of syllable duration (transformed into modulation frequency) and the modulation spectrum of the Japanese material shown in Figure 1(a), computed for the octave region between 1 and 2 kHz. Adapted from [1].

understand speech under a broad range of conditions that distort many of the acoustic–phonetic properties of the signal via such interference conditions as reverberation and background noise, and (2) the remarkable degree of pronunciation variation observed at the phonetic level in everyday speech [10]. These two signatures of "real-world" speech—acoustic distortion and pronunciation variability—render untenable many popular models of speech recognition, as well as wreak havoc with current-generation automatic (machine) speech recognition systems. An alternative theoretical formulation is required, one capable of accounting for the patterns of pronunciation variation in casual speech [10][11], and that provides a principled mechanism for the stability of intelligibility under the broad constellation of acoustic conditions characteristic of the real world. Moreover, the theoretical formulation should be capable of accounting for the importance of visible speech information, particularly under conditions of acoustic interference and non-native familiarity with the language spoken.

1.   The Doors of Perception

One means by which to delineate the essential cues for understanding spoken language is to artificially distort the speech signal and measure its impact on intelligibility. Such distortions may be used to expose chinks in the perceptual armor which normally shield the brain from the deleterious effects of reverberation and other forms of acoustic interference.

The perceptual studies described in this chapter are all linked in some fashion to the low-frequency (3–20 Hz) modulation spectrum. The modulation spectrum reflects fluctuations in energy associated with articulatory dynamics pertaining to the movement of the lips, jaw and tongue during the production of speech. The modulation of energy at such low frequencies is inherently tied to the syllable, the linguistic unit most closely associated with articulatory gestures. The duration of syllables varies greatly, and is reflected in the modulation pattern of the speech signal. Moreover, the structure of syllables, both in terms of phonetic constituents, as well as prosodic prominence, is reflected in syllabic duration and hence in the modulation spectrum.

2. Syllable Duration and The Modulation Spectrum

Syllable duration varies by roughly ten-fold in stress–timed languages such as English, ranging between 50 and 500 ms [10]. Even in Japanese, a language noted for its even tempo, syllables vary in length between 50 and 300 ms [1]. Figure 1(a) illustrates the distribution of syllable duration for English and Japanese spontaneous material. Overall, the distributions are similar – the characteristic distinguishing among the two languages pertains to the proportion of syllables longer than 300 ms. In English, approximately 15% of the syllables are longer than this limit [10], while Japanese contains many fewer syllables (ca. 1–2%) longer than 300 ms [1]. In this sense the distinction between a stress–timed and syllable–timed language is relatively subtle – a matter of the proportion of syllables whose duration exceeds a specific interval of time. This limit reflects two specific properties of English syllable structure that is encountered in Japanese to a far lesser degree: (1) a profusion of consonant clusters, particularly at syllable onset, and (2) syllable lengthening, particularly in the vocalic nucleus, associated with prosodic prominence [14][16].

Figure 1(b) illustrates the close relationship between syllable duration and modulation spectrum. The bandwidth of the modulation spectrum is quite broad, encompassing frequencies between 3 and 20 Hz, consistent with the broad variation in syllable duration observed. Because of the intimate relationship between energy dynamics, speech production and syllable structure, there is an intrinsic correlation between syllable duration and the modulation of the signal's waveform. The core of the syllable is the nucleus, which is almost always vocalic and usually voiced. The nucleus contains the greatest overall energy within the syllable, serving as the foundation upon which the onset and coda constituents lie. A syllable is only a syllable by virtue of its nucleic core. The onset and coda are optional. In many languages, such as Japanese, the nucleus is the dominant constituent of the syllable. The amplitude of the onset and coda is generally lower than that of the nucleus and conforms to an "energy arc" in which the sound pressure rises and falls gradually over time [11]. This energy gradient is the principal reason why the modulation spectrum of speech is dominated by frequencies in the 3–10 Hz region rather than by components higher than 20 Hz [11].

The relation between syllable structure and the modulation spectrum is manifest in prosodic prominence. In all languages certain syllables are more linguistically and perceptually prominent than others. In stress–timed languages syllable duration (particularly of the nucleus) plays a particularly important role [4]. However, even in non-stress languages, duration is likely to play some part in the specification of prosodic accent that is reflected in the modulation spectrum.

Figure 2 illustrates the relationship between prosodic prominence, word duration and the modulation spectrum for American English. The material is derived from a corpus of spontaneous telephone dialogues (SWITCHBOARD – [7]) that was phonetically and prosodically annotated by trained linguistic transcribers [10]. In this corpus most

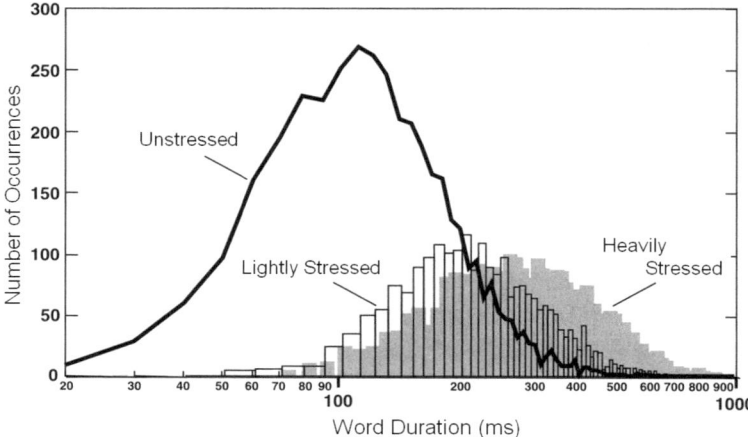

Figure 2. Word duration as a function of stress–accent level. Frequency histograms of words (n = 10,001) associated with a range of stress–accent levels are shown. Eighty percent of the words are mono-syllablic. For those containing more than a single syllable, a word is deemed as stressed if it contains at least one syllable of that accent level (the most heavily accented syllable in the word determining its stress–accent pattern). Unstressed words are entirely without stress in any syllable. The solid black curve represents the histogram for unstressed words (n = 3946). The histogram associated with lightly stressed words (n = 2484) is represented by unfilled black columns. Heavily stressed words (n = 3571) are shown in grey. The bin width for lexical duration is 10 ms.

words contain only a single syllable, so that word duration and syllable length are largely coterminous.

Words without accent (i.e., unstressed) are generally *shorter* than 200 ms, while heavily accented words are usually *longer* than this interval (Figure 2). More importantly, the distributions associated with unaccented and accented lexical forms overlap only to a slight degree (Figure 2), suggesting that these represent two separate classes (at least with respect to duration).

Given the relation between syllable duration and the modulation spectrum, one may infer that the lower branch of the spectrum (< 4 Hz) is largely associated with heavily accented syllables, while the upper branch (> 5 Hz) is most closely associated with unaccented forms. The central core of the modulation spectrum, between 4 and 5 Hz, pertains to syllables spanning a range of accent levels (i.e., represents the convergence of accented and unaccented forms).

3. The Perceptual Significance of The Modulation Spectrum

A variety of studies have shown that intelligibility depends on the integrity of the low-frequency modulation spectrum [2][3][5][13][21]. Within reverberant environments the greatest impact of acoustic reflections is between 2 and 6 Hz [18]. In an overly reverberant environment the acoustic reflections combine with the original signal to reduce the amount of modulation apparent in the waveform. The consequence of such reflections is to reduce the magnitude of the modulation spectrum at its peak, as well as to reduce the spectral peak from 4–5 Hz to ca. 1–2 Hz. If the amount of modulation attenuation is not too severe the speech signal is still intelligible, if somewhat distorted in quality. However, significant attenuation of the modulation spectrum results in a drastic decline in intelligibility, akin to speech broadcast over a poor-quality public address system as often occurs in a bus depot or other large enclosure with reflective surfaces.

Houtgast and Steeneken demonstrated many years ago that the modulation spectrum was a good predictor of speech intelligibility over a broad range of acoustic environments [18]. More recently, Drullman and colleagues have shown that the key portion of the modulation spectrum for intelligibility lies below 8 Hz [5], a result confirmed for Japanese [3] and for English [2]. Thus, it is clear that the integrity of the modulation spectrum is both essential for understanding spoken language and that its general characteristics reflect something important about syllables with respect to their structure or segmentation (or both).

But what precisely in the modulation spectrum is so important for understanding spoken language? And how can such knowledge be used for developing technology capable of benefiting large numbers of people? Perceptual studies may provide certain insight of potential utility for speech technology and as well as for scientific knowledge.

4. Spectral Asynchrony's Impact on Intelligibility and Its Relation to Reverberation

One effect of reverberation is to jumble the spectral content of the acoustic signal across both time and frequency, particularly that portion of the spectrum below 1500 Hz. Although reverberation is known to interfere with intelligibility, particularly among the hearing impaired, the basis for its deleterious impact is not well understood.

In order to gain some insight into reverberation's impact on intelligibility the following experiment was performed. The spectrum of spoken sentences (American English, the TIMIT corpus) was partitioned into 19 quarter-octave channels and quasi-randomly jittered in time. The jittering algorithm insured that adjacent channels were desynchronized by a minimum interval of time (at least one quarter of the maximum interval) and that the mean temporal jitter across channels was equal to precisely one half of the maximum jitter interval. Using such an algorithm provides a convenient means of comparing the amount of cross-spectral jitter imposed with durational properties of important linguistic units such as the phonetic segment and the syllable.

In order to assess the impact of time jitter on the ability to understand spoken language, the amount of (maximum) spectral asynchrony was varied systematically between 20 and 240 ms, and the effect on intelligibility measured (in terms of the proportion of words correctly reported). But this relation alone does not provide much insight into the underlying mechanisms responsible for understanding speech presented under such distorted conditions. For this reason modulation spectra were also computed for the sentence material used. The modulation spectra were computed for delimited spectral regions ("sub-bands") rather than across the entire frequency range (6 kHz) of the acoustic signal. Three of the four sub-bands were an octave wide, while the lowest contained all frequencies below 750 Hz. The highest sub-band encompassed 3–6 kHz, while the other octave bands ranged between 1.5–3 kHz and 0.75–1.5 kHz. In this fashion it was possible to compute the modulation spectrum for each sub-band and relate this pattern to the decline of intelligibility. In order to provide a simple, quantitative metric relating the modulation spectrum and acoustic frequency to intelligibility, the

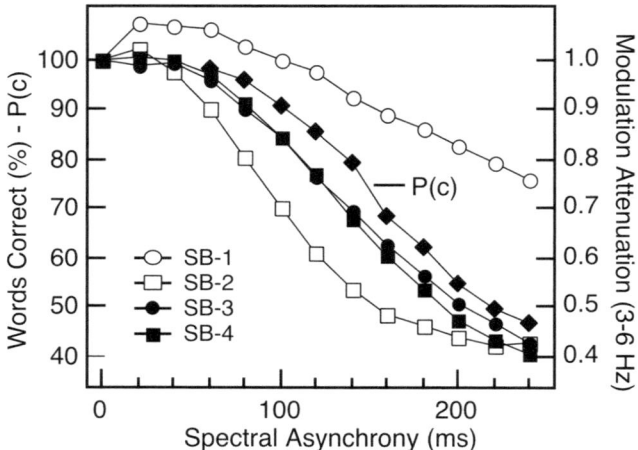

Figure 3. Intelligibility (P(c)) of de-synchronized spectral channels as a function of the amount of maximum cross-spectral asynchrony imposed. This function is compared with the magnitude of the modulation spectrum in the range of 3–6 Hz for four separate sub-bands for the 40 TIMIT sentences used in Experiment 1. From [2].

magnitude of the modulation spectrum in the crucial 3–6 Hz region was computed for each sentence and time–jitter condition. This information was normalized relative to the original, undistorted signal for each sentence and the results plotted on the same scale as the data pertaining to intelligibility for the 27 listeners participating in the experiment.

The results of this study are shown in Figure 3. Intelligibility declines progressively with increasing amounts of cross-spectral jitter. The surprising aspect of these data concerns the relatively modest impact on intelligibility exerted by significant amounts of cross-spectral time jitter. Even when the spectral asynchrony encompasses a (maximum) range of 140 ms (i.e., a mean jitter interval of 70 ms), 75% of the words are accurately reported by listeners. This jitter interval is equivalent to the average duration of a phonetic segment, and implies that the auditory system (and the brain) is exceedingly tolerant of spectro–temporal distortion in the speech signal.

This tolerance of spectral asynchrony is precisely what one would expect of a processing mechanism that has evolved to decode acoustic signals propagating through environments of variable (and unpredictable) nature. In particular, such robustness to cross-spectral time jitter would be quite useful in reverberant environments, where acoustic reflections are commonplace, and would help to instill some measure of perceptual stability amidst a highly variable background.

The intelligibility data also suggest that listeners rely on different parts of the acoustic spectrum for decoding speech, depending on the specific background conditions. When there is relatively little cross-spectral jitter the data imply that frequencies below 1.5 kHz play a particularly important role in decoding the signal. As the amount of spectral asynchrony increases, the decline in intelligibility closely mirrors the fall-off of the modulation spectrum in the channels above 1.5 kHz. To the extent that such jitter simulates the distortion imposed by reverberation, this result implies that the high-frequency portion of the spectrum plays a particularly important role in decoding speech under reverberant conditions.

This spectrally adaptive strategy could be important for understanding the frequency–selective nature of intelligibility deficits among the hearing impaired. In quiet listening conditions such individuals rarely experience a significant problem understanding speech. However, in reverberant and noisy conditions their ability to comprehend declines markedly.

The data in Figure 3 provide a potential explanation for this selective deficit. The effects of reverberation and other common background noise are particularly pronounced below 1.5 kHz.

Normal–hearing individuals may shift their listening strategy under such conditions to rely on spectral information above 1.5 kHz that is largely redundant with the low frequencies in quiet. The hearing–impaired rarely possess the luxury of such redundant processing capacity given their deficit's concentration in channels above 1.5 kHz. Thus, it is likely that in reverberant conditions, these individuals would be less able to extract useful information from the high-frequency channels to aid in decoding the speech signal. Under such conditions, they may rely on visual cues (i.e., "speechreading") to a large extent [8]. In the absence of such visual cues, the hearing impaired are likely to experience extreme difficulty understanding speech associated with reverberant and other noisy environments. Visual supplementation of the acoustic speech signal could be extremely important under such circumstances and is addressed in Section 9.

5. How Much of the Acoustic Spectrum is Required to Understand Spoken Language?

The intelligibility data described in Section 5 imply that the auditory system (and by extension, the brain as a whole) is remarkably insensitive to time jitter across the spectrum. However, this assumption was not *directly* tested in Experiment 1 because of the nature of the signals used. In that study the signal spectrum was 6 kHz wide as well as continuous, comprising much of the frequency information utilized for speech decoding under favorable listening conditions. In such circumstances there is considerable redundancy in the signal that listeners may exploit to decode the speech signal. Exploitation of such redundancy could potentially foil the experimental design's intent through temporal correlation of modulation patterns distributed across the (tonotopic) spectrum. If listeners were capable of selectively focusing on just a few channels broadly distributed across the frequency spectrum whose modulation patterns are largely in sync (relative to the original, undistorted signal), the auditory system's "true" sensitivity to cross-spectral jitter may have been grossly underestimated.

A statistical analysis of the cross-spectral time–jitter patterns used in Experiment 1 is consistent with this intuition. If only four channels are chosen from the nineteen used in the experiment, and these four are distributed across the frequency spectrum so that one channel comes from the lowest sub-band (< 750 Hz), one from the highest sub-band (3–6 kHz) and the remaining two from the other sub-bands (0.75–1.5 kHz and 1.5–3 kHz), then it is possible to ascertain the time jitter of four such channels *relative to each other* as a means of estimating the potential magnitude of temporal correlation across frequency. Such an analysis shows that ca. 10% of the 448 potential 4-channel combinations exhibit very little time jitter across the spectrum [13]. Thus, if the brain were capable of decoding the speech signal from just four channels widely distributed across the acoustic spectrum, and if it were possible to determine which of the 19 channels were

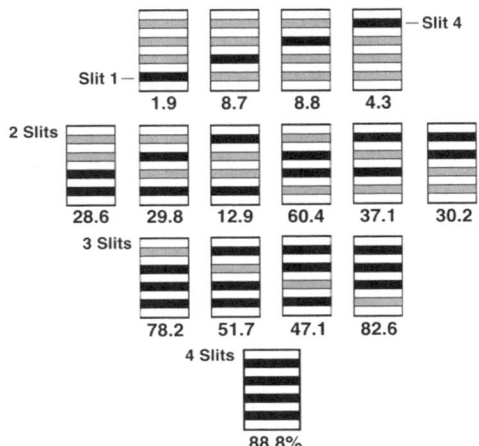

Figure 4. Intelligibility of sparse–spectrum sentences under 15 separate listening conditions. Baseline word accuracy is 88.8% (4-channel condition). The intelligibility of the multiple-channel signals is far greater than would be predicted on the basis of word accuracy (or error) for individual channels presented alone. The region between 750 and 2400 Hz (slits 2 and 3) provides the most important intelligibility information. From [13].

synchronized to each other, then it would be possible, in principle, to decode the speech signal through some form of frequency–selective listening.

In order to test this possibility a second perceptual experiment was performed. In contrast to the original set of signals, in which all frequencies below 6 kHz were presented to the listener, sentences were filtered into narrow (1/3-octave) channels and most of the spectral information discarded. Listeners were asked to report the words heard when one, two, three or four channels were presented concurrently (and in synch with each other). The lowest channel was centered ca. 335 Hz, the second ca. 850 Hz, the third ca. 2135 Hz and the fourth ca. 5400 Hz. Intelligibility depends on the number of channels presented, as well as their position within the frequency spectrum (Figure 4). The most pertinent result is the intelligibility associated with four concurrently presented channels. Under such conditions ca. 90% of the words are accurately reported. This result is important, for it demonstrates that a detailed spectro–temporal representation of the speech signal is not required for the acoustic signal to be intelligible. Three quarters of the spectrum was discarded without a significant decline in the ability to correctly specify the words spoken. Note, that for the example shown in Figure 5, the modulation pattern associated with the four-channel signal is remarkably similar to that of the original waveform (except for a scaling factor), suggesting that sparsely sampling the spectrum in this fashion is capable of capturing the essence of the sentence's modulation properties. To the extent that intelligibility is derived from such modulation patterns, it is perhaps not so surprising that virtually all of the words spoken are accurately reported. The experimental results also provide a stable baseline with which to measure the impact of various signal manipulations (as described below).

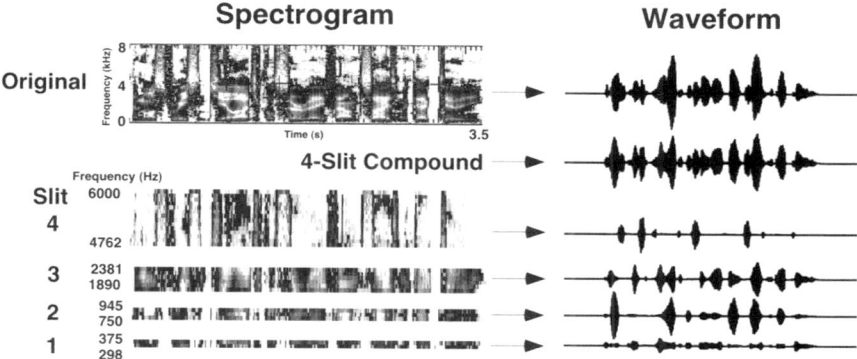

Figure 5. Spectrographic and time–domain representations of a representative sentence ("The most recent geological survey found seismic activity") used in the study. The channel waveforms are plotted on the same amplitude scale, while the scale of the original, unfiltered signal is compressed by a factor of five for illustrative clarity. The frequency axis of the spectrographic display of the channels has been non-linearly compressed for illustrative tractability. Note the quasi-orthogonal temporal registration of the waveform modulation pattern across frequency channels. From [13].

6.   Measuring the Auditory System's "True" Sensitivity to Spectral Asynchrony

Using a performance baseline for various combinations of sparse spectral sentences one can measure intelligibility when the channels are desynchronized relative to each other – this is the basis of Experiment 3. Listeners were presented only a small proportion of the spectrum with which to decode the sentential material. Because the listening task is intrinsically difficult – listeners are rarely able to accurately report all of the words presented – it encourages subjects to use all of the spectral information provided. Thus, when some of the spectral information is removed or desynchronized relative to other

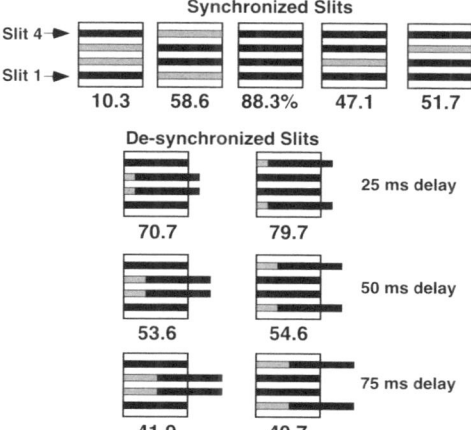

Figure 6. Intelligibility (percent words correct) of sparse spectral sentences containing four narrowband (1/3 octave) channels as a function of channel asynchrony. Note the relatively symmetrical decline in intelligibility associated with the central channels leading or lagging the lateral channels. 16 subjects. Adapted from [13].

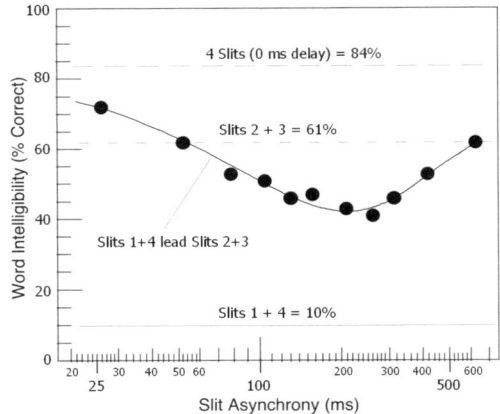

Figure 7. Intelligibility of sparse spectral sentences containing four narrow–band (1/3 octave) channels as a function of slit asynchrony. Note that intelligibility goes below baseline (slits 2+3) when the slit asynchrony exceeds 50 ms). 27 subjects. Adapted from [21].

channels, a reliable estimate can be made of the contribution to intelligibility made by each of the channels involved. It is thus possible to estimate the contribution of each portion of the spectrum to overall intelligibility, as well as to measure how sensitive the auditory system is to cross-spectral time jitter imposed on the modulation patterns associated with each spectral channel. For the present discussion we focus on one form of channel asynchrony, in which the two central channels either lead or lag the lateral channels in time (in a separate experiment, also shown, a single central channel was desynchronized relative to its counterparts).

Figure 6 shows how desynchronizing one or both of the two central channels relative to their lateral counterparts affects intelligibility for various degrees of asynchrony. When the channels are jittered by 25 ms the impact on intelligibility is small, ranging between 10 and 20%. For greater amounts of asynchrony the impact is profound – intelligibility falls to 60% or less. Increasing the cross-spectral asynchrony lowers intelligibility for jitter intervals up to ca. 250 ms (Figure 7). Beyond this limit additional delays result in a slight *improvement* in intelligibility overall (but is quite variable across listeners and sentential material). Such results imply that the auditory system is quite sensitive to spectral asynchrony – it is necessary only to use a sufficiently sensitive assay in order to expose the chinks in the brain's perceptual armor. Moreover, when asynchrony across channels exceeds 50 ms, intelligibility descends below performance baseline for the two central channels presented alone (ca. 60%), suggesting that there is active interference among channels under such conditions. Clearly, the auditory system is far less tolerant of cross-spectral asynchrony than implied in Experiment 1. The *apparent* tolerance of cross-spectral jitter in the first experiment is probably the result of redundancy among channels that affords numerous opportunities for modulation information to be combined across the spectrum for optimum decoding of linguistic information contained in the speech signal. Such redundancy masks the exquisite sensitivity of the auditory system to cross-spectral time jitter.

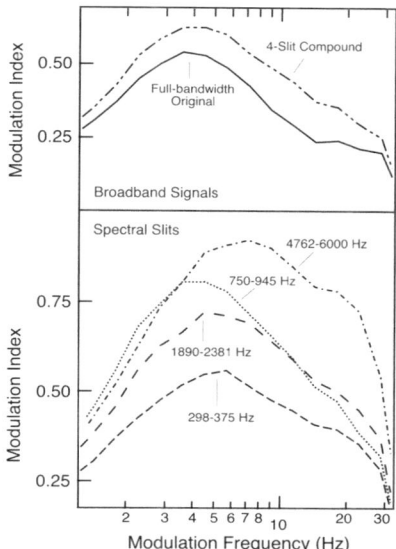

Figure 8. The modulation spectrum (magnitude component) associated with each 1/3-octave channel, as computed for all 130 sentences presented in Experiment 2 [bottom panel]. The peak of the spectrum (in all but the highest channel) lies between 4 and 6 Hz. Its magnitude is considerably diminished in the lowest frequency slit. Also note the large amount of energy in the higher modulation frequencies associated with the highest frequency channel. The modulation spectra of the 4-channel compound and the original, unfiltered signal are illustrated for comparison [top panel]. From [13].

7. The Importance of Modulation Phase for Intelligibility

The results described in Section 7 imply that the relation between intelligibility and the low-frequency modulation spectrum is more complex than the formulation proposed by Houtgast and Steeneken using their Speech Transmission Index (STI) [18]. According to the STI, intelligibility is largely predictable from the contour and magnitude of the modulation spectrum. However, the results of Experiments 2 and 3 imply otherwise. If the modulation spectrum (as conventionally represented) was the primary determinant of intelligibility then each of the channels presented in isolation would be highly comprehensible, as each is associated with a modulation spectrum that fits the conventional profile for intelligible speech (Figure 8). Clearly, this is not the case, suggesting that some property of the acoustic signal other than the conventional modulation spectrum is essentialfor understanding spoken language. for understanding spoken language.

The results of Experiment 3 suggest that the *phase* of the modulation spectrum may be crucial for understanding spoken language. The temporal relation of the modulation patterns across the spectrum appear to be extremely important for decoding the speech signal. It is as if the underlying representation in the signal was derived from a complex topography of peaks and valleys distributed across frequency and time [14]. Both the phase and magnitude of the modulation spectrum would be required to reconstruct the topography with precision.

If this were the case, then it should be possible to scramble the phase of the modulation spectrum using a different method and achieve a result comparable to that of Experiment 3.

In a fourth experiment this objective was accomplished using a full-spectrum version of the speech signal. Local time reversal of the signal's waveform, as shown in Fig-

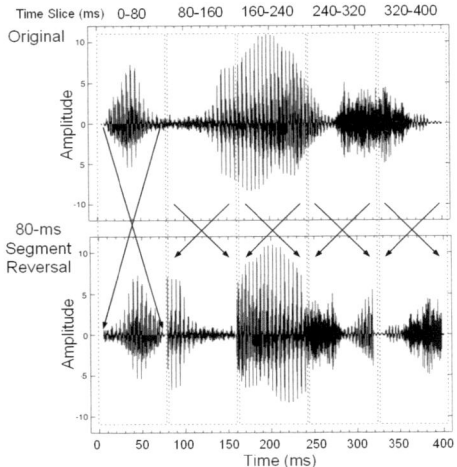

Figure 9. The stimulus–processing procedure, as illustrated for a brief portion of a single sentence. Each segment was "flipped" on its horizontal axis, preserving all other temporal properties of the signal. In this example the reversed–segment duration is 80 ms. From [12].

ure 9, provides a convenient means with which to dissociate the phase and magnitude components of the modulation spectrum. The experimental paradigm is loosely based on a study published by Saberi and Perrott [20]. Waveform segments of variable (and uniform) length were flipped on their horizontal axes and the intelligibility measured after such signal manipulations were imposed. As the length of the waveform interval increases, the amount of modulation–phase dispersion across the frequency spectrum increases substantially (relative to the original, undistorted signal), even though the impact on the magnitude component of the modulation spectrum is somewhat less dramatic. In fact, the magnitude of the modulation spectrum below 9 Hz actually *increases*

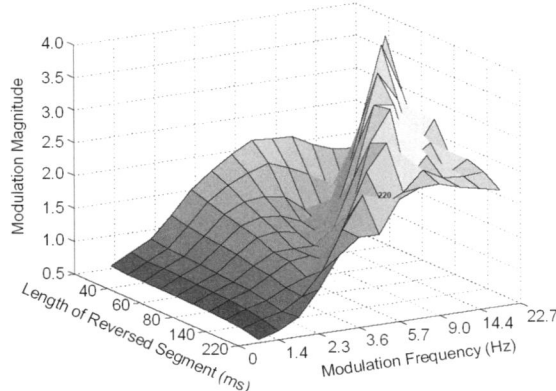

Figure 10. The magnitude component of the modulation spectrum computed for all 40 sentences used in the experiment as a function of reversed–segment duration. Note that there is a slight decline in magnitude in the key, 3–9 Hz region for reversed–segment lengths of 20–50 ms, followed by a steep increase in magnitude for longer reversed–segment intervals. From [12].

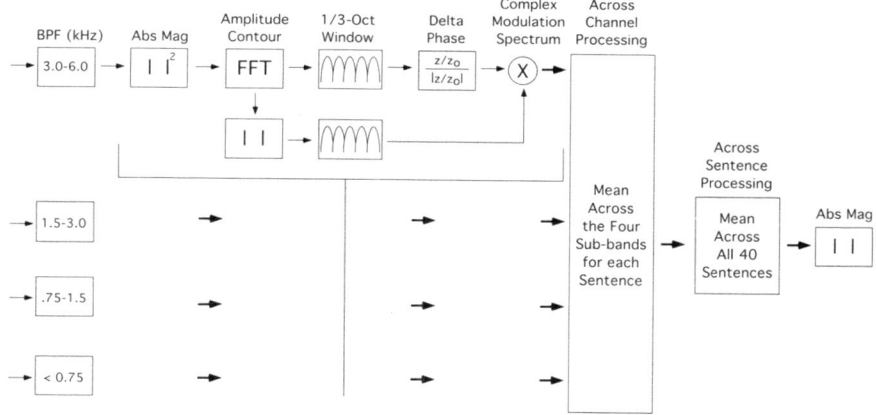

Figure 11. Signal–processing procedure for computing the complex modulation spectrum of the sentential material. The magnitude and phase components of the modulation spectrum are initially computed separately for each of the four sub-bands. The delta–phase (relative to the original signal) is computed for each one–third–octave interval of the modulation spectrum and then combined with the commensurate amplitude component to obtain the *complex* modulation spectrum (phase and amplitude combined) as illustrated in Figure 12. From [12].

for reversed waveform lengths of 50 ms or longer (Figure 10).

When the phase and magnitude components are combined into a single representation ("complex modulation spectrum" – [12]) the relation to intelligibility becomes much clearer. In this representation the magnitude of the modulation spectrum at each frequency depends on the phase coherence relative to the original signal. When modulation phase across the acoustic spectrum is coherent, the associated magnitudes sum linearly. Phase scrambling results in a diminution of complex modulation magnitude because the vectors associated with the magnitude component tend to cancel. Figure 11 illustrates the computation of the complex modulation spectrum.

Figure 12 illustrates the relationship between intelligibility and the length of time reversal in the waveform along with its association with the *complex* modulation spectrum. Intelligibility progressively declines as the reversal interval increases from 20 ms to 100 ms. Clearly, the decline in intelligibility does not parallel modulation–spectrum *magnitude*, a result consistent with Experiments 2 and 3 using sparse spectral signals.

The complex modulation spectrum progressively diminishes as the length of the waveform–reversal increases, and is closely paralleled by a concomitant decline in intelligibility (Figure 12). Thus, the ability to understand spoken language appears to depend on *both* the magnitude and phase of the modulation spectrum distributed across the frequency spectrum.

In some sense the fine acoustic–phonetic detail that figures so importantly in conventional accounts of the speech chain may merely reflect the modulation pattern distributed across the acoustic (tonotopic) frequency axis. This is hardly a novel concept, dating back to the development of the VOCODER in the late 1930s [6]. However, the importance of modulation seems to be have been largely forgotten over the intervening years.

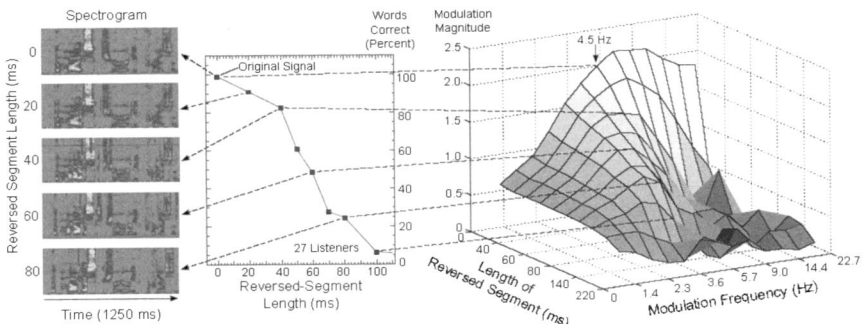

Figure 12. Relation of intelligibility of locally time–reversed sentences (center) to the complex modulation spectrum (right) for reversed–segment durations between 20 and 100 ms (as well as the original signal). Spectrograms of a sample sentence are shown on the left. As the reversed–segment duration increases beyond 40 ms, intelligibility declines precipitously, as does the magnitude of the complex modulation spectrum. The spectro–temporal properties of the signal also degrade under such conditions. From [12].

8. The Role of Visual Information in Understanding Spoken Language

Despite the importance of the complex modulation spectrum for speech intelligibility, something else is missing from our formulation, namely the role played by the visual motion of the tongue, lips and jaw (as well as other facial features) in decoding spoken language.

The salient properties of auditory–visual integration commonly used by both normal and hearing–impaired listeners in the speech–decoding process is described in detail elsewhere [8]. This section focuses on an experiment that provides additional insight into the underlying mechanisms that enable the brain to proceed from sound to meaning over a wide range of acoustic conditions.

In this experiment, the visual component of the speech signal (a talker producing short, simple sentences) was presented in tandem with a sparse spectral version of the same sentential material [9]. In this study only two acoustic channels were presented, one centered at 335 Hz, the other centered at 5400 Hz. The sentences were similar to (but distinct from) those used in Experiments 1–4. The two acoustic channels presented by themselves (A alone) are associated with an intelligibility of ca. 20%. The visual information by itself (V alone) results in only ca. 10% of the words being accurately reported. When the two modalities are combined (A–V) and presented synchronously, intelligibility rises to 63% overall for the nine listeners tested. The conditions described are associated with a 44–53% dynamic range in intelligibility. We can exploit the experimental paradigm to ascertain the temporal limits to A–V integration for decoding the speech signal by desynchronizing the audio and visual streams and then measuring this manipulation's effect on intelligibility. The impact of modality desynchronization is highly asymmetric and depends on which information stream (visual or audio) leads the other. When the audio signal is presented in advance of the video the intelligibility declines progressively with increasing amounts of asynchrony (Figure 13). Except for a difference in baseline performance, the intelligibility function is similar to that of the acoustic–only condition described in Experiment 3 (in which the two central channels

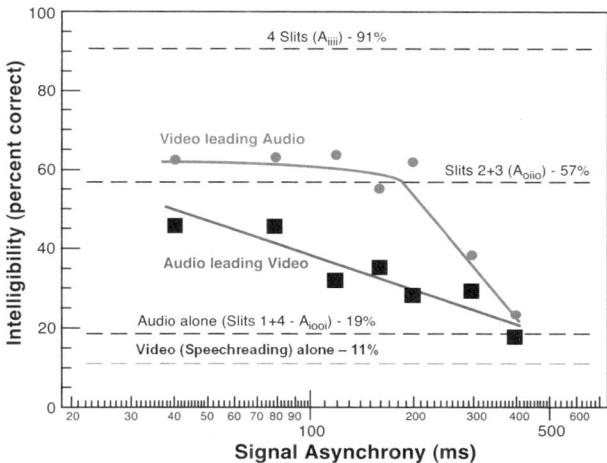

Figure 13. *Average* intelligibility (for 9 subjects) associated with audio—visual speech recognition as a function of bimodal signal asynchrony. The audio—leading—video conditions are marked in blue, the video—leading—audio conditions shown in red. Baseline audio—only conditions are marked in black, dashed lines, and the video—alone condition is shown in orange. From [9].

are desynchronized relative to their lateral counterparts). The performance functions run parallel to each other, suggesting that the mechanisms underlying the decoding of the speech signal under these two conditions are similar.

On the other hand, when the visual signal leads the audio, intelligibility remains unchanged overall until the two streams are desynchronized by more than 200 ms (Figure 13). For larger amounts of asynchrony, intelligibility declines to baseline performance for intervals of 400 ms or longer. This is an intriguing result, as it implies that when the visual stream arrives first the brain is remarkably tolerant of asynchrony between acoustic and visual modalities (but not vice versa). What is the basis of this asymmetry? And can it provide additional insight into the mechanisms enabling the brain to decode spoken language?

A variety of potential "explanations" for this perceptual asymmetry come readily to mind.

A physical explanation, based on the disparate transmission speeds of acoustic and optical signals, does not account for the perceptual data observed. The speed of light is virtually instantaneous (299,792,458 m/s) while sound travels much more slowly, roughly one foot per millisecond (or 331.5 m/s). In the current experiment listeners were wearing headphones and viewing the visual stream on a monitor from a distance of a few feet. Thus, the physical time disparity between the arrival of audio and visual signals was a few milliseconds at most, nowhere close to the disparities observed in the experimental data.

A second form of prospective explanation pertains to the differential processing speeds of acoustic and visual information in the brain. If visual input is processed more slowly than the acoustic signal, then the early arrival of the visual signal could compensate for the differential processing speed, insuring that the two streams are internally processed in sync. Irrespective of the validity of this assumption (that visual information is processed more slowly than auditory), this hypothesis would imply that the intelligibility functions would be offset, but parallel to each other. However, the performance functions are of very different shapes, and therefore differential neural processing speed *by itself*, is unlikely to provide a full explanation for the perceptual asymmetry observed.

A third explanation combines elements of the first two hypotheses. Because the brain has evolved to process and decode information contained in sensory streams that are often of variable temporal relation to each other, it must have evolved mechanisms that are tolerant to A–V asynchrony. Although this hypothesis is appealing, it fails to account for the asymmetry observed in intelligibility. Some other factor must be at work. What might this be?

It has been shown by Grant and by others that much of the phonetic information contained in speechreading cues pertains to "place of articulation" – the characteristics distinguishing [p] from [t] and [k], or [b] from [d] and [g] (see [8]). Such place cues reflect the locus of articulatory constriction during consonantal (particularly stop, fricative and nasal segments) production and are quite important for lexical discriminability (particularly at word onset). Such articulatory information is concentrated in the spectral region between 800 and 3000 Hz, and is often embedded in the dynamic patterns associated with formant transitions binding consonants and vowels. In this sense, place–of–articulation cues are inherently trans-segmental, spanning two or three phonetic segments in time [11].

Perhaps the perceptual asymmetry observed in Experiment 4 reflects "priming" properties of place–of–articulation cues contained in the visual stream? If this were so, then one would anticipate that under certain conditions having the visual stream lead the audio would result in intelligibility that is even better than when the two streams are synchronized. This is precisely what happens for eight of the nine listeners in this experiment. Having knowledge of the visual signal in advance of the audio stream actually improves intelligibility slightly for asynchronies ranging between 80 and 120 ms. Why should this be so?

9. Prosody's Role in Decoding the Phonetic Properties of The Syllable

A salient property of speechreading information is the opening and closing of the jaw. When the opening ("aperture") is relatively wide the syllable nucleus is likely to contain a vowel of low height, such as [a] or [ae], while when the aperture is small the vowel is more likely to be a high vowel such as [I] or [u]. Low vowels tend to be long, while high vowels tend to be short. Moreover, low vowels tend to contain more energy than their high vocalic counterparts [17]. These sorts of acoustic distinctions among vowels are extremely useful for determining the prominence of syllables [17] and can be used to automatically classify such syllables with human-like precision [16].

Foreknowledge of a syllable's prominence can potentially facilitate the phonetic decoding of speech. In English, there is a systematic relationship between vocalic identity, vowel height and prominence [17] (Figure 14). High vowels tend to occur in unaccented syllables while heavily accented syllables generally contain vowels of low or mid height [17]. Moreover, the phonetic manifestation of many consonants is correlated with the syllable's prominence. Heavily accented syllables tend to be canonically pronounced [14][15], with most phonetic constituents carefully articulated (Table 1). The

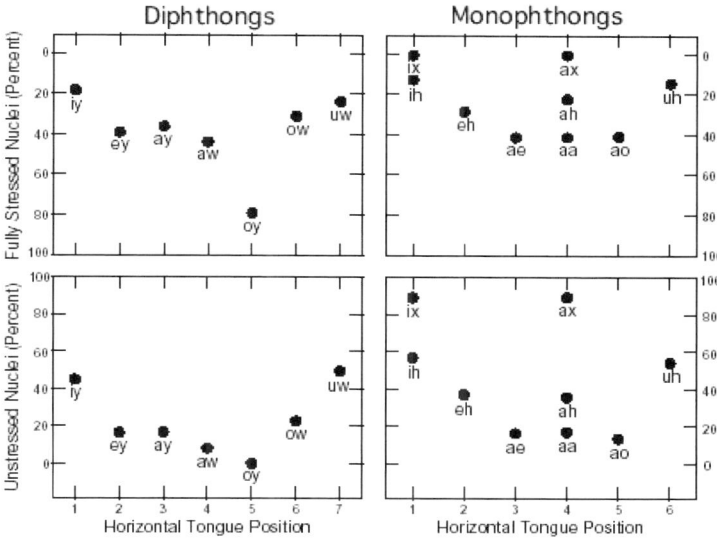

Figure 14. The proportion (in percent) of tokens for each vocalic class labeled as either completely accented (level—1 accent, top panels) or entirely unaccented (level—0 accent, bottom panels), partitioned into two broad classes, diphthongs and monophthongs (for clarity of illustration). Note reversal of scale for the ordinates associated with the top and bottom panels. Adapted from [17].

onset and nucleus segments tend be significantly longer than the same constituents in accented syllables. There is a much higher probability of segmental deletion (particularly among coronals) within syllable codas associated with unaccented syllables relative to their accented counterparts (Table 1).

For such reasons, *a priori* knowledge of articulatory dynamics related to syllable prominence derived from speechreading can facilitate and enhance the interpretation of the acoustic signal. The visual stream is potentially helpful in estimating the number of syllables in an utterance, as well as providing information germane to syllable structure and segmentation. Moreover, as mentioned above, speechreading can also provide important information about place–of–articulation of consonantal constituents that facilitates lexical discrimination, possibly through frequency–selective cues associated with the articulatory dynamics of production.

10. What is the Essence of Spoken Language?

Traditional models of spoken language focus on the phonetic segment (and its abstract representation, the phoneme) as the principal building block of words. However, the studies described in this chapter suggest that the syllable is likely to play a far more important role than the phone in the lexical decoding process. The time intervals over which speech can be distorted and still be understood are more compatible with the syllable than the phone. Moreover, articulatory gestures associated with visible speech cues are syllabic rather than phonetic in nature. And yet the phone has figured importantly in models of speech for many decades. How can this be so if the phonetic segment plays a relatively minor role in lexical decoding?

Segments	Stress Par	Syllable Onset								Syllable Coda							
		Heavy		Light		None		Total		Heavy		Light		None		Total	
		Can	Tran	Can	Tran	Can	Tran	Can	Tran	Can	Tran	Can	Tran	Can	Tran	Can	Tran
Anterior Constriction	N	857	851	1301	1244	1491	1212	3649	3307	261	235	357	331	372	264	990	830
[p, b, m, f, th, dh, y]	%	37.8	36.7	43.2	40.8	45.7	41.2	42.7	39.8	15.3	17.9	13.9	17.8	13.3	15.4	14.0	17.0
Central Constriction	N	818	831	962	965	1110	1017	2890	2813	1154	766	1828	1121	2127	1186	5106	3073
[t, d, dx, n, nx, s, z]	%	36.1	35.9	31.9	31.6	34.0	34.6	33.8	33.9	67.7	58.4	71.2	60.1	76.3	69.2	72.4	62.8
Posterior Constriction	N	590	635	752	840	665	713	2007	2188	289	310	383	412	289	265	961	987
[k, g, ng, sh, ch, zh, jh, q]	%	26.0	27.4	24.9	27.6	20.4	24.2	23.5	26.3	17.0	23.6	14.9	22.1	10.4	15.5	13.6	20.2
All Consonants	N	2265	2317	3015	3049	3266	2942	8546	8308	1704	1311	2568	1864	2788	1715	7060	4890

Table 1. The impact of stress accent (heavy, light, none), syllable position (onset, coda) and place of articulation (anterior, central, posterior) on the likelihood of canonical pronunciation (canonical vs. transcribed). In instances where the number of canonical and transcribed instances are similar, the pronunciation is generally realized as canonical. Percentages pertain to the proportion of segments associated with a specific place of articulation (anterior, central, posterior. The place "chameleons" ([h], [l], [r]) are excluded from analysis. Abbreviations: Can – Canonical; Tran – Transcribed. Percentages and parameter labels are indicated in **bold** characters. From [15].

Studies of pronunciation variation in spontaneous speech provide a potential explanation. Although words are commonly presented in terms of their phonetic constituents, oftentimes these phones are transformed in everyday utterances to something other than their canonical identity. The patterns of pronunciation variation provide important clues as to the underlying relation of the phone to the syllable.

The initial consonant(s) in a word (and syllable) are usually pronounced canonically (i.e., as represented in a dictionary) and such onsets are usually stable under a wide range of speaking styles and dialectal conditions. In contrast, vocalic nuclei of the same words vary a lot. Such variation is conditioned by such factors as speaking style, geographical dialect, socio-economic status, emotionality and so on. Despite the enormous range of vocalic realization conditioned by such factors, certain principles apply that constrain the specific sorts of variation observed (at least in American English). Generally, pronunciation variants are of the same (or proximal) height as the canonical form, and it is rare that front and back variants are interchanged [14]. In other words, the basic "value" of a vowel remains preserved, even when its phonetic realization changes from a diphthong to a monophthong. The basic "place" within the articulatory vowel space remains relatively stable.

The final (coda) consonants lie somewhere in between the onset consonants and vocalic nuclei with respect to stability. In English, 75% of the coda consonants are coronals (mostly [t], [d] and [n]) [15]—such constituents manifest a propensity for "deletion" or "reduction" in spontaneous speech, particularly in unaccented syllables. This tendency is also common among syllable–final liquids ([l] and [r]) (though these constituents act more like vowels than consonants in many respects, and should therefore be considered as the terminal portions of the nucleus). Otherwise, coda consonants are relatively stable, like their onset counterparts. The specific behavior of constituents with the syllable is largely conditioned by the syllable's prominence. Constituents within heavily accented syllables are usually canonically pronounced, providing some measure of support to the phonemic framework for spoken language. But such syllables are in the minority (at least for American English). The phonemic perspective appears to be, in part, a reflection of how words are *supposed* to be articulated under "ideal" (i.e., canonical) conditions. But there is more to the phonemic perspective than merely canonical pronunciation.

The three major articulatory dimensions for spoken language are voicing, place and manner of articulation. Manner of articulation (i.e., the distinction in the mode of production characterizing stops, nasals, fricatives, vowels, etc.) is temporally isomorphic with the concept of the phonetic segment [11]. The interval over which articulatory manner pertains also applies to the segment. Under virtually all conditions in which a pronunciation variant occurs there is stability in the *inferred* manner of articulation. For vocalic variants the manner is also preserved. In the case of coda deletions there is often the *implication* of a final constituent by virtue of the formant patterns remaining in the terminal portion of the vowel [15] as well as the fall in energy often associated with that segment. In this sense, manner of articulation can be used to deduce the number (and often the identity) of the "underlying" segments, even when they are acoustically absent. In this sense, the concept of the phone (and phoneme) is largely grounded in manner of production.

Within this framework, manner is coterminous with the segment, while voicing and place of articulation are not. Voicing is, according to this perspective, a syllabic feature, driven by prosodic factors, that can vary its temporal range across and within the conventional segment [11]. Thus, certain constituents are partially or entirely devoiced, while others exhibit more or less voicing than is typical of the canonical form. Place of articulation serves to bind the vocalic nucleus with onset and coda constituents, and in this sense is inherently trans-segmental [11]. It serves as the articulatory basis of the diphone and demi-syllable concepts used in speech synthesis. Place, like its articulatory counterparts manner and voicing, is sensitive to prosodic factors, and is particularly apparent in the visible speech cues used to decode the speech signal [8][11].

The syllable serves as the organizational unit through which the articulatory dimensions of voicing, place and manner interact with each other and with prosodic information to shape the phonetic form of words within an utterance. Ultimately, such factors reflect the underlying information (both linguistic and paralinguistic) contained in the signal used by listeners to deduce the meaning associated with speech. The time constants associated with these processes are likely to be variable, ranging from ca. 10 ms for micro–phonetic phenomena to ca. 3000 ms for prosodic information. However, the core of processing for speech intelligibility ranges between 40 ms and 400 ms, and largely reflects syllables and the articulatory constituents contained within.

Acknowledgements

The research described in this chapter was supported by the Learning and Intelligent Systems Initiative of the National Science Foundation as well as the U.S. Department of Defense. Hannah Carvey, Shuangyu Chang, Leah Hitchcock, Joy Hollenback and Rosaria Silipo contributed to some of the work described. This chapter is adapted from an article that appears in the IEICE Transactions on Information and Systems (Vol. E87, pp. 1059–1070).

References

[1] Arai, T. and Greenberg, S. "The temporal properties of spoken Japanese are similar to those of English." *Proc. 5th Euro. Conf. Speech Comm. Tech. (Eurospeech-97)*, pp. 1011—1014, 1997.

[2] Arai, T. and Greenberg, S. "Speech intelligibility in the presence of cross-channel spectral asynchrony." *Proc. IEEE Int. Conf. Acoust. Speech Sig. Proc.*, pp. 933—936, 1998.

[3] Arai, T., Pavel, M., Hermansky, H. and Avendano, C. "Syllable intelligibility for temporally filtered LPC cepstral trajectories." *J. Acoust. Soc. Am*. 105: 2783—2791, 1999.

[4] Beckman, M. *Stress and Non-Stress Accent*. Dordrecht: Fortis, 1986.

[5] Drullman, R., Festen, J.M. and Plomp R. "Effect of temporal envelope smearing on speech reception." *J. Acoust. Soc. Am*. 95: 1053—1064, 1994.

[6] Dudley, H. "Remaking speech." *J. Acoust. Soc. Am*. 11: 169—177, 1939.

[7] Godfrey, J.J., Holliman, E.C. and McDaniel, J. "SWITCHBOARD: Telephone speech corpus for research and development." *Proc. IEEE Int. Conf. Acoust. Speech Sig. Proc.*, pp. 517—520, 1992.

[8] Grant, K.W. "Auditory supplements to speechreading." *IEICE Workshop on Speech Dynamics by Ear, Eye, Mouth and Machine,* Kyoto, 2003.

[9] Grant, K.W. and Greenberg, S. "Speech intelligibility derived from asynchronous processing of auditory—visual information." *Proc. Workshop Audio-Visual Speech Proc.,* pp. 132—137, 2001.

[10] Greenberg, S. "Speaking in shorthand—A syllable-centric perspective for understanding pronunciation variation." *Speech Communication* 29: 159—176, 1999.

[11] Greenberg, S. "Pronunciation variation is key to understanding spoken language." *Proc. 15th Int. Cong. Phon. Sci.,* pp. 219—222, 2003.

[12] Greenberg, S. and Arai, T. "The relation between speech intelligibility and the complex modulation spectrum." *Proc. 7th Eur. Conf. Speech Comm. Tech.,* pp. 473—476, 2001.

[13] Greenberg, S., Arai, T. and Silipo, R. "Speech intelligibility derived from exceedingly sparse spectral information." *Proc. 5th Int. Conf. Spoken Lang. Proc.*, pp. 74—77, 1998.

[14] Greenberg, S., Carvey, H., Hitchcock, L. and Chang, S. "Beyond the phoneme – A juncture-accent model for spoken language." *Proc. 2nd Int. Conf. Human Lang. Tech. Res.*, pp. 36—43, 2002.

[15] Greenberg, S., Carvey, H., Hitchcock, L. and Chang, S. "The phonetic patterning of spontaneous American English discourse." *Proc. ISCA/IEEE Workshop Spont. Speech Proc. Recog.*, pp. 35—38, 2003.

[16] Greenberg, S., Chang, S. and Hitchcock, L. "The relation between stress accent and vocalic identity in spontaneous American English discourse." *Proc. ISCA Workshop on Prosody Speech Recog. Understanding*, pp. 51—56, 2001.

[17] Hitchcock, L. and Greenberg, S. "Vowel height is intimately associated with stress accent in spontaneous American English discourse." *Proc. 7th Eur. Conf. Speech Comm. Tech. (Eurospeech-2001),* pp. 79—82, 2001.

[18] Houtgast T. and Steeneken H. "A review of the MTF concept in room acoustics and its use for estimating speech intelligibility in auditoria." *J. Acoust. Soc. Am*. 77: 1069—1077, 1985.

[19] Marslen-Wilson, W.D. and Zwitserlood, P. "Accessing spoken words: The importance of word onsets." *J. Exp. Psych.: Human Percept. Perf*. 15: 576—585, 1989.

[20] Saberi, K. and Perrot, D. "Cognitive restoration of reversed speech." *Nature* 398: 760, 1999.

[21] Silipo, R., Greenberg, S. and Arai, T. "Temporal constraints on speech intelligibility as deduced from exceedingly sparse spectral representations." *Proc. 6th European Conf. Speech Comm. Tech.*, pp. 2687—2690, 1999.

[22] Stevens, K.N. "Toward a model for lexical access based on acoustic landmarks and distinctive features." *J. Acoust. Soc. Am*. 111: 1872—1891, 2002.

Using Dynamics in Speech Applications

Dynamics of Speech Production and Perception
P. Divenyi et al. (Eds.)
IOS Press, 2006

Using Dynamics in Speech Applications

Malcom SLANEY
YAHOO! Laboratories
Mountain View, California, USA
and
CCRMA, Stanford University
Stanford, California, USA

Speech, as described throughout this book, is certainly a dynamic process. The chapters in this section investigate the effect that dynamics has on a number of different speech applications, including recognition and learning.

Nobody working on speech thinks that speech is a static process. Synthetic vowels without formant or pitch variation do not sound like speech. It's only when the sound changes is it perceived to be speech. Another example are "white vowels" first demonstrated by Manfred Schroeder and colleagues. A sentence is filtered so that one phoneme has a perfectly flat spectrum. There are no formants at that point in time. Yet, when the entire sentence is played to a listener, they clearly hear normal speech.

Even the white vowel is perceived correctly. (Part of this is due to the language context, but certainly some of it is caused by our ability to recognize the changes in the spectrum as speech.)

Yet, it's easier to think about and build systems for static sounds. Even HMM's, which do a great job of modeling many aspects of speech, model the signal as a set of static states. It's only natural. We must stand before we walk, let alone run.

Now 55 years after the first speech-recognition engine, it's time to start thinking about how we can better incorporate the dynamic aspects of speech into our systems.

The chapters in this section all take a very different approach to modeling and using the dynamics of speech.

The chapter by Les Atlas directly addresses dynamic aspects of speech by characterizing the modulation spectrum of speech. Here we are not interested in spectral slices, but instead we want to measure how the information in auditory bands change over time. Atlas measures the spectrum of the slow modulations in each channel, a modulation spectrogram. He can use this information to separate two speakers based on their separate modulations.

Hynek Hermansky ties this all together by describing the convergence between successful statistical approaches to speech recognition and that which is already known about human perception. In one case, a statistical method for linearly discriminating between different classes of data (LDA) derives a set of basis functions that approximate the spectral resolution of the human auditory system (RASTA). Hermansky uses this knowledge to build a two-stage feature analyzer that transforms the input waveforms into a set of cross-frequency and cross-time features. These new features are used as input to a conventional hidden-Markov model (HMM) recognizer.

Chin-Hui Lee advocates a different approach to the same problem. His work describes the difficulties that speech recognizers have with many simple speech-discrimination tasks. These difficulties are caused by only looking at static spectral slices, while many interesting speech phenomena are dynamic. A good example is the time between the end of a plosive and the start of voicing, the voice-onset time. This is not a measure that is captured by conventional representations like MFCC, but yet is relatively easy to measure. Prof. Lee suggests there are many such opportunities, all of which lead to a knowledge-based approach to speech recognition.

Peter Mihajlik and his collagues address the problem of getting training data for speech recognition systems. High-quality training data is the key to modern speech-recognition systems, and this data-collection effort is made all the more difficult because speech is so dynamic. Even when reading, speakers have speech disfluencies, and use alternate pronunciations. They would love to have a fully automated approach to generating speech-recognition training data. Even though Hungarian has a relatively straightforward mapping between the orthographic representation and phonemes, still much manual work is needed to get the right labels for each utterance. Still, a combination of automatic and manual segmentation and labeling does almost as well as a fully manual method.

Klara Vicsi considers the dynamics of speech for a different purpose: the training students to speak better. His work helps students improve their speech by visualizing different aspects of the speech they produce. This is a difficult problem because the dynamics of speech are important, and doubly hard because the students are often children. Cartoon displays are used to display the loudness, rhythm, dynamics, intonation and even the spectrogram to students. By turning speech-production training into a game, children consistently learned to speak a speech sound in a shorter period of time.

Finally, Victor Sorokin talks about the difficulty, the mathematics, and the solutions possible when discovering the articulatory positions that represent any particular speech waveform. This is clearly a mapping that humans learn: with training we can shape our mouths to produce any needed sound. Computationally, this is an ill-posed problem— there are many positions of the articulators that can produce nearly identical sounds. Again the dynamics of the speech-production process are an important constraint when finding an optimal solution to this speech-inversion problem.

Dynamics of Speech Production and Perception
P. Divenyi et al. (Eds.)
IOS Press, 2006

Modulation Frequency Filtering of Speech

Les ATLAS
Department of Electrical Engineering
University of Washington
Seattle, Washington, USA

Abstract. Recent auditory physiological evidence points to a modulation frequency dimension in the auditory cortex. This dimension exists jointly with the tonotopic acoustic frequency dimension. Thus, audition can be considered as a relatively slowly-varying two-dimensional representation, the "modulation spectrum," where the first dimension is the well-known acoustic frequency and the second dimension is modulation frequency. We have recently developed a fully invertible analysis/synthesis approach for this modulation spectral transform. A general application of this approach is removal or modification of different modulation frequencies in audio or speech signals, which, for example, causes major changes in perceived dynamic character. A specific application of this modification is single-channel multiple-talker separation. While the approach we describe can offer novel means for modifying and separating speech, modulation frequency filtering is not yet a principled approach like standard linear time-invariant filtering. First steps toward this goal are described.

Keywords. Modulation spectrum, speech coding, talker separation

Introduction

Zadeh first proposed that a separate dimension of modulation frequency could supplant the standard concept of system function frequency analysis [1]. His proposed two-dimensional system function had two separate frequency dimensions—one for standard frequency and the other a transform of the time variation. This two-dimensional bi-frequency system function was only defined, but was not analyzed. Kailath followed up nine years later [2] with the first analysis of this joint system function. More recently, Gardner (e.g. [3][4]) greatly extended the concept of joint frequency analysis for cyclostationary systems. These cyclostationary approaches have been widely applied for parameter estimation and detection. However, transforms that are used in compression and for many pattern recognition applications usually have a need for invertibility. Cyclostationary analysis does not provide an analysis/synthesis framework.

   Evidence for the value of modulations in the perception of speech quality and in speech intelligibility has come from a variety of experiments by the speech community. For example, the concept of an acoustic modulation transfer function [5] has also been successfully applied to the measurement of speech transmission. More direct studies on speech perception [6] demonstrated that the most important perceptual information lies at modulation frequencies below 16 Hertz. More recently, Greenberg and Kingsbury [7] showed that a "modulation spectrogram" is a stable representation of speech for automatic recognition in reverberant environments. This modulation spectrogram provided a time-frequency representation that maintained only the 0 to 8-Hertz range of modulation frequencies (uniformly for all acoustic frequencies), and emphasized the 4-Hertz range of modulations.

While these examples strongly suggest the important potential of modulation filtering, we also observe some remaining undesired artifacts. We will thus conclude by describing how an ideal and artifact-free modulation filtering system should behave.

1. A Modulation Spectral Model

For further progress to be made in the understanding and applications of modulation spectra, a foundation for the concept of modulation frequency analysis/synthesis needs to be established. In this section we will propose a foundation that is based upon a set of necessary conditions for a two-dimensional acoustic frequency versus modulation frequency representation. By "acoustic frequency" we mean an exact or approximate conventional Fourier decomposition of a signal. "Modulation frequency" is the dimension that this section will begin to strictly define.

The notion of modulation frequency is quite well understood for signals that are narrowband. A simple case consists of an amplitude modulated fixed–frequency carrier

$$s(t) = m(t) \cos \omega_c t$$

where the modulating signal $m(t)$ is non-negative and has an upper frequency band limit suitable for its perfect and easy recovery from $s(t)$. It is straightforward that the modulation frequency for this signal should be the Fourier transform of the modulating signal only

$$M(e^{j\omega}) = F\{m(t)\} = \int_{-\infty}^{\infty} m(t)e^{-j\omega t} dt$$

But what is a two-dimensional distribution of acoustic versus modulation frequency? Namely, how would this signal be represented as the two-dimensional distribution $P(\eta, \omega)$, where η is modulation frequency and ω is acoustic frequency?

To begin answering this question, we can further simplify the model signal to have a narrowband cosinsoidal modulator

$$s(t) = (1 + \cos \omega_m t) \cos \omega_c t$$

In order to allow unique recovery of the modulating signal, the modulation frequency ω_m is constrained to be less than the carrier frequency ω_c. The additive offset allows for a non-negative modulating signal. Without loss of generality we assume that the modulating signal is normalized to have peak values of ± 1 allowing the additive offset to be 1.

The process of amplitude demodulation, whether it is by magnitude, square–law, Hilbert envelope, cepstral or synchronous detection, or other techniques, is most generally expressed as a frequency shift operation. Thus, a general two-dimensional representation of $s(t)$ has the dimensions acoustic frequency versus frequency translation. For example, much as in the bilinear formulation seen in time–frequency analysis, one dimension can simply express acoustic frequency ω and the other dimension can express a symmetric translation of that frequency via the variable η :

$$S(\omega - \eta/2)S^*(\omega + \eta/2)$$

where $S(\omega)$ is the Fourier transform of $s(t)$

$$S(\omega) = F\{s(t)\} = \int_{-\infty}^{\infty} s(t)e^{-j\omega t}dt$$

and $S^*(\omega)$ is the complex conjugate of $S(\omega)$. This representation is similar to the denominator of the spectral correlation function described by Gardner [4].

Note that there is a loss of sign information in the above bilinear formulation. For analysis/synthesis applications, such as in the approaches discussed later in this paper, phase information needs to be maintained separately.

In the same spirit as previous uses and discussions of modulation frequency, an ideal two-dimensional representation $P_{ideal}(\eta, \omega)$ for $s(t)$ should have significant energy density only at only six impulsive points in the (η, ω) plane

$$P_{ideal}(\eta, \omega) = \delta(0, \omega_c) + \delta(\omega_m, \omega_c) + \delta(-\omega_m, \omega_c) + \delta(0, -\omega_c) + \delta(\omega_m, -\omega_c) + \delta(-\omega_m, -\omega_c)$$

Where $\delta(\eta, \omega)$ is the standard Dirac delta function. For the above ideal two-dimensional representation, the desired terms are jointly at the carrier and modulation frequencies only, with added terms at the carrier frequency for DC modulation, to reflect the above additive offset of the modulating signal. However, going strictly by the definitions above, the Fourier transform of the narrowband cosinsoidal modulator $s(t)$ is

$$S(\omega) = F\{s(t)\} = F\{(1 + \cos\omega_m t)\cos\omega_c t\}$$

$$= \frac{1}{2}\{\delta(\omega - \omega_c) + \delta(\omega + \omega_c)\} + \frac{1}{4}\{\delta(\omega + \omega_c + \omega_m) + \delta(\omega + \omega_c - \omega_m)\}$$

$$+ \frac{1}{4}\{\delta(\omega + \omega_c + \omega_m) + \delta(\omega + \omega_c - \omega_m)\}$$

This transform, when expressed as a bilinear formulation $S(\omega - \eta/2)S^*(\omega + \eta/2)$ has much more extent in both η and ω than desired. A comparison of the ideal and actual two-dimensional representation is shown in Figure 1.

The solid lines of Figure 1 represent the support regions of both $S(\omega - \eta/2)$ and $S^*(\omega + \eta/2)$. Thicker lines represent the double area under the carrier–only terms relative to the modulated terms. The small dots, including the one hidden under the large dot at $(\eta = 0, \omega = \omega_c)$, represent the support region of the product $S(\omega - \eta/2)S^*(\omega + \eta/2)$. The three large dots represent the ideal representation, $P_{ideal}(\eta, \omega)$, of modulation frequency versus acoustic frequency.

It can be observed from Figure 1 that the representation, $S_2(\omega + \eta)S_2^*(\omega - \eta)$, has more impulsive terms than the ideal representation. Namely, the product $S_2(\omega + \eta)S_2^*(\omega - \eta)$ is underconstrained. To approach the ideal representation, two conditions need to be added: 1) A kernel which is convolutional in ω and 2) a kernel

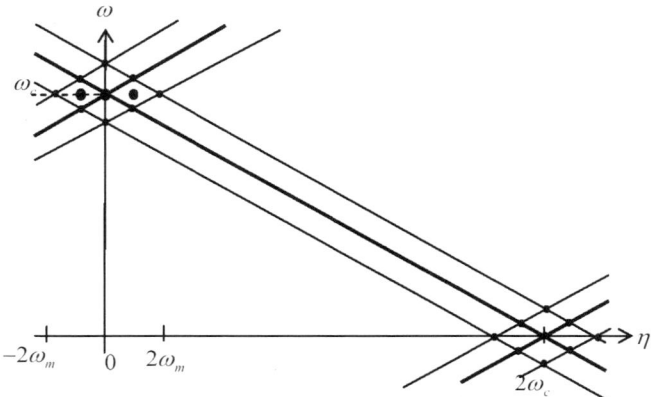

Figure 1. Two-dimensional representation of cosinusoidal amplitude modulation.

which is multiplicative in η. Thus, a sufficient condition for the ideal modulation frequency versus acoustic frequency distribution is

$$P_{ideal}(\eta, \omega) = \left\{ S(\omega - \eta/2)S^*(\omega + \eta/2)\phi_m(\eta) \right\} * \phi_c(\omega)$$

It is important to note that the above condition does not require that the signal be simple cosinusoidal modulation. In principle, any signal

$$s(t) = m(t)c(t)$$

where $m(t)$ is non-negative and band limited to frequency $\omega < |\omega_m|$ and $c(t)$ has no frequency content below ω_m can have a modulation frequency versus acoustic frequency distribution in the form of the above ideal distribution.

An example of an implicitly convolutional effect of $\phi_c(\omega)$ is the limited frequency resolution that arises from a transform of a finite duration of data, e.g. the windowed time analysis used before conventional short–time transforms and filter banks. The multiplicative effect of $\phi_m(\eta)$ is less obvious. Commonly applied time envelope smoothing has, as a frequency counterpart, low pass behavior in $\phi_m(\eta)$. As will be seen in the next section, other efficient approaches can arise from decimation already present in critically–sampled filterbanks. Note that the non-zero terms centered around $\eta = \pm 2\omega_c$, which are well above the typical pass band of $\phi_m(\eta)$, are less troublesome than the typically much lower frequency quadratic distortion term(s) at $\eta = \pm 2\omega_m$. Thus, broad frequency ranges in modulation will be potentially subject to these quadratic distortion term(s).

2. A Modulation Spectral Analysis/Synthesis System

The analysis approach described above provides a foundation for 2 frequency variables

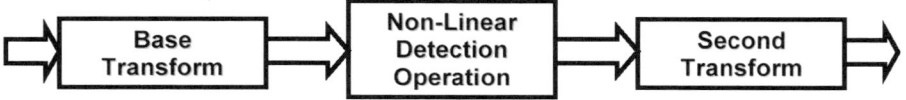

Figure 2. Generic transform approach to joint acoustic/modulation frequency analysis.

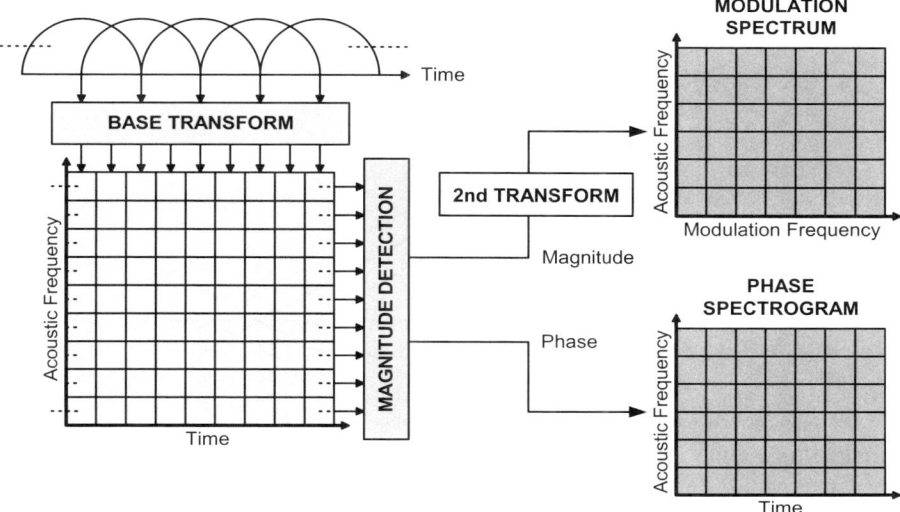

Figure 3. A specific example of a modulation spectral analysis (from [8]).

which represent acoustic and modulation frequency. Filtering in modulation spectra can be considered as analysis, some modification, followed by synthesis. Figures 2 and 3 show a general and specific approach to analysis, respectively.

Starting with Figure 2, the non-linear detection operation can be a magnitude envelope or a magnitude of a Hilbert envelope. A main goal of the detection operation is to find the real part of the complex first or "base" transform, thus demodulating the modulation component in each base transform acoustic frequency sub-band. The synthesis operation is simply the reverse of these operations, where original base transform phase is used with the inverse base transform.

Figure 3 shows a modulation spectral analysis system which has been applied to audio coding [8]. The system in figure 3 employs a time domain aliasing cancellation (TDAC) filter bank [9] as the first or "base" transform. The TDAC filter bank possesses the desirable properties of producing complex outputs and providing 50% overlapping in time while maintaining critical sampling. The TDAC filter bank uses alternating modified–discrete cosine transforms (MDCT) and modified–discrete sine transforms (MDST). Two neighboring MDCT and MDST transform blocks are temporally aligned and combined to form a single complex transform block. The MDCT coefficients are taken as the real part and the MDST coefficients are taken as the imaginary part of the complex coefficients. A magnitude detection operation is performed on the complex transform blocks, which are then arranged into a time–frequency distribution.

The second transform then converts the time evolution into modulation frequency, potentially compacting energy into the lowest modulation frequencies for audio coding. As will be seen in the section below, this joint acoustic/modulation frequency representation is potentially useful for separating sources in the signal

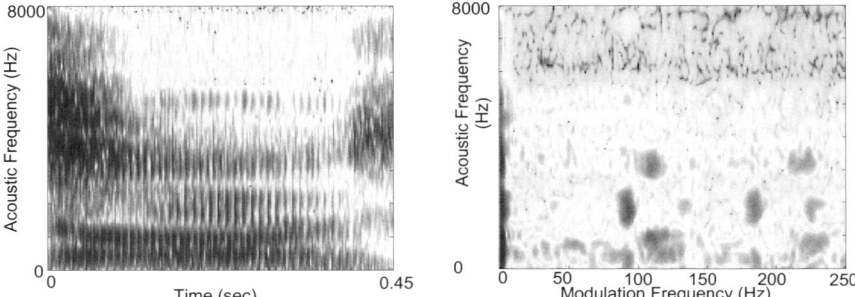

Figure 4. Spectrogram (left) and joint acoustic/modulation frequency representation (right) of the central 450 milliseconds of "two" (talker A) and "dos" (talker B) spoken simultaneously and by two speakers and recorded monourally. The y-axis of both representations is standard acoustic frequency. The x-axis of the right panel representation is modulation frequency, as from a Fourier second transform.

3. Talker Separation

The problem of talker separation is also called "co-channel speech interference." One past approach to the co-channel speech interference problem is blind signal separation (BSS) that approximately recovers unknown signals or "sources" from their observed mixtures [10]. Typically, these mixtures are acquired by a number of sensors, where each sensor receives a different combination of the source signals.

However, a different and perhaps complementary approach can utilize modulation spectra. Figure 4 shows a joint acoustic/modulation frequency transform as applied to two simultaneous speakers. Talker A is saying "two" in English while talker B is saying "dos" in Spanish. This data is from [11].

The right side of Figure 4 shows distinct and isolated regions of acoustic information associated with the fundamental pitch along with its first and aliased higher harmonics of the two distinct speakers. These pitch energy locations are both in modulation frequency (at the respective speaker's pitch rate and its harmonics) and in acoustic frequency (at the respective speaker's resonant frequencies). For example, it is clear that for the signal duration analyzed in Figure 4, the higher pitch (about 100–130 Hz modulation frequency) talker B has a first formant at less than 1 kHz acoustic frequency and a second formant at 3–4 kHz acoustic frequency. Since it is possible to arbitrarily modify and invert this transform [8], the clear separability of the regions of sonorant sounds from different simultaneous talkers can be used to design talker–separation mask filters.

Figure 5 illustrates an example of an application of a talker-separation mask filter. Typically, several 450 millisecond segments are processed in this matter. The segments are overlapped and the mask is independently chosen for each new segment.

Even though the reconstruction used the phase of the original two-talker speech, the English talker greatly dominates the reconstructed speech and little Spanish speech remains. However, these practical problems remain:

1. There is potential overlap between modulation spectral regions representing the two talkers. If the talkers' pitches where closer than seen in the example above, the overlap would be greater. Having graded (non-binary) talker

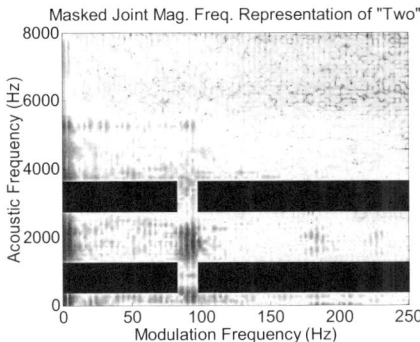
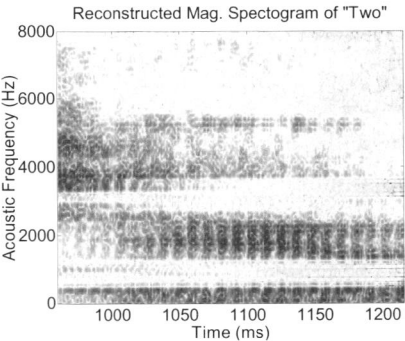

Figure 5. Example of application of a talker separation modulation mask filter. The left panel is the same modulation spectrum as seen in the right panel in figure 4, with a multiplicative mask overlaying areas which are set to zero. These zero-mask areas are assumed to represent mainly the speech of the Spanish talker. The right panel represents a spectrogram of the reconstructed speech from this masked modulation spectrum.

removal masks, which would allow for partial removal in areas of overlap, would potentially ameliorate this problem.

2. The talker removal mask areas change with time. While this change is relatively slow, about 4 times per second, automatic determination of the talker removal mask is an unsolved problem. In our own examples we visually inspected the modulation spectrum and found that it was easy for a human observer to determine the mask regions. However, this does not imply that it would be easy to automate this task. Further investigation is needed to determine automated schemes to determine talker removal masks and the relation between these masks and automatic pitch estimates.

This masking approach is related to the modulation maps proposed by Meyer *et al.* [12]. In their approach, modulation spectra were used to segregate concurrent vowels for machine recognition. The approach described above, being an analysis/synthesis approach, also offers modified speech output where undesired talkers are masked out.

4. Speech Modification

Psychoacoustic evidence [13] indicates that the shape of perceptual modulation filters approximately imitate a constant–Q bandwidth. Also, results in speech recognition studies point to advantages of a modulation wavelet transform in automatic speech recognition [14]. For audio coding purposes, we recently have proposed the use of an octave–band non-uniform modulation transform to mimic the spacing of modulation filter subbands of the human auditory system [15]. This non-uniform second stage transform is depicted in the structure of Figure 6. The use of a non-uniform second transform leads to a resulting representation which generates three dimensions: acoustic frequency, modulation scale, and modulation time–shift. This approach preserves phase, which has previously been found to be important [16], of the modulation spectrum, via a potentially decimated (the amount of decimation depends upon the scale) modulation time–

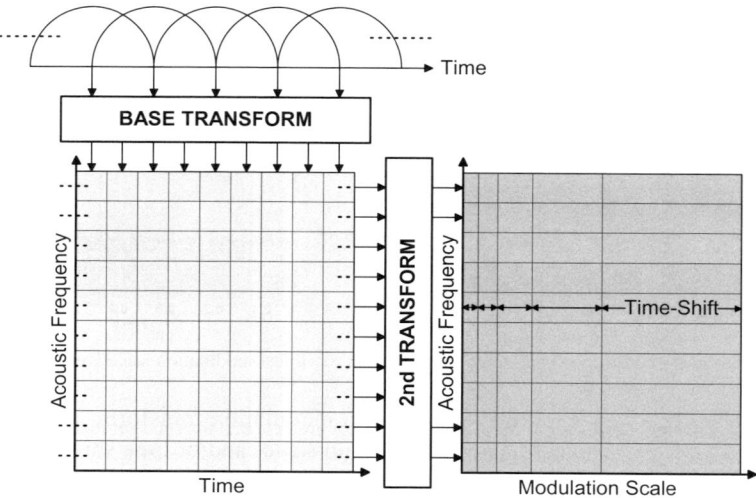

Figure 6. Structure of the proposed non-uniform modulation transform resulting in three dimensions: acoustic frequency, modulation scale, and modulation time–shift. Note that the second transform is only on the magnitude of the base transform.

shift waveform.

A hierarchical lapped transform (HLT) [17] is used for the second stage transform of Figure 6. The HLT is a multi-resolution transform which maintains good time localization for high frequency components and good frequency resolution for low frequency components.

The HLT is similar in structure to a quadrature–mirror filter bank (QMF) and the wavelet filter bank. The HLT is applied on the magnitude values in each acoustic frequency sub-band of the time–frequency representation as shown in Figure 3. Note that the HLT second transform is not performed on the phase values from the base transform.

Figure 7 shows an example of the above modulation spectrum applied to the spoken letter "k." Note that the plosive burst is clearly seen at the finer scales of modulation.

Filtering in modulation spectra can be effected by simply masking chosen coeffi-

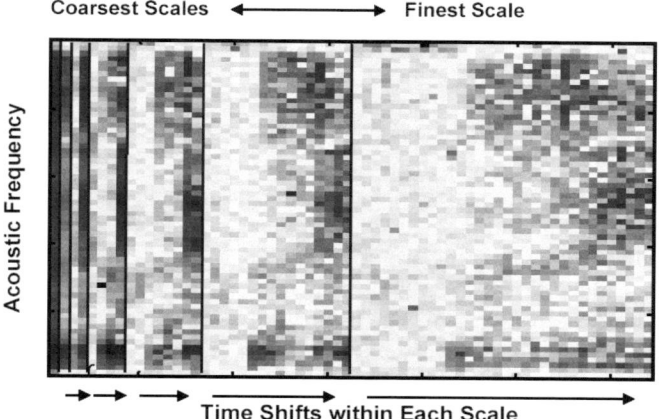

Figure 7. The non-uniform modulation transform.

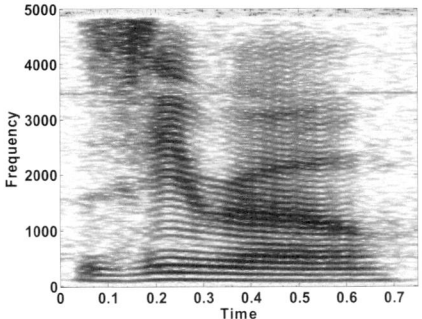 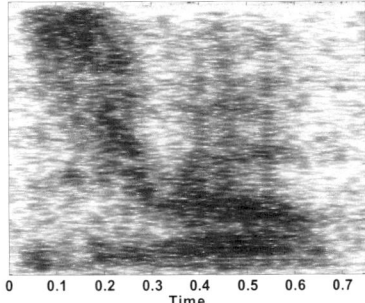

Figure 8. Spectrograms before (left) and after (right) all but the finest modulation scale were removed from the spoken sound "zero."

cients which result after the above non-uniform modulation transform, if the mask is chosen to only have dependency upon modulation scale (and/or time shift). For example, Figure 8 shows spectrograms of the spoken sound "zero" before and after filtering out all modulation scales except for the finest scale. (All time shifts for this finest modulation scale were retained.) Quite notably, the filtered sound is highly intelligible yet virtually all sensation of pitch is removed. This observation raises questions about the kind of basis functions which are appropriate for the modulation dimension. It also suggests a highly redundant representation across modulation scales.

Figure 9 shows the effect of severe lowpass filtering in modulation. As expected, speech transitions were blurred in time. Harmonic structure was maintained and unvoiced and mixed voiced regions were extended in time. A negative observation seen in the artifacts present at about 0.4, 1.6, and 2.8 seconds. These audible artifacts were due to the filtered transform time envelopes becoming negative. While the analysis

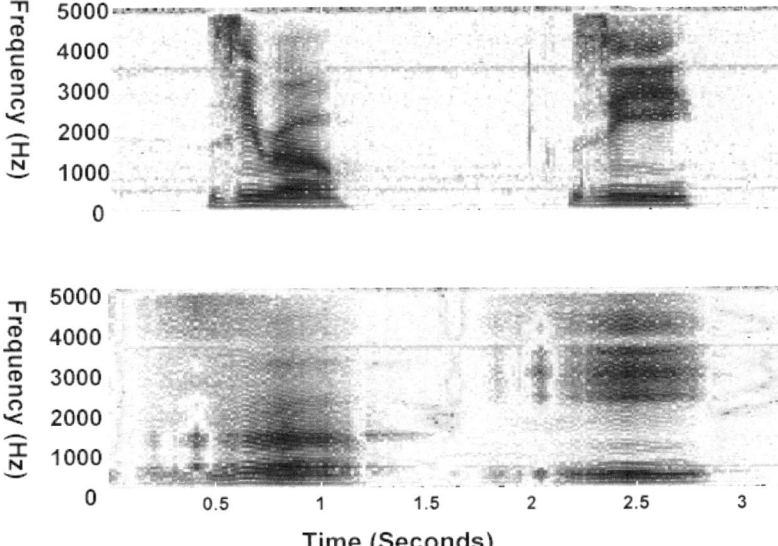

Figure 9. Spectrograms of speech before (top panel) and after (bottom panel) severe lowpass modulation filtering of the spoken sound "zero" then "zee."

assumes that the time envelope for each transform index is non-negative, the use of an arbitrary filter in modulation does not ensure non-negativity. While it may be possible under some conditions to restrict modulation filter choices to one which ensures non-negativity, a more general approach would be to define temporal envelopes to be more general negative and even complex functions.

5. Conclusions

We have described the underlying conditions for an invertible modulation spectral transform. This transform, with linear spacing in modulation frequency, was applied to single–channel talker separation. We then extend the transform to a non-uniform (or scale) spacing in modulation and demonstrate its potential to represent and modify speech in new ways.

The current understanding of what is meant by "modulation spectral filtering" is incomplete. For example, Drullman *et al.* [6] take a vocoding type of view where envelopes of sub-bands are smeared. Yet we take an alternative transform–based view in this paper and in our previous audio coding work (e.g. [15]). While we would argue that the transform approach can provide a more distortion-free solution, distortion still exists. For example, as shown in the spectrogram of the modulation low passed signal in Figure 9, severe lowpass filtering in modulation causes the supposedly positive envelope of the reconstructed signal to attempt to go negative.

It is clear that results of modulation filtering depend upon sub-band widths and transform window sizes. For example, if the base transform used in Figure 2 is doubled in length, while maintaining the same amount of overlap, the frequency resolution increases and the boundary point between lower modulation frequency and higher acoustic frequency is decreased by ½. Similar observations hold for vocoding types of approaches, but are mathematically more complex when sub-bands are not of uniform width. However, even with an assumption of this boundary, we still need a single definition of modulation frequency and modulation filtering. This chapter suggests that modulation filtering and frequency provide new approaches to speech manipulation and representation, respectively. However, if these approaches are to gain the design power and utility of standard frequency filtering, deeper foundations and definitions of modulation frequency be needed.

Acknowledgements

This research was supported by the Office of Naval Research. We'd like to thank Drs. Shihab Shamma and Steven Greenberg for their helpful discussions and Somsak Sukittanon, Jeff Thompson, Qin Li, and Steven Schimmel for their helpful discussions and figures.

References

[1] Zadeh, L. "Frequency analysis of variable networks." *Proc. IRE* 38(3): 291–299, 1950.
[2] Kailath, T. "Channel characterization: Time–variant dispersive channels." In *Lectures on Communication System Theory*, E. Baghdady (ed)., New York: McGraw-Hill, pp. 95–123, 1961.
[3] Gardner, W. *Statistical Spectral Analysis: A Non-probabilistic Theory.* Englewood Cliffs, NJ: Prentice-Hall, 1987.

[4] Gardner, W. "Exploitation of spectral redundancy in cyclostationary signals." *IEEE Signal Processing Magazine*, April, pp. 14–36, 1991.

[5] Houtgast, T. and Steeneken, H. "The modulation transfer function in room acoustics as a predictor of speech intelligibility." *Acustica* 28: 66–73, 1973.

[6] Drullman, R., Festen, J., and Plomp, R., "Effect of temporal envelope smearing on speech reception," *J. Acoust. Soc. Am.* 95, 1053–1064, 1994.

[7] Greenberg, S. and Kingsbury, B.E.D., "The modulation spectrogram: In pursuit of an invariant representation of speech." *Proc. ICASSP*, pp. 1647–1650, 1997.

[8] Vinton, M. and Atlas, L. "A scalable and progressive audio codec." *Proc. ICASSP*, 2001.

[9] Princen, J. and Bradley, A. "Analysis/synthesis filter bank design based on time domain aliasing cancellation." *IEEE Trans. Acoust., Speech, and Signal Processing*, 34: 1153–1161, 1986.

[10] Lee, T., Bell, A. and Lambert, R., "Blind separation of delayed and convolved sources." In *Advances in Neural Information Processing Systems*, Vol. 9, Cambridge, MA: MIT Press, pp. 758–764, 1997.

[11] www.cnl.salk.edu/~tewon/Blind/blind_audio.html.

[12] Meyer, G.F., Plante, F. and Berthommier, F. "Segregation of concurrent speech with the reassigned spectrum." *Proc. ICASSP*, pp. 1203–1206, 1997.

[13] Houtgast, T. "Frequency selectivity in amplitude–modulation detection." *J. Acoust. Soc. Am.* 85: 1676–1680, 1989.

[14] Okada, K., Arai, T., Kanedera, N., Momomura, Y. and Murahara, Y., "Using the modulation wavelet transform for feature extraction in automatic speech recognition," *Proc. ICSLP*, pp. 337–340, 2000.

[15] Thompson, J. and Atlas, L. "A Non-uniform modulation transform for audio coding with increased time resolution." *Proc. IEEE ICASSP*, Hong Kong, 2003.

[16] Greenberg, S. and Arai, T. "The relation between speech intelligibility and the complex modulation spectrum." *Proc. Eurospeech* , pp. 473–476, 2001.

[17] Malvar, H. *Signal Processing with Lapped Transforms*. Boston: Artech House, 1992.

Dynamics of Speech Production and Perception
P. Divenyi et al. (Eds.)
IOS Press, 2006

Data-Driven Extraction of Temporal Features from Speech

Hynek HERMANSKY

IDIAP Research Institute, Martigny, Switzerland
and
Ecole Polytechnique Fédérale de Lausanne, Switzerland

Abstract. Conventional features in automatic recognition of speech describe the instantaneous shape of a short-term spectrum of speech and the pattern classification module is relying on information extracted from large amounts of acoustic and text training data. The article describes an alternative approach where the feature extraction module is trained on data. These data-derived features are consistent with auditory-like frequency resolution and with temporal properties of human hearing. The features describe instantaneous likelihoods of sub-word classes and are derived from temporal trajectories of band-limited spectral densities in the vicinity of the given instant. The paper presents some rationale behind the data-driven approach, briefly describes the technique, points to relevant publications and summarizes results achieved so far.

Keywords. Model of hearing, temporal aspects of speech perception, automatic speech recognition, class-posterior based speech features, auditory perception and properties of speech signal

Introduction

Machine that automatically decodes the linguistic information remains an elusive engineering goal for many decades. Workers in automatic recognition of speech (ASR) face a similar challenge as human cognitive system does, i.e. to decode the information in the one-dimensional signal. In spite of that, ASR processing of a speech signal is different from the way the speech signal is handled in human speech communication. This is partly because many aspects of human information processing are becoming to be known only recently and many are still shrouded in mystery.

Limited knowledge of human speech communication process did not stop successful and profitable engineering applications of speech processing. In speech coding, the genius of inventors of telephony was in emulating the actions of the outer and middle ear and in converting the changes in the acoustic pressure into changes in electric current. The electric signal then could be transmitted and/or stored and used for reconstruction of the acoustic signal that closely resembles the original. Over the years, various techniques of digitizing and of efficient coding of the digitized electric signal evolved and are in daily use. Most of efficient speech coding techniques first convert speech signal to a sequence of short-term spectral vectors, each vector describing frequency content of a single short segment of speech. Aspects of these short-term spectral vectors are extracted and transmitted to the receiver, where the speech is reconstructed.

Since ASR evolved from speech coding, the feature extraction module in ASR typically resembles techniques from speech coding. The speech signal is first chopped into a short segments and the shape of the short-term spectral density is derived to yield data for the subsequent pattern classification. Thus, the one-dimensional speech signal is converted into a sequence of short-term spectral vectors, each vector describing frequency content of a single short segment of speech. This short-term spectral vector is typically transformed by series of ad-hoc transformations into the feature vector for the subsequent pattern classification. The local spectral dynamics in included by use of the first (delta) and the second (delta-delta) temporal derivatives of the feature trajectory in the vicinity of the current element [14].

In the currently dominant stochastic ASR, the sequential pattern classification module is applied to decode the information in feature vectors. This is done by first obtaining likelihoods of sub-word elements (states of the stochastic hidden Markov model), used in the search for the best fitting hypothesis about the uttered sound sequence. The information is decoded by finding the most likely path through the lattice of these discrete elements while respecting the prior knowledge about the possible distribution of the elements. The global dynamics of speech is emulated by sequential organization of the elements.

The pattern classification module is relying on information extracted from large amounts of acoustic and text training data. Elaborate ASR systems, capable of acquiring and summarizing the information contained in large amounts of training data, have been developed. Still, existing ASR-based human-machine interfaces are inadequate, fragile and unreliable in many realistic situations and environments encountered in human-human interactions. This prevents the wide acceptance of ASR technology by general public.

Most of techniques employed in ASR are in many aspects inconsistent with hearing. We believe that improved understanding of the ways human perceptual system processes cognitive signals such as speech and images and of the methods of emulating such human-like processing by the machine would to necessary improvements of the human-machine communications. Given the knowledge about human auditory system, we would like to question some of the aspects of the current approach, and to suggest possible alternatives, more in line with the current knowledge of human hearing.

Why should the knowledge of human hearing help in ASR? The human perceptual system appears to be optimally suited for decoding the information conveyed by sensory signals [3][36]. Following human-like strategies in processing the cognitive signals is therefore a reasonable engineering approach towards improvements of human-machine interface. Some of the aspects of hearing such as the nonlinear (critical-band like) frequency resolution or compressive nonlinearity between acoustic stimulus and its percept are well accepted by speech engineering community. Several times in the career of the author it happened that optimizing the ASR system resulted in processing that is consistent with human hearing. Some of this experience is summarized in the sections below.

1. Short-term Spectrum of Speech

An important (and well accepted) model of human speech communication uses a concept of resonance frequencies of the vocal tract (formants). The formants show in the short-term spectrum as peaks of the short-term spectral envelope. Accurate emulation of time-varying formants yields intelligible speech [30, 8]. Over the years, the concept of a linear model of speech production and the emphasis on short-term spectral envelopes of speech dominate the field and finding the spectral envelopes of speech forms basis of many speech coding techniques.

As discussed above, most current ASR devices use stochastic pattern matching of features, which are derived from short-term spectral envelopes of speech sounds. The short-term spectral envelope is usually modified by nonlinear warping of its frequency (Mel or Bark scale) and amplitude axes (logarithm) and projected on cosine spectral basis (computation of so-called cepstrum) that decorrelate the feature space.

A single frame of short term spectrum does not contain all the information that is necessary for decoding the phonetic value of a given segment of speech. This is because the neighboring speech sounds influence the short-term spectrum of the current sound. The mechanical inertia of human speech production organs (coarticulation) results is significant spreading of linguistic information in time (our current estimates are of the order of several hundreds of ms [44]). Given the typical phoneme rate of about 15 phonemes per second, this means that at any given time, at least 3-5 phonemes interact. Some studies indicate that the within class variability is comparable in magnitude to the across-class variability among phoneme classes [32]. The coarticulation effects, combined with many additional sources of nonlinguistic variability such as speaker identity and the effects of the acoustic environment, all contribute to high within-phoneme variability of the instantaneous spectral envelope. Subsequently, coding of linguistic information in a single short-term spectrum of speech appears to be rather complex.

ASR attempts to classify phonemes from individual slices of the short-term spectrum and needs to deal with this within-class variability. This is often done by increasing number of sounds to be classified, e.g. by introducing so called context-dependent phonemes and by sub-dividing phonemes into several parts, each of which is emulated by a separate model. Both techniques lead to more complex ASR models. However, human listeners appear to be able to identify phonemes independently of their context [12] in spite of large variability introduced by the coarticulation with the neighboring phonemes. This observation suggests that the coarticulation effects, while clearly evident in temporal evolution of spectral envelopes, may not present the same problem in human speech perception that they do in current ASR.

While there is no doubt that the auditory periphery is frequency selective, it is not clear that its main purpose is the deriving short-term spectrum of the acoustic signal. Even though for steady sounds it may be possible to find some correlation between the shape of the sound spectrum and the level of activity on the auditory nerve, this correlation weakens when the sound intensity approaches levels encountered in speech communication [40]. It seems more likely that (consistently with color separation in vision) the selectivity of hearing is used for separating the reliable (high SNR) part of the signal from the unreliable ones. This is supported by the findings that for normal sound levels, temporal aspects of the sound need to be explored in order to account for the sound spectral shape in mammalian hearing [45].

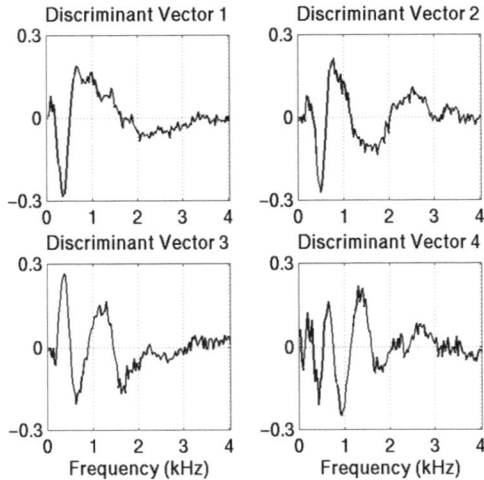

Figure 1. Spectral basis vector derived by data-driven LDA technique.

2. Spectral Aspects of Information in Speech Signal

ASR community is currently settled on two dominant and similar spectral processing techniques, the Mel cepstrum [38][10] and PLP [16]. Both techniques employ auditory-like warping of short-term spectrum of speech, yielding higher spectral resolution at lower frequencies. The need for such non-uniform spectral resolution in ASR seems well established through years of comparative experiments. To measure the benefit of one particular spectral warping optimal requires running a number of ASR experiments. Such optimization is costly and there is no guarantee that the solutions obtained will not be specific to a given ASR system. Therefore, we use a data-based optimization, which avoids using a specific ASR paradigm. Such a technique is based on linear discriminant analysis (LDA), which is a stochastic technique that attempts to optimize the linear dis-criminability between classes in the presence of undesirable within-class variability (see e.g. [25][5] for some examples of previous use of LDA in ASR).

LDA, applied to short-term spectral vectors from FFT analysis of OGI Stories data-base (OGI Stories contain about 3 hours of fluent American English telephone-quality speech from more than 200 adult speakers of both genders, hand-labeled by phonemes) yields the spectral basis illustrated in Figure 1. Notice that these spectral bases oscillate around zero faster at lower frequencies. Subsequently, speech analysis that employs such spectral basis has higher spectral resolution at lower frequencies. [35][36] show that the spectral resolution implied by spectral basis in Figure 1 is very similar to spec-tral resolution of auditory-like Bark frequency scale. This finding supports earlier results [43] that derived auditory-like frequency warping by minimizing differences between speeches from different talkers.

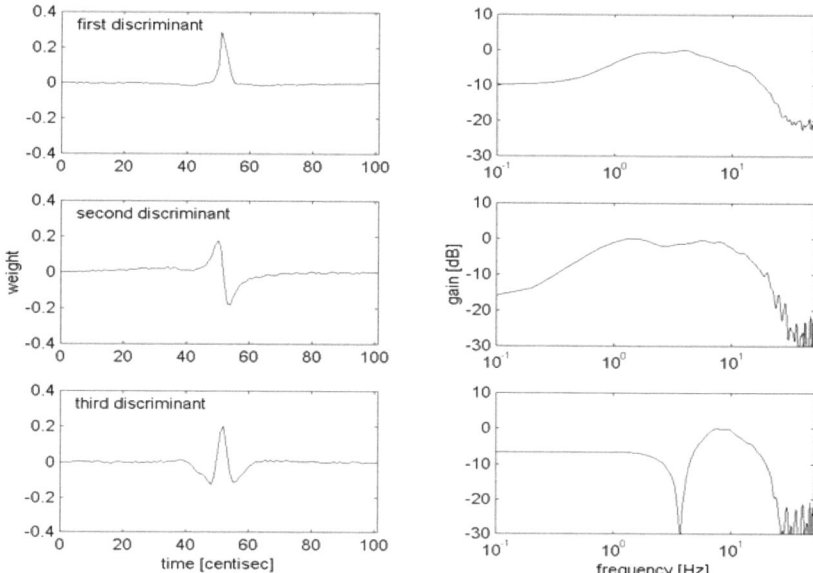

Figure 2. Impulse and frequency responses of the first three discriminant vectors from the LDA-derived discriminant matrix. The filters for the 5 Bark frequency channel are shown here. Filters for the other carrier frequencies studied (between 1 and 14 Bark) are very similar.

3. Temporal Aspects of Information in the Speech Signal

The relatively fast changes in the acoustic pressure (20-20000 Hz) are merely the carrier of the acoustic information that is to be extracted from the signal. In human speech, the fast changes are caused by action of voice source (e.g. vocal cords in the case of voiced sounds). The slower modulations of the speech signal that carry the actual linguistic information result from movements of vocal tract. Therefore the information that we are interested in machine recognition of speech is mostly encoded in the relatively slow modulations (below 50 Hz and likely not much higher than 10 Hz) of the acoustic wave [33]. Many perceptual phenomena such as forward masking, growth of loudness, detection of constant energy stimuli, or binaural release from masking, exhibit time constants of several hundreds of milliseconds. As discussed later in this article, such time constants most likely originate at higher levels of neural systems. Thus, the human hearing apparatus seems to have right properties for decoding the slow modulation changes.

3.1 Data-guided design of RASTA-like filters

RASTA processing filters the time trajectories of speech features to attenuate the features with rate-of-change that is not expected for speech. The initial ad hoc form of the RASTA filters [24] was optimized on a relatively small series of ASR experiments with noisy telephone digits. We later realized that it is possible to structure the LDA problem in such a way that the LDA solution can be interpreted as a set of FIR RASTA-like filters, which are applied on time trajectories of spectral energies. This happens when the labeled vector space for LDA analysis is created by extracting temporal vectors cut out from trajectories of logarithmic critical-band spectral energy over a relatively long (typically about 1 second) span of time. Each vector typically spans much more than a single phoneme, and is labeled by the phoneme at the center of the vector.

Having formed such 101-dimensional (each vector spans about 1 s at 100 Hz sampling frequency) vector space with vectors labeled by their respective phoneme classes, LDA analysis yields a 101 X 101 scatter matrix, decomposed into its principal components. Then the principal vectors represent FIR filters, which most efficiently (with respect to the within-class and the across-class variability) map the 101-dimensional input space to several points of the output space.

Frequency responses of the first three FIR filters derived from OGI Stories database are shown in Figure 2. Filters for different frequency channels are similar. The frequency characteristic (shown at in the right part of the Figure) are generally consistent with RASTA [24], and delta, and double-delta feature of speech [14]. However, the impulse responses of the data-derived filters shown in the upper left part of the figure suggest preference for the zero-phase filters. Effective parts of the impulse responses appear to span at least 250 ms.

The general characteristics of the data-derived RASTA filters appear to be relatively independent of the particular database used for their design. The most important processing involves a mild temporal lateral inhibition in which the average of several spectral values around the current time instant is subtracted from the weighted average of spectral values from surrounding past and future contexts. This gives a mild band-pass filter as shown in the upper right of the figure. The second discriminant vector computes the difference between weighted averages from left and right contexts of the current frame (the first derivative of the first discriminant vector). The third discriminant vector is an aggressive mexican hat temporal lateral suppression (the second derivative of the first discriminant vector) implying quite narrow band-pass filter with 12 dB/oct slope. Such dynamics-enhancing functions are hypothesized to be important for scene interpretation by human visual system [37]. These three vectors correspond to RASTA filtering with subsequent computation of the first (delta) and the second (delta-delta) dynamic features [14].

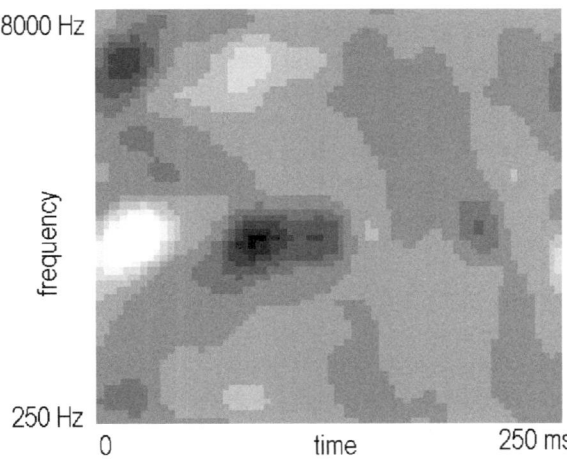

Figure 3. A cortical receptive field, observed in the auditory cortex of ferret (courtesy of David Klein).

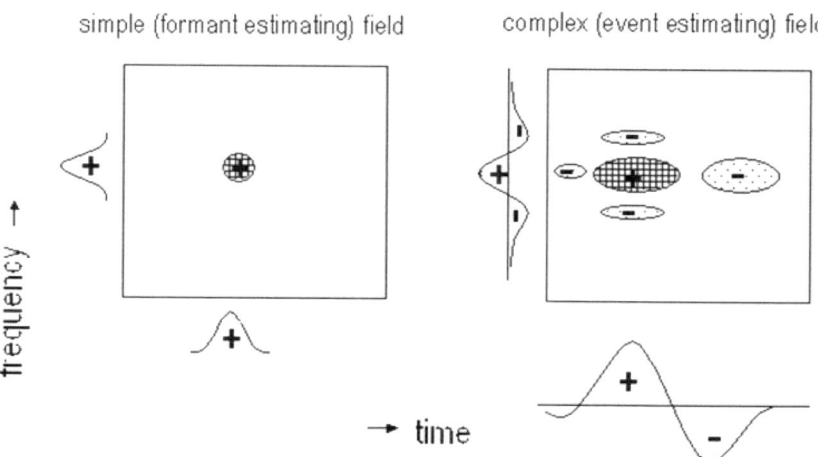

Figure 4. Schematic examples of simple and more complex receptive fields.

4. Spectro-temporal Aspects of Auditory Processing

The current knowledge about cortical responses to acoustic stimuli (cortical receptive fields) [e.g. 11, 31, 9] suggests that the auditory system is most likely to produce responses to specific time-and-frequency localized combinations of spectral densities in the time-frequency plane (acoustic events). One cortical field is shown in Figure 4 (1). It shows the spectro-temporal pattern of the auditory stimulus that is most likely to cause firing of the particular cortical neuron. The neuron merely detecting energy at the given time and frequency (e.g. the formant in speech) would have receptive field with a single high region at the given frequency and close to beginning of the temporal axis, the rest of the field would be close to zero. Such neurons do exist, but most cortical neurons have receptive fields far more complex than that. The length of a typical receptive field is up to several hundreds of milliseconds, thus easily spanning the time span of speech coarticulation. Both the time and the frequency resolution of the individual receptive fields vary rather widely with medians somewhere around 200 ms and 1 octave [9].

These relatively recent findings about the physiology of auditory cortex may have important implications in ASR. Since neurons in the auditory cortex respond best to certain kinds of acoustic signals (e.g. [31]), they seem to act as a kind of two-dimensional matched filter that detects the existence of a particular pattern (acoustic event) in the incoming signal. Then, just as a certain combination of formants indicate certain steady vowel sound; a certain combination of particular events could indicate certain dynamic acoustic event such as realistic dynamic phoneme of the language.

To elaborate this notion further, think about a vowel formant as one particular type of an acoustic event, characterized by a rather trivial time-frequency localized pattern consisting of high vocalic energy at the given time instant and at frequencies in the neighborhood of the formant frequency. A receptive filed responding to the instantaneous formant position is shown in the left part of Figure 4.

Typical cortical receptive field is more complex than a single short excitatory region. As described earlier, the cortical receptive fields span up to several hundreds of ms and up to several octaves and exhibits not only excitatory but also inhibitory regions. Cortical neurons associated with such receptive fields would optimally respond to complex acoustic events.

Thus, to account for such complexity we need to replace formants by more complex spectro-temporal events as carriers of linguistic information in speech. Such broadly defined events are characterized by complex time-frequency patterns, involving times other than the current instant.

5.   ASR Based on Complex Spectro-temporal Patterns

Now, how do we use this notion of complex time-frequency acoustic events in an automatic speech recognizer? First, we need to realize the needs of state-of-the-art stochastic recognizers. Ideally, the ASR system expects within state uncorrelated and normally distributed features every 10 ms or so. Further, the feature vectors should be low-dimensional so that the subsequent pattern classifier is also small and could be trained on a finite amount of training data. The smallest set of features for classification is posterior probabilities of the classes to be classified [13]. So we need a module capable examining relatively long spans of speech signal within various frequency bands to deliver every 10 ms or so posterior probabilities of particular temporal events within such bands and to convert these posteriors to a small set of uncorrelated and normally distributed features.

5.1 TRAP-TANDEM technique

A step in this direction is the TRAP-TANDEM and related techniques [18, 20]. A schematic picture of the TRAP-TANDEM techniques is shown in Figure 5. The TRAP (standing for TempoRAl Pattern) refers to a particular way in which the linguistic information is extracted from the speech data. In a conventional speech analysis, the spectral shape of full-band spectrum a short segment (about 10-20 ms) of speech signal is used to provide evidence for the subsequent stochastic recognition techniques. In TRAP, the evidence is derived from a relatively long (500-1000 ms) and frequency-localized (1-3 Bark) overlapping time-frequency regions of the signal. The TANDEM refers to a way of converting the frequency-localized evidence to features for the HMM-based ASR system. The name TANDEM reflects the fact that the classifier is used in tandem with

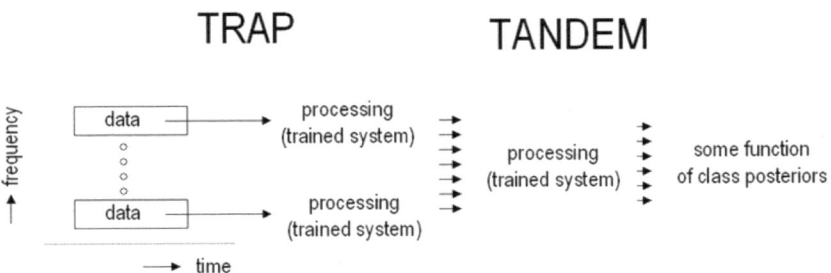

Figure 5. TRAP-TANDEM feature extraction

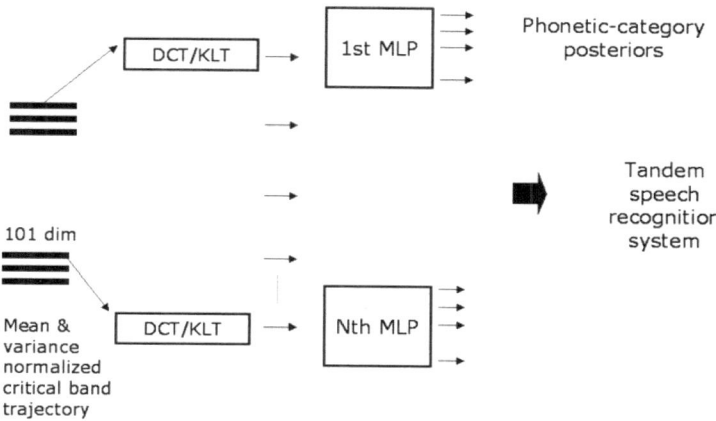

Figure 6. TRAP module

the conventional HMM-based classifier. Both the TRAP and the TANDEM modules are trained on development data.

Why would we attempt to derive speech features from time intervals as long as 1 s? Because the information about the underlying sub-word classes (phonemes) spreads at least over the interval of 200-300 ms. This has been demonstrated by Bilmes [4] and confirmed by Yang et al. [44]. Since the derived features will be used for classification into phoneme-like classes, it makes sense to collect the evidence from all the data points which carry the information, hence at least 300 ms. But why even longer time interval? Because we want to remove the information about slowly varying noise (subtract the mean) from the data. This harmful information is in modulation spectrum below 1 Hz [33], hence 1 s.

Why should we abandon the short-term spectrum of speech? First, the envelope of the short-term spectrum is notoriously unreliable in presence of common distortions such as the distortions caused by frequency response of communication equipment or by frequency localized noise. Fletcher [12] (and many after him) demonstrated that uncorrelated noise outside the critical band has only a negligible effect on detection of the signal within the critical band. He further proposes that errors in human recognition of nonsense syllables within relatively narrow articulatory spectral bands (each articulatory band spanning about 2 critical bands) are independent. Hence, the first stage of processing of acoustic signals seems to happen on frequency-localized regions of the signal.

Why do we need to train the analysis module to derive features that will then be used in another trained stochastic system? Because the more knowledge we build into the feature extraction module, the less we need to train the subsequent stochastic recognizer. Our knowledge about coding of information in speech signal is still incomplete. As evidenced by the success of data-driven stochastic pattern classification and language modeling methods (see e.g. [29] for details), using incorrect prior knowledge may be worse than using no prior knowledge at all, and rather to derive all the required knowledge a posteriori from the data. Enough speech data, labeled with respect to the targeted linguistic message (either by hand or by forced alignment procedures) is available and can provide the feature extraction module with speech-specific knowledge.

5.2 Details of the technique

5.2.1 TRAP

At the moment, the time-frequency spectral density plane uses the front end module from PLP analysis [16]. It does the short-time spectral analysis of the speech signal with a subsequent Bark-like summation of the spectral components. However, there is a recently emerging interesting alternative for estimating temporal evolution of critical band spectral density that completely eliminates the short-term spectral analysis is the frequency domain linear prediction [2].

The input to the TRAP estimator is formed from time trajectories of critical-band energies. Some benefits are seen when more than one time trajectory is used as an input. The PCA analysis of the data suggests in this case, that to preserve most of the variability in the multiple-trajectory data, the data from the individual trajectories should be averaged and differentiated, in effect crudely describing the spectral shape in the vicinity of the frequency of interest [28, 15]. The most successful dimensionality reduction has been so far the cosine transform that typically allows for at least 50% reduction of the input data.

The TRAP technique is depicted in Figure 6. Figure 7 schematically shows a few principal bases, resulting from the PCA analysis on three concatenated trajectories of critical band spectral densities. As seen in the figure, the lower KLT bases represent cosine transform on averaged temporal trajectories; some higher ones represent cosine transform on differentiated trajectories. It is interesting, that even though the differentiating bases account for relatively little variability, their elimination results in noticeable worsening of the performance [28, 27].

TRAP estimators, using multi-layer perceptrons, deliver vectors of posterior probabilities of sub-word acoustic events, each estimated at the particular individual frequency. The events targeted by TRAP estimators are most common American English phonemes clustered into 6 broad phonetic classes [1, 27] and a separate estimator is trained for each frequency region of interest. More recently, there are efforts to derive a single "universal" estimator, which could be used at all frequencies of interest [19]. This would be much more in line with our "event" concept outlined above.

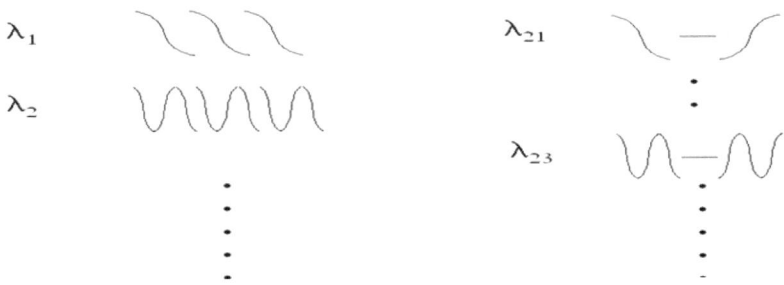

Figure 7. Schematic illustration of basis functions of the KLT transform derived for the three-band TRAP input

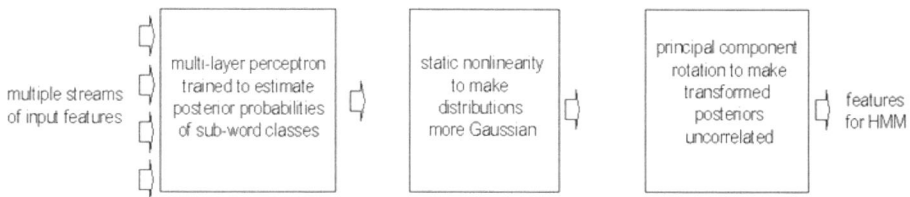

Figure 8. TANDEM technique for deriving features for HMM-based ASR

5.2.2 TANDEM

Techniques based on optimal rotation of feature space such as linear discriminant analysis (LDA) have been used in feature extraction in ASR for quite some time [25, 5]. A nonlinear alternative to LDA is a multi-layer Perceptron (MLP) trained in one-high, rest-low paradigm. When properly trained, such MLP estimates posterior probabilities of classes of interest [6, 7].

The MLP posterior probability estimates are gaussianized by a static nonlinearity and whitened by the KL transform derived from training data. Such gaussianized and whitened posterior probabilities form the feature vector for the subsequent HMM recognizer.

Thus, in TRAP-TANDEM we are replacing the conventional features derived from a spectral density vector representing the spectral envelope, by a matrix of transformed posteriors of acoustic events (in the original concept the events were context-independent phonemes). If the targeted events are independent, the output of the trained TANDEM MLP could represent an estimate of the efficient low-entropy statistically-independent code, hypothesized in perceptual processing [3, 34].

The events targeted by the TRAP estimators may be but do not need to be the same at the events targeted by the TANDEM estimator. At the moment, the events targeted by the TRAP are broad phonetic classes where the targets for the TANDEM estimator are typically context-independent American English phonemes. Also, TRAP estimators can be (and often are) trained on different database than the database used in training the TANDEM estimator. Both the TRAP and the TANDEM estimators are nonlinear feed-forward Multi-Layer Perceptron (Quicknet [26]) discriminative classifiers. Hierarchical classification schemes in TANDEM estimator were also investigated [42].

The TRAP-TANDEM features have been so far found most useful in combination with the conventional spectrum-based (PLP, Mel Cepstrum,..) features. Thus, e.g. the system with TRAP-TANDEM module was shown to perform the best among all presented feature extraction techniques (including the official standard accepted by European Telecommunications Standards Institute) on the small vocabulary Aurora task [1]. More recently, the TRAP-TANDEM features were successfully used in DARPA EARS program, where they brought about 10% relative improvement in error rate [39].

On the small vocabulary continuous OGI Numbers task, the three-band TRAP-TANDEM system yields the same (5%) word error rate as the best system with the conventional (PLP+delta+ddelta) features [27, 28]. In phoneme-string recognition without use of any language model on TIMIT database, using TRAP features in the PLP-HMM hybrid system gave about 10% relative improvement in phoneme error rate, comparing to the best multiframe Mel cepstral features [41].

6. Discussion and Conclusions

Short-term spectrum of speech and its spectral envelopes have been basis of features for ASR since its beginning. Gradually, auditory-like modifications of is frequency resolution [38] and of its amplitude axis [16], together with attempts for describing temporal dynamics of spectral envelopes [14] have emerged and been accepted by the engineering community. The current article shows that these modifications are supported by the character of speech signal. Namely, the nonlinear (critical-band like) spectral resolution as well as the description of spectral dynamics by local temporal derivatives emerges from the phoneme-based linear discriminant analysis of speech spectro-temporal plane. Moreover, these analyses also show the dominance of low (1-12 Hz) modulation frequencies in coding the phoneme-related information in speech with the subsequent need for relatively long (up to 1 second) segments of the speech signal when extracting this information from the signal. Further speculative reasoning then leads to abandoning the spectral envelope altogether, replacing it by frequency-specific posterior probabilities of speech-related events. That all then leads to a new data-driven feature extraction technique called TRAP-TANDEM which derives ASR features related to posterior probabilities of context-independent phoneme classes.

In several aspects, TRAP-TANDEM represents a significant conceptual departure from the current practice in feature extraction for ASR.

- The knowledge used for feature extraction is not coming from beliefs and convictions of the designer but is derived from development data. The goal here is to derive and to put into the feature extraction module the speech-specific but task-independent knowledge. In this way, the subsequent pattern classification module needs to learn only the task-specific knowledge, possibly reducing the need for the re-learning the same knowledge again and again each time the task changes.

- Derived features do not represent the shape of the short-term spectral envelope of speech. Instead, in the early stages of the feature extraction, the frequency-localized evidence is converted to frequency-localized estimates of posterior probabailities of speech events (the TRAP part). These estimates are then used in later stages of the feature extraction (the TANDEM part). In that way, many vulnerabilities of the short-term spectral envelope of speech (discussed earlier in this paper) are alleviated.

- Evidence used for deriving the features does not come from relatively short segments of speech representing a short part of the underlying sub-word class (phoneme). Instead the time span employed covers the typical coarticulation span of the phoneme. In that way, each feature vector carries most of the available information about the underlying phoneme.

- Final features represent estimates of posterior probabilities of sub-word classes postulated in the subsequent HMM-based pattern classification. In that way, the feature set can be smaller and the burden on the subsequent HMM classifier is reduced.

The TANDEM-TRAP technique is still evolving and in order to get the most out of it, it may require some evolution in the existing ASR approach. However, it is already beneficial for the existing mainstream HMM-based ASR. Unlike the conventional feature extraction approaches, it is consistent with the current knowledge of higher cognitive levels of mammalian auditory perception. We hope that it receives critical attention of the ASR community.

Acknowledgements

The insights presented in this chapter come from research of many of my colleagues, most of them hopefully acknowledged through references to their works. Works of my former students Sangita Sharma, Pratibha Jain, and Sunil Sivadas are particularly relevant. Writing of the paper was supported by Swiss National Center of Competence in Research on Interactive Multimodal Information Management, by DIRAC Integrated Project in the 6th Program of the European Commission, and by DARPA GALE program. The text greatly benefited from a critical review by Malcolm Slaney.

References

[1]   Adami, A., Burget, L., Dupont, S., Garudadri, H., Grezl, F., Hermansky, H., Jain, P., Kajarekar, S., Morgan, N. and S. Sivadas, S. "QUALCOMM-ICSI-OGI Features for ASR." *Proc. Int. Conf. Spoken Lang. Proc.,* 2002.

[2]   Athineos, M. and Ellis, D. "Frequency-domain linear prediction for temporal features." *Proc. IEEE Workshop Automatic Speech Recognition and Understanding,* 2003

[3]   Atick, J.J. "Could information theory provide an ecological theory of sensory processing?" *Network: Computation in Neural Systems* 3: 213-251, 1992

[4]   Bilmes, J. "Maximal mutual information based reduction strategies for cross-correlation based joint distributional modeling." *Proc. Int. Conf. Spoken Lang. Processing,* 1998

[5]   Brown, P. *The Acoustic-Modeling Problem in Automatic Speech Recognition.* PhD Thesis, Computer Science Department, Carnegie Mellon University. 1987.

[6]   Bourlard, H. and Wellekens, C. "Links between Markov models and multilayer perceptrons." *IEEE Transactions on Pattern Analysis and Machine Intelligence* 12: 1167-1178, 1990

[7]   Bourlard, H.and Morgan, N. *Connectionist Speech Recognition - A Hybrid Approach,* Boston: Kluwer, 1994

[8]   Cooper, F.S., Liberman, A.M.. and Borst, J.M. "The interconversion of audible and visible patterns as a basis for research in the perception of speech. *Proc. Nat. Acad. Sci. (USA),* 37(5): 318-325, 1951.

[9]   Depireux, D.D., Simon, J.Z., Klein, D.J., Shamma, S.S. "Spectro-temporal response fields characterization with dynamic ripples in ferret primary auditory cortex." *J. Neurophysiol.* 85: 1220-1234, 2001

[10]   Davis, S.B. and Mermelstein, P. "Comparison of parametric representations for monosyllabic word recognition in continuously spoken sentences." *IEEE Trans. Acoust., Speech, Sig. Proc.* 28: 357-366, 1980

[11]   deCharms, C.R., Blake, D. and Merzenich, M.M. "Optimizing sound features for cortical neurons." *Science* 280, 1998

[12]   Fletcher, H. *Speech and Hearing in Communication.* New York: Van Nostrand, 1953. [reprinted 1995 by the Acoustical Society of America]

[13]   Fukunaga, K. *Statistical Pattern Recognition.* San Diego: Academic Press, 1990.

[14]   Furui, S. "Cepstral analysis technique for automatic speaker verification." *IEEE Trans. Acoust. Speech Sig. Proc.,* 29: 254-272, 1981

[15]   Grezl, F. and Hermansky, H. "Local averaging and differentiating of spectral plane for TRAP-based ASR." *Proc. Eurospeech,* 2003.

[16]   Hermansky, H. "Perceptual linear predictive (PLP) analysis of speech." *J. Acoust. Soc. Am.* 87: 1738-1752, 1990.

[17] Hermansky, H. "The modulation spectrum in the automatic recognition of speech." IEEE *Workshop on Automatic Speech Recognition and Understanding Proceedings,* 1997
[18] Hermansky, H. and Sharma, S. "TRAPS Classifiers of Temporal Patterns." *Proc. Int. Conf. Spoken Lang.,* 1998,
[19] Hermansky, H. and Jain, P. "Band-independent speech event categories for TRAP-based ASR." *Proc. Eurospeech,* 2003.
[20] Hermansky, H. "Should recognizers have ears?" *Speech Communication* 25: 3-27, 1998
[21] Hermansky, H., Ellis, D.P.W. and Sharma, S. "Connectionist Feature extraction for conventional HMM systems", *Proc. Int. Conf. Spoken Lang. Processing,* 2000
[22] Hermansky, H. and Sharma, S. "Temporal patterns (TRAPS) in ASR of noisy speech." *Proc. Int. Conf. Spoken Lang. Processing,* 1999
[23] Hermansky, H. and Malayath, N. "Spectral basis functions from discriminant analysis." *Proc. Int. Conf. Spoken Lang. Processing,* 1998.
[24] Hermansky, H and Morgan, N. "RASTA processing of speech." IEEE Trans. Speech Audio Processing, 2 (4): 578-589, 1994.
[25] Hunt, M.J. "A statistical approach to metrics for word and syllable recognition." *J. Acoust. Soc. Am.* 66: S35(A), 1979.
[26] www.icsi.berkeley.edu/speech/faq/ICSI_SPEECH_FAQ
[27] Jain, P., *Temporal Patterns of Frequency-Localized Features in ASR.* PhD. thesis, Department of Electrical and Computer Engineering, OGI School of Oregon Health & Sciences University, Portland, Oregon, 2003
[28] Jain, P. and Hermansky, H. "Effect of combining temporal patterns from critical-bands on ASR." *Proc. Eurospeech,* 2003
[29] Jelinek, F. *Statistical Methods for Speech Recognition.* Cambridge, MA: MIT Press, 1998
[30] Kempelen, W. von *Mechanismus der menschlichen Spraeche.* Vienna: J.B. Degen, 1791.
[31] Klein, D.J., Depireux, D.A., Simon, J.Z., Shamma, S. "Robust spectro-temporal reverse correlation for auditory system: Optimizing stimulus design." *J. Comp. Neuroscience* 9: 85-111, 2000.
[32] Kajarekar, S. and Hermansky, H. "Analysis of information in speech and its application in speech recognition." *Proc. Workshop Text, Speech and Dialogue,* 2000.
[33] Kanedera, N., Arai,, T., Hermansky, H. and Pavel, M. "On the relative importance of various components of modulation spectrum for automatic speech recognition." *Speech Communication* 28: 43-55, 1999.
[34] Lewicki, M.S. "Efficient coding of natural sounds." *Nature Neuroscience,* 5(4): 356-363, 2002
[35] Malayath, N. and Hermansky, H. "Bark resolution from speech data." *Proc. Int. Conf. Spoken Lang. Process.,* 2002.
[36] Malayath, N. and Hermansky, H. "Data-driven spectral basis functions for automatic speech recognition," *Speech Communication* 40: 446-466, 2003.
[37] Marr, D. *Vision,* San Francisco: W.H. Freeman, 1982
[38] Mermelstein, P. "Distance measures for speech recognition, psychological and instrumental." In *Pattern Recognition and Artificial Intelligence,* R.C.H. Chen (ed.), New York: Academic Press, pp. 374-388, 1976.
[39] Morgan, N., Zhu, Q., Stolcke, A., Sonmez, K., Sivadas, S., Shinozaki, T., Ostendorf, M., Jain, P., Hermansky, H., Ellis, D. Doddington, G., Chen, B., Cretin, O., Bourlard, H. and Athineos, M. "Pushing the envelope - aside." *IEEE Signal Processing Magazine,* 22 (5): 81- 88, 2005
[40] Sachs, M. and Young, E. "Encoding of steady state vowels in the auditory nerve: Rrepresentation in terms of discharge rate." *J. Acoust. Soc. Am.* 66: 470-479, 1979
[41] Schwarz, P., Matejka, P. and Cernock, J. "Recognition of Phoneme strings using TRAP technique." *Proc. Eurospeech,* 2003
[42] Sivadas, S. and Hermansky, H. "Hierarchical tandem feature extraction." *Proc. Int. Conf. Acoustics, Speech Sig. Process.,* 2002.
[43] Umesh, S., Cohen, L. and Nelson, D. "Frequency warping and speaker normalization." *Proc. IEEE Int. Conf. Acoust. Speech Signal Process.,* 1997.
[44] Yang, H.H., Sharma, S., van Vuuren, S. and Hermansky, H. "Relevance of time-frequency features for phonetic and speaker/channel classification," *Speech Communication,* 2000
[45] Young, E. and Sachs, M. "Representation of steady-state vowels in the temporal aspects of the discharge patterns of population of auditory nerve fibers." *J. Acoust. Soc. Am* 66: 1381-1403, 1979.

Dynamics of Speech Production and Perception
P. Divenyi et al. (Eds.)
IOS Press, 2006

Back to Speech Science - Towards a Collaborative ASR Community of the 21st Century

Chin-Hui LEE
School of Electrical and Computer Engineering
Georgia Institute of Technology
Atlanta, Georgia, USA

Abstract. We present an historic perspective on the development of automatic speech recognition (ASR) technologies and discuss the role speech science played in the past and would likely to assume in the future. First we introduce the prevailing data-driven, pattern recognition approach to ASR. Then we show that some speech knowledge sources could be integrated into ASR to enhance the capabilities and overcome many of the limitations of current ASR systems. In order to promote a wide applicability of knowledge integration, we need to address the following four major issues, namely: (1) the need of an ASR paradigm that facilitates an easy knowledge integration; (2) an objective evaluation methodology that allows quality and robustness assessment of existing and development of new knowledge sources; (3) the necessity of enhancing ASR capabilities over the state-of-the-art systems; and (4) an open, plug-'n'-play software development and common evaluation platform to lower ASR entry barriers and promote research collaboration. Finally, to circumvent the above difficulties, we propose a new paradigm that combines data- and knowledge-driven approaches to ASR. Under the new framework we expect researchers from all diverse areas in speech production, perception, analysis, coding, synthesis and recognition could work collaboratively towards establishing an ASR Community of the 21st Century.

Keywords. Automatic speech recognition, acoustic phonetics, speech perception and production, robustness

Introduction

At the dawn of the 21st Century the automatic speech recognition community is at a crossroads. On one hand, we have learned a great deal about how to build practical speech recognition systems for almost any spoken languages without the need of a detailed understanding of the language. Data-driven, machine learning techniques, such as *hidden Markov model* (HMM) [78] and *artificial neural network* (ANN) [40][12][50], are becoming so prevailing that numerous software packages and development kits have been developed and made available to the public (e.g. [97][11]) to develop their own applications with ease. With the vast collections of speech and language corpora sponsored by many business- and government-funded projects in many countries, it is now quite straightforward to demonstrate *automatic speech recognition* (ASR) capabilities of new tasks for almost any spoken languages. Advances in hardware, algorithms and data structures have also made implementation of large vocabulary, continuous speech recognition (LVCSR) systems affordable.

On the other hand, these systems are often so restrictive that their users have to follow a very strict set of protocols to effectively utilize spoken language applications. The technology is so fragile that careful designs have to be rigorously practiced to hide technology deficiencies. Furthermore, the ASR accuracies often degrades dramatically in adverse conditions to an extent that it becomes unusable even for cooperative users. When compared with *human speech recognition,* or HSR, the state-of-the-art ASR systems usually give much larger error rates even for rather simple tasks operating in clean environments [67]. In highly noisy conditions, such as those in moving vehicles, ASR sometimes gives an error rate more than one order of magnitude higher than HSR. Such a performance gap is unacceptable for users and difficult for application designers. There remain a number of fundamentals about the ASR technology to which the research community has yet to address.

It is clear that speech is one of the most complex signals that we need to deal with. The inherent complexity of the speech production mechanism and the complicated interactions among speech, language and acoustics make it difficult to model the speech communication process exactly and analytically. The speech signals, even when produced by the same person for multiple utterances of the same sequence of words, already exhibit some degree of variability. In addition to these intra-speaker variations, speech is influenced by cross-speaker variation, transducers used to capture the signal, channels in which the signal is transmitted, and speaking environments that can add distortion to the speech signal or change the way the signal is produced in very noisy and reverberant conditions. As a result, ASR systems could function very well in one instance but then fail miserably in a slightly different situation. This so-called *robustness* problem severely limits the widespread deployment of applications and services.

There have been attempts to find a set of *distinctive features* of speech (e.g. [27][92]) which are invariant to changes in speakers and speaking environments. By organizing such acoustic cues in a systematic manner, speech recognition can (in theory) be performed by first identifying the sequence of features, then mapping them into the corresponding sounds in speech, and finally decoding the corresponding words in speech using lexical access to a dictionary of words based on task syntax and semantics. This has been repetitively demonstrated in *spectrogram reading* by trained experts who can visually segment and identify speech sounds based on knowledge in acoustic-phonetics [99]. These features are not widely used in ASR due to the fact that they could not be reliably detected in continuous speech, especially in adverse acoustic conditions. Some effort on ASR, through generating phone lattices [68][100] first and followed by lexical access, has been attempted. A *phonological parsing* paradigm for ASR has been proposed by assuming all the distinctive features could be exactly detected [17]. The missing link lies in designing a bank of "perfect" feature detectors. We argue that such deterministic detectors are hard, if not impossible, to realize. They should be stochastic in nature and the success we enjoyed in data-driven modeling in state-of-the-art systems could be extended to a bottom-up detection approach to ASR in which speech attribute detection and knowledge integration play key roles.

The rest of the paper is organized as follows. In Section 2 we present a historic perspective of ASR technology advances in the last forty years. In Section 3 we briefly review the most successful data-driven, pattern matching approach to ASR in state-of-the-art systems implementations. To demonstrate the applicability of speech science, we next describe three examples of incorporating knowledge into current ASR systems to improve performance in Section 4. We then present a knowledge-based, data-driven paradigm aiming at enhancing ASR capabilities and mitigating ASR limitations in Section 5. Finally in Section 6 we propose an open platform for knowledge sharing and objective technology evaluation at both the system and the component levels. This is critical towards lowering barrier entries to ASR and establishing a *Collaborative ASR community of the 21st Century.*

1. ASR Approaches – A Historic Perspective

It is instructive to examine key developments in ASR technology in the past and contemplate on potential new directions. Textbooks and reference books [80][44][22][31] [62] are good sources for ASR fundamentals.

Before the 1960's the dominating approach to ASR was based on sound classification rules developed by speech scientists. In the 1970's we saw an intensive study in applying acoustic and linguistic knowledge sources to speech recognition in the ARPA Speech Understanding Project [53]. Many notable examples were documented [83][56]. Due to the implied rule-based scenario, expert knowledge is often required to even design a simple task. Robustness to adverse conditions in this setting was never addressed in a serious manner. Much of the knowledge accumulated in these studies was left in the background since then. Instead we saw an emergence of HMM-based continuous speech recognition in the *Dragon System* [9].

Moving on into 1980's and 1990's we witnessed the maturity of data-driven learning approaches to speech modeling. A number of techniques, including vector quantization [37], HMM [78], *self-organizing map* (SOM) [54], and ANN [12], have been successfully adopted. This *knowledge ignorance modeling* paradigm relies on collecting a large amount of task-specific speech and text examples and learning the corresponding model parameters without the need of using detailed knowledge embedded in the speech data. Using the knowledge hierarchy in the linguistic structure of acoustics, lexicon, syntax and semantics, it is possible to approximate some of the above knowledge sources and compile them into a single finite state network composed of acoustic HMM states, grammar nodes, and their connections [66]. ASR is then performed by matching the input feature sequence to all the possible acoustic state sequences and finding the most likely word string by traversing the above knowledge network using *dynamic programming* (DP) [71] and *heuristic search* [72]. These two collections of techniques, namely data-driven model learning and structural search over knowledge integration networks, have contributed greatly to the fast progress in the speech recognition technology.

In the meantime in the 1990's a significant portion of ASR research has gone into studying practical methods for implementation of large vocabulary spoken language systems. Much of this effort has been stimulated by the ARPA Human Language Technology Program, on three LVCSR projects, namely the Naval Resource Management (RM), the Air Travel Information System (ATIS) and the North American Business (NAB, previously known as the Wall Street Journal or WSJ) tasks. Along with large

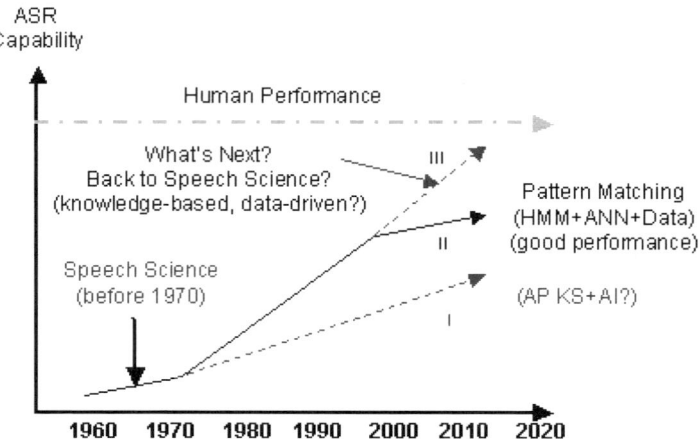

Figure 1. S-curve limits ASR technology advances.

data collection efforts and algorithm development, objective technology evaluation methodology also played a key role. A recent summary of ASR tests on all past bench-marking evaluations can be found in [76]. Furthermore, there is a worldwide activity in multi-lingual LVCSR for applications to voice-interactive database access, communications services [18], voice dictation [43] and continuous speech recognition (e.g. [36]), conversational systems [101], spoken document retrieval [69] and limited-domain spoken language translation (e.g. [91][95]). For more detail the reader is referred to a recently published special issue of the *Proceedings of the IEEE* [47]. A conceptual view of ASR advances in the last four decades of the 20th Century is depicted in Figure 1.

Curve II in Figure 1 illustrates the slow progress we started in the 1960's, followed by 30 years of fast progress based on the pattern matching paradigm shift. It is also clear that technology improvement has slowed down somewhat recently. If we were to follow the knowledge-driven paradigm (shown in Curve I in dashed line because it never took place), we might have also enhanced some ASR capabilities, but probably at a slower pace than those achieved by using data-driven approaches. It is interesting to project the future directions the community might take us into the 21st Century. It seems clear that the performance gap between ASR and HSR would have taken a long time to bridge if we would follow Curve II. Could we instead ride on Curve III in Figure 1 in which a knowledge-based, data-driven paradigm shift would take place and lead to a family of next-generation ASR approaches that eventually surpass human performance in some tasks? What should be the new paradigm? What roles could the speech science community play? What role could data-driven, machine learning approaches play to enhance knowledge-driven, rule-based approaches? A recent NSF Symposium to explore new directions in next generation ASR is documented in [60].

2.   Data-driven Pattern Matching Paradigm

To date, the prevailing approach to ASR is to treat speech as a stochastic pattern and adopt a statistical pattern matching paradigm. Assume a source-channel speech genera-

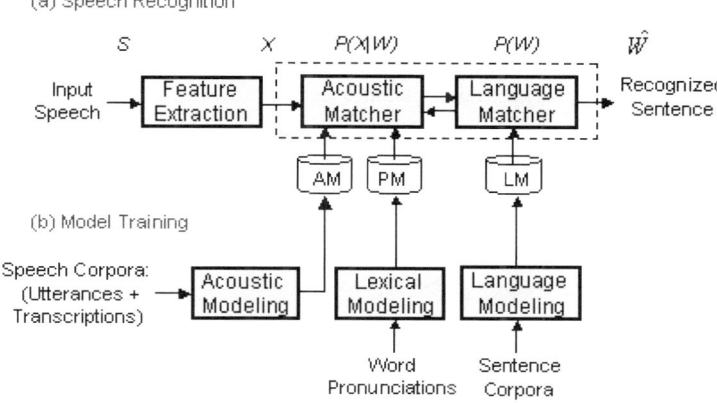

Figure 2. Data-driven pattern matching approach to ASR: (a) MAP decoding; and (b) Training of models.

tion model [7] in which the message source produces a sequence of words, W. Because of uncertainty and inaccuracy in converting from W to an observed speech signal, S, we model the process as a noisy channel. ASR is then formulated as a *maximum a posteriori* (MAP) decoding problem, as shown in Figure 2.

Instead of working with speech, S, directly, one can convert S to a sequence of acoustic vectors, X, and formulates the speech decoding problem as:

$$\hat{W} = \mathbf{argmax}_W P(W|X) = \mathbf{argmax}_W P(W|X)P(W) \qquad (1)$$

in which the recognized sentence is obtained by searching the set of all permissible sequences of words. $P(X|W)$, often referred to as an *acoustic model* (AM), is the conditional probability of the feature, X, for a given W. A comprehensive review of and some critical look at acoustic modeling and its interactions with the MAP decision rule in Eq. (1) can be found in [63]. $P(W)$ is the *a priori* probability of generating the sentence W, known as a *language model* (LM) [51][8][85][10]. *Pronunciation model* (PM) can also be built from word pronunciation examples to model lexical variation in spoken languages [84][30].

Instead of providing a detailed model for each of the intermediate channels of message to sentence generation, speech production, speaker variability, speaking environments, and transmission channels, they are collectively characterized in a *knowledge ignorance channel model*, $P(X|W)$. Since it is not feasible to have an exact and complete specification about such a noisy channel, the statistical learning approach often assumes particular parametric forms for $P(X|W)$ and $P(W)$. All model parameters needed to evaluate the acoustic and language probabilities, are estimated from a huge collection of speech and text corpora given by a large user population.

The most widely used and successful modeling approach to ASR is HMM [78]. Since it is capable of jointly characterizing both the temporal and spectral varying nature of the speech signal, many algorithms for model training have been proposed. They mainly aim at two key objectives, namely: (1) model accuracy in estimating the feature distributions (e.g. [45][75][61]); and (2) model discrimination for minimizing

Application	Input	Output	P(I)	P(O|I)
Optical Char. Recognition	Actual Letters	Noisy Letters	Character (Letter) LM	OCR Error Model
Bioinformatics	DNA Sequence	Noisy DNA Sequence	LM of Nucleotides	Bio-genetic Model
Machine Translation	Source Sentence	Target Sentence	Source LM	Translation Model
Text Understanding	Semantic Concept	Word Sequence	Concept LM	Semantic Model
Part-of-Speech Tagging	POS Tag Sequence	Word Sequence	POS Tag LM	Tagging Model
Parsing	Parse Tree	Word Sequence	LM of Derivations	Parsing Model

Table 1. Data-driven approaches to related problems

the recognition error rate (e.g. [46][49]).

2.1 Generalization to Other Recognition Tasks

The same channel decoding paradigm discussed above for ASR has been successfully extended to dealing with many other similar pattern recognition problems in text and multimedia applications, as shown in Table 1. For example, in row 4, machine translation can be formulated as a decoding problem similar to Eq. (1) [15], in which W can interpreted as the unknown *target* sentence to be translated into from the observed *source* sentence X. *Translation models* need to be developed from parallel text training corpora in order to compute a *translation probability*, $P(W|X)$. HMM is again used to model hidden structures in signal patterns.

2.2 The Robustness Problem

The most serious drawback of the statistical modeling approaches is the implied mismatch caused by unseen data. This is clearly illustrated in Figure 3. The pattern mis-

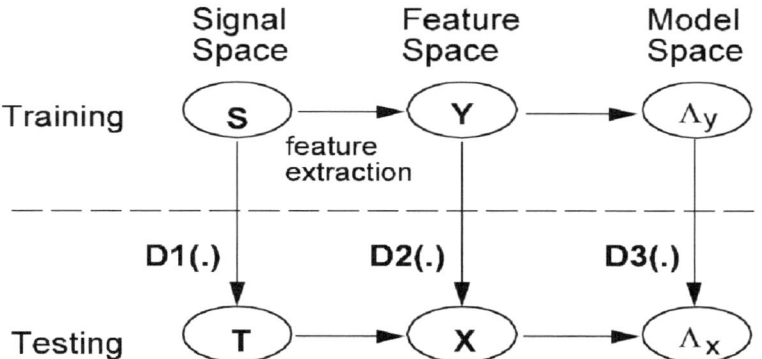

Figure 3. Data-driven approaches to related problems Robustness: Signal, feature and model mismatches between training and testing conditions.

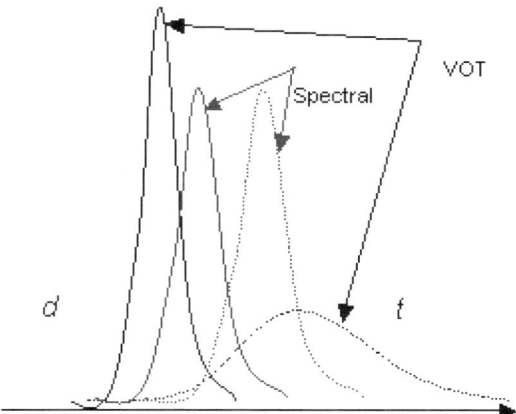

Figure 4. Sound-specific event detectors: A single VOT parameter is better than 39 cepstral features in discriminating voiced "d" against unvoiced stop "t".

match between training and testing conditions often results in a significant degradation in ASR performance. Comprehensive reviews of compensation methods to reduce mismatches and consequently to improve ASR performance can be found in [58][48]. These techniques include *feature compensation* [1], parallel model combination [32], *model adaptation* [35][41][63], maximum likelihood linear regression [65], *stochastic matching* [86][93], and *robust decision* [42], etc.

With so many possible combinations of speech variability factors, it is not possible to collect a large training set to cover every single condition and train a set of focused models that works well in all cases. Therefore it seems clear that the robustness problem could not be solved with only data-driven top-down approaches. It has been argued that human beings perform speech recognition by integrating multiple knowledge sources from the bottom up [5]. This inspires a new ASR paradigm to solve the robustness problems by "divide and conquer". It enables us to take advantage of the vast body of literatures developed outside the ASR community [16][29][27][53][74][39][92]. Knowledge in speech production (e.g. [26][23][14][77][33]) and auditory processing and perception [38][87][13][88][6][24] can also been applied to bottom-up, detection-based ASR. We will come back to address these issues later.

3. Three Knowledge-based ASR Examples

Before introducing the detection-based approach to ASR, it is useful to examine how knowledge sources developed in the speech science community can be effectively incorporated into state-of-the-art HHM-based systems to enhance ASR capabilities. In this following we give three examples.

3.1 Sound-Specific Speech Features

Cepstral parameters, computed at every 10 msec, have been the chosen feature vectors in almost all the state-of-the-art ASR systems (e.g. [36]). It is well-known that temporal

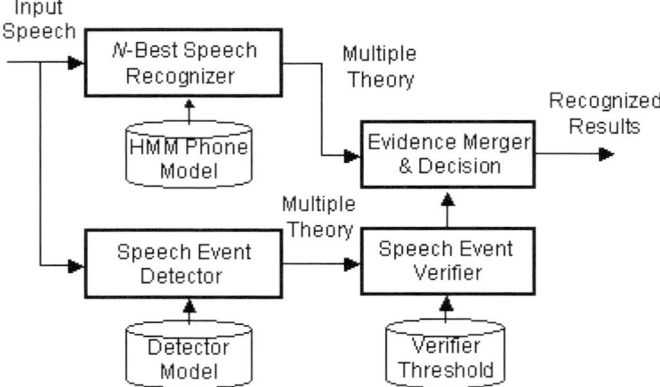

Figure 5. A two-stage speech recognizer incorporating sound-specific event detectors.

features are critical in detecting some speech sounds. In [73], it was shown that *voice onset time*, or VOT, is an ideal parameter for discriminating a voice stop, like "d", against the corresponding unvoiced stop, "t". In Figure 4 we plot the distributions of the likelihood ratio for "d" and "t" based on 39 cepstral parameters and a single VOT. Clearly, the VOT temporal feature produces a pair of curves that better discriminate themselves (with more separation between them) than those obtained with spectral features.However, it is not effective to concatenate the VOT feature with the cepstral features in the HMM-based systems to form new feature vectors because the additional parameter contributes very little to evaluating the likelihood of the overall feature vectors. However, we can design a two-stage recognizer as shown in Figure 5. In the first stage, a conventional recognizer is used to produce a list of multiple candidates. To further discriminating some of the minimum pairs such as the English letters, D and T, a VOT-based detector [73], can be used in the second stage to provide a detailed discrimination. By re-ordering candidates according to VOT, the two-stage recognizer gave an error rate 50% less than that obtained in a state-of-the-art ASR system [82]. The same notion has been applied to natural number recognition in which resolving the "teen-ty" confusion is critical. By discriminating nasal sounds against others, the confusion rate was reduced by 46% using a two-stage speech recognizer (in an unpublished report).

3.2 Key-Phrase Spotting Mimicking Foreign Ears

Recently several spoken dialogue systems have been evaluated in real-world applications. These systems use finite state grammars to accept typical user utterances, because there is not enough data available to train *N*-gram language models for the specific tasks. The use of such rigid grammars is effective for typical *in-grammar* (IG) utterances. However, in *spontaneous* speech, we have observed a wide utterance variation that is not covered by the task grammars intended for a large population, although they had been iteratively tuned by developers during a trial period. Even in apparently simple sub-tasks such as asking for date or time, a large portion of the user utterances turned out to be *out-of-grammar* (OOG). These samples include extraneous speech, such as hesitations, repetitions, and unexpected expressions. We even observe many totally

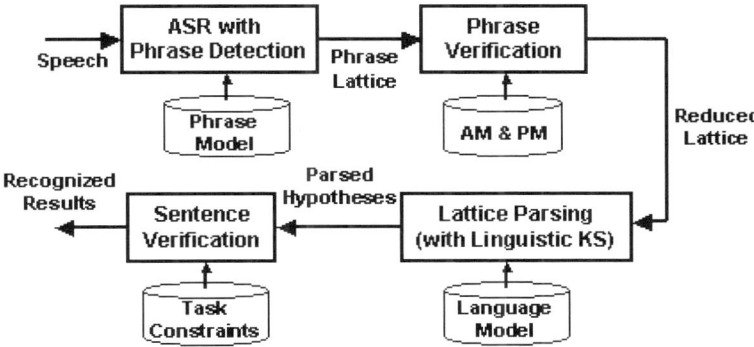

Figure 6. ASR by mimicking "foreign ears" with combined key-phrase detection and verification.

irrelevant or *out-of-task* (OOT) utterances.

Most of such spontaneous utterances contain some key-phrases that are task-related and may lead to partial or full understanding. It is well-known that human listeners are very good in picking up relevant keywords, even when they are buried in utterances in a foreign language. This suggests a detection approach to mimic keyword spotting by "foreign ears". By relaxing the grammatical constraints and focusing on the key-phrases, it will accept a wider variety of utterances than rigid grammars. Combined with a flexible dialogue manager, the detection-based approach realizes partial understanding and disambiguation of the unclear portions through human-like follow-up dialogue interactions. Since words and phrases are relatively stable units to detect in continuous speech, we use them as detection units and follow the approach shown in Figure 6.

This combined recognition and verification strategy [52], incorporating both phrase detection networks and utterance verification into the system, maintained a good accuracy for IG utterances and greatly reduces semantic errors for OOG and OOT sentences. In contrast, for decoding with rigid grammars, the conventional system only worked well for IG speech inputs but failed miserably for ill-formed, spontaneous utterances, often encountered in human-machine dialogues.

3.3 A Knowledge-Based Front-End for LVCSR

We have just demonstrated the effectiveness of the detection paradigm using large units, like key-phrases. Next we show how to combine top-down and bottom-up approaches. Here we implemented an LVCSR system [55] based on features derived from speech attributes. These "knowledge-based" features were then used to train a set of context-dependent phone HMMs in a data-driven fashion as shown in Figure 2. Based on a set of known techniques, the system offers the following: (1) data-driven ANN-based detectors that measure the presence or absence of speech cues directly from short-time, mel-frequency cepstral coefficients (MFCCs) [19] as shown in Figure 7; and (2) features that can be used directly in HMM-based systems. With these non-linear detectors, we intend to simulate activity levels between 0 and 1 (in a probabilistic sense) of acoustic-phonetic attributes and use them as feature vectors in an ASR front-end. Furthermore we can combine multiple ASR systems (having different error patterns at the word level) to improve word recognition performance.

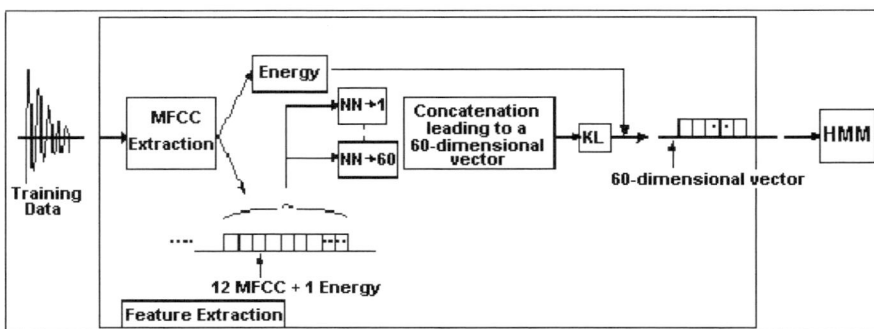

Figure 7. ANN-based feature vectors for HMM.

Experiments were performed on the WSJ task using the standard 5K and 20K Nov-92 tests. For the language models, we used the trigram provided by NIST. First, we built an MFCC baseline system, leading to the word error rates (WERs) listed in the second row of Table 2. In the third row the WERs, for the system based on the 61-dim feature vectors (1 energy + 60 KL-transformed), computed as in Figure 7, are listed. While the performance is significantly worse than the MFCC baseline, we observed that the error patterns are more meaningful, suggesting that the two systems could be combined. Instead of using speech attributes, we also used the 44 phone labels adopted in the HMM-based system as features, using the same technique described above. The WER results are given in the fourth row of Table 2. Again, we found that the error patterns are different from those obtained above.

Based on this outcome, we combine the results of our systems using ROVER [28], which essentially corresponds to a majority vote decision, illustrated in Figure 8 (@ denoting null). We first merged the two systems built on the (60+1) speech attributes and the (44+1) phone-based features. The obtained results are given in the fifth row of Table 2, labeled "Combination without Baseline". Such a system is marginally better than the baseline MFCC system, but is significantly better than our best system built either on the (60+1) or (44+1) features.

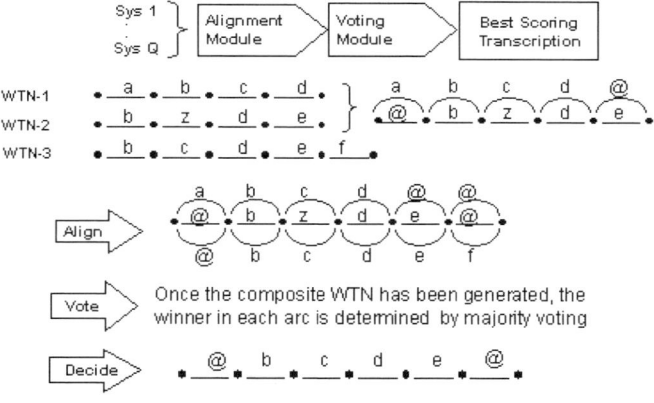

Figure 8. Combining multiple results by ROVER.

Features	Test 5k	Test 20k
1. Baseline (MFCC)	4.6	11.8
2. 60 Phonetic Attributes	7.6	16.8
3. 44 Phone Features	5.6	13.0
Combination w/o Baseline	4.4	11.8
Combination with Baseline	3.7	10.6

Table 2. Word error rates of the Nov-92 WSJ test in different features and system configurations.

Finally we included our baseline results into the ROVER combination, leading to the best results in the bottom row of Table 2. These represent about 20% and 10% relative WER reduction over our best baseline MFCC system, on the 5K and 20K tasks, respectively. The set of encouraging results seems to suggest that acoustic-phonetic features are useful and they could be integrated into our best HMM-based recognizer to produce even better accuracies. It also indicates that knowledge-based features, produced with the same MFCC, provide extra information. A better understanding of feature usage is needed.

4. Knowledge-based, Data-driven Paradigm

It has long been postulated that a human determines the linguistic identity of a sound based on detected evidences that exist at various levels of the speech hierarchy, from acoustics to pragmatics. For example, Klatt [53] studied the so-called *acoustic land-marks*. Stevens [92] and Fant [27] have consistently advocated the approach of distinctive features from an acoustic-phonetic theoretical viewpoint. Indeed, people do not continuously convert a speech signal into words as an ASR system would; instead, they detect *acoustic* and *auditory* evidences, weigh them and combine them to form *cognitive* hypotheses, and then *validate* the hypotheses until satisfactory decisions are reached. Along with the discussions in [5], this human-based model of speech processing suggests a candidate framework for developing next generation speech technologies that will go beyond the current limitations. Instead of the top-down, network decoding paradigm discussed earlier in Section 3, we propose a bottom-up event detection and

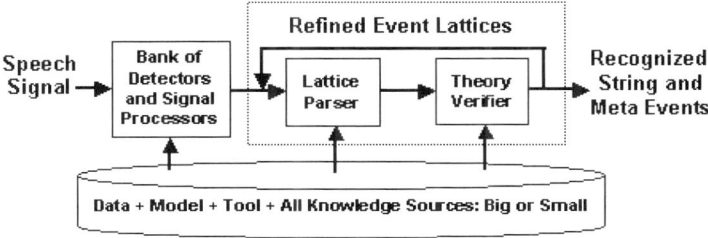

Figure 9. Bottom-up ASR based on speech attribute detection, event merging and evidence verification.

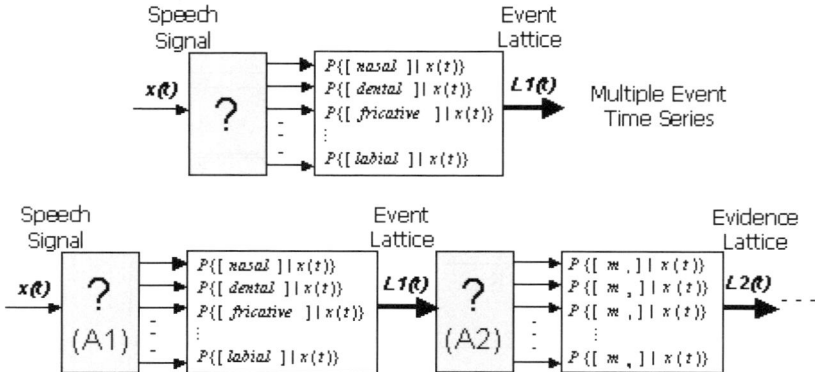

Figure 10. An auditory perception perspective of acoustic-phonetic event detection and combination.

evidence combination paradigm for ASR as shown in Figure 9.

The speech signal is first processed by a bank of speech attribute detectors, followed by a sequence of verifiers, validating evidences at every level of the linguistic knowledge hierarchy to recognize speech and other human information embedded in speech. An event or attribute can be the presence of a particular acoustic-phonetic cue, such as "voicing" as a function of time. It can also characterize a speaking environment, such as an estimated confidence of how likely the noise background stays at a prescribed signal-to-noise (SNR) level, say 10dB, over time. Sometimes it can be used to represent the presence of important speech parameters, such as the gender, accent, and emotional state according to a *speaker's profile*. At the physiological response level, firing of a neuron can also be interpreted as an event. As discussed above, a properly designed score function of the detector can also be used to model the *a posteriori* probability of the event, given the observed speech signal. One key feature of the detection-based approach is that the outputs of the detectors do not have to be synchronized in time and therefore it is flexible to allow a direct integration of both short-term detectors, e.g., for detection of VOT, and long-term detectors, e.g., for detection of pitch, syllables, and particular word sequences.

An *event detector* converts an input speech signal $x(t)$ into a time series, which describes the level of presence (or *level of activity*) of a particular property (or *attribute*) in the input speech utterance over time. This function can be computed as the *a posteriori* probability of the particular attribute, given the speech signal, within a proper time window, or the *likelihood ratio* which involves calculation of two likelihoods, one pertaining to the target model and the other the contrast model. The bank of detectors consists of a number of such attribute detectors, each being individually and best designed for the detection of a particular property. These properties are often stochastic in nature and are relevant to information needed to perform ASR.

The *event merger* takes the set of detected events as input and attempts to infer the presence of higher level attributes (e.g., a phone or a word) which are then verified by the *event verifier* to produce a refined and partially integrated lattice of event hypotheses. This new lattice of hypotheses is then fed back for further knowledge integration. This iterative information fusion process always uses the original event activity functions as the raw evidence. A terminating strategy can be instituted by exhausting all the

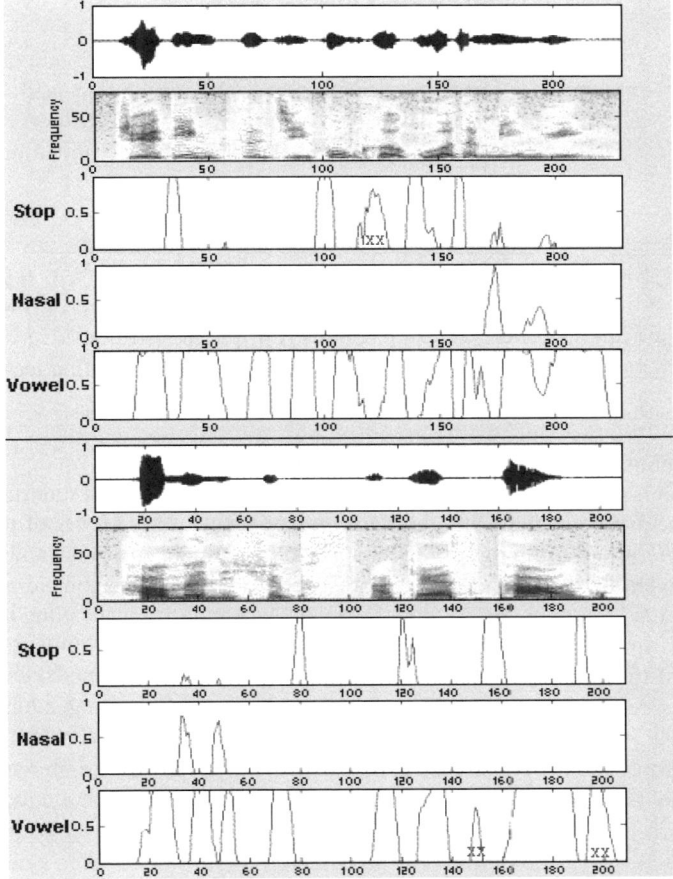

Figure 11. Detectors trained on Mandarin speech: (top) Tested on an unseen Mandarin utterance; and (bottom) Tested on an English utterance, spoken by a non-native speaker using a different microphone.

supported attributes. The procedure produces the evidence for a final decision or the recognized sentence itself, depending on the desired application.

The proposed approach, when applied to auditory processing, attempts to simulate the human auditory process by assuming that the speech signal is first converted to a collection of auditory response patterns (feature detection), each modeling the probabilistic activity level of a particular acoustic-phonetic event of interest (shown in the A1 module in Figure 10). Detection of the next level of events or evidences, such as phones, is accomplished by combining relevant features from A1 (as shown in the A2 module in Figure 10). Each activity function can be modeled by a corresponding neural system, or neuron. Both the activation level and firing rates have been used in neural encoding (e.g. [20]). ANNs provide a convenient mathematical tool to model neuron combinations. *Feedforward neural networks* have been used to model the encoding and decoding of temporal neural information. *Recurrent neural networks* have also been used to provide feedback loops to simulate neural processing. Simulating perception of temporal events is of particular interest in auditory perception of speech (e.g. [25][70]).

4.1 Detection of Speech Attributes and Landmarks

For the proposed detection paradigm shown in Figure 9, it is a "divide and conquer" strategy that a community effort is required to come up with the best bank of detectors. It was argued earlier that the ASR robustness problem could not be solved by simply collecting a large training set attempting to cover all possible combinations of speech variation.

However it is possible for the speech science community to work together with the speech processing community in a collaborative manner to provide the best detectors for all speech attributes of interests. A large body of literature already exists for pitch tracking, formant estimation, voicing detection, and many other related problems. Recent efforts in classification of nasal and stop sounds [2][3] demonstrated advantages of integrating speech knowledge sources, and signal processing and modeling techniques (e.g. [79]).

In a preliminary experiment, we show in Figure 11 that language-independent detection of broad acoustic-phonetic sound classes is feasible. First, we designed a set of ANN-based stop, nasal and vowel detectors, using about 40,000 Mandarin utterances, spoken by 80 talkers, from different regions across China, each contributing about 500 phonetically balanced utterances (database collected in the *863 National Project*; published in Chinese in 1999).

In the top of Figure 11, we show a good detection performance for an unseen Mandarin utterance from a new speaker. Only a significant false alarm of stop, labeled "XX", is observed in the middle panel. We then tested the same three detectors using an English utterance spoken by a non-native speaker via a different type of microphone from the one used in the training set. The detection results are displayed in the bottom part of Figure 11. It is interesting to note that the four stops and the two nasals are all correctly detected. There were two false alarms of vowels shown in the bottom panel, both labeled "XX". Note that the error at the end of the sentence was caused by a mispronunciation.

Although we still have a long way to go before realizing a collection of high performance event detectors, knowledge and experience acquired in the speech science and speech processing communities can definitely contribute to this collaborative effort.

4.2 Verification of Speech Events and Evidences

The plug-in MAP decoder to recognize W in Eq. (1) is a choosing-one-of-the-above scenario. However there are many practical difficulties with the formulation. First of all, the candidate set, is usually of a finite size and it is not possible to cover all possible sentences and therefore it results in recognition errors if the sentence is not part of the set. Second, the quality of the recognition result is not properly quantified because the RHS of Eq. (1) is only computing relative likelihood differences of competing word strings. Since speech sounds are inherently ambiguous, we need to ask the question "why should we accept W as the recognized string?" and "can we assign a value to measure the confidence of our acceptance?"

These two issues lead researchers to study three new but closely related topics not existing in conventional ASR, namely: (1) keyword recognition and non-keyword rejection ([96]); (2) utterance verification (at both the string and word levels (e.g. [90][81]);

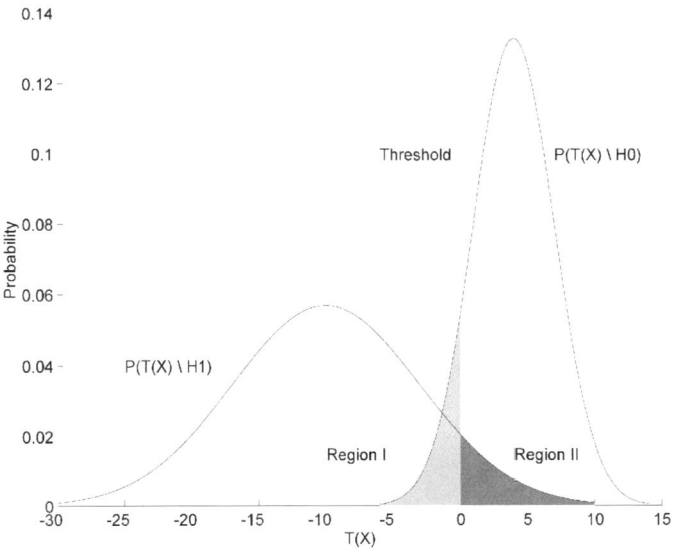

Figure 12. Distributions of target and its corresponding alternative for evidence verification.

and (3) confidence measures (e.g. [59]). Although the above three research areas can not directly be solved with the classification formulation shown in Eq. (1), the theory of hypothesis testing provides a framework to tie these three topics in a unified manner [59] as shown below.

Verification of patterns, or detected events, is often formulated as a statistical hypothesis testing problem. There are plenty of techniques available in the literature for designing optimal tests, if the distributions of the null and alternative hypotheses, $P(X|H_0)$ and $P(X|H_1)$, are known exactly. However, for most practical verification problems, we use a set of training examples to estimate the distributions.

Due to its overlapping nature, shown in Figure 12, of the two competing distributions, $P(X|H_0)$ on the right and $P(X|H_1)$ on the left, two categories of verification error thus exist. First, one could have decided that X was not generated from the signal source while it was indeed coming from the source. Second, one could have verified the given signal X as coming from the source while it was actually from a different source. The former, often referred to as *type I error* (area of Region I in Figure 12), is the error of *false rejection* or *missed detection*, and the latter, known as *type II error* (area of Region II in Figure 12), is the error of *false acceptance* or *false alarm*. The verification performance is often evaluated as a combination of type I and II errors.

In many general speaker verification (SV) and utterance verification (UV) problems, H_1 assumes that X is not generated by the known source, which often means H_1 is a *composite* hypothesis as opposed to being a simple hypothesis which makes the design of optimal tests much more involved. In real-world practice, we form a test statistic, $T(X)$, such that we accept the assumed target event if $T(X)$, where is a verification threshold. The *receiver operating characteristic*, or ROC, curve of a test provides a way of tuning the desired performance, according to the choice of threshold values. Following the Neyman-Pearson lemma (e.g. [64], [21]), a *probability ratio* or *likelihood ratio* (LR) test is often performed. Likelihood functions of the distributions of the null and alternative hypotheses need to be evaluated for any input X. For verification of long *temporal* events, such as in utterance verification, consisting of a sequence of smaller events, a string-based log likelihood ratio (LLR) statistic is usually decomposed into a sum of a sequence of word-based LLR statistics, i.e.

$$T(X) = \text{LLR}(X|W) \approx \sum_i \text{LLR}(X_i|w_i)$$

$$= \sum_i \left[\log f(X_i|\lambda_w) - \log f\left(X_i|\lambda_{\overline{w}_i}\right) \right]$$

(2)

Each word LLR in turn is computed as a sum of LLR statistics for phones, which is evaluated from a set of pairs of phone and its anti-model $\{\lambda_p, \lambda_{\overline{p}}\}$, i.e.

$$\text{LLR}(X_i|w_i) \approx \sum_k \text{LLR}(X_{ik}|p_{ik})$$

$$= \sum_k \left[\log f\left(X_{ik}|\lambda_{w_i}\right) - \log f\left(X_{ik}|\lambda_{\overline{w}_i}\right) \right]$$

(3)

4.3 Combination of Evidences

Consider a set of K multiple time series, each representing an activity function for an event, say a "voiced" attribute, $v(t)$, or a "stop" attribute, $p(t)$, detected over time on input speech, $s(t)$, by the event detectors in the ensemble, as shown in Figure 9. To combine these stochastic evidences to form a higher-level evidence, which is also an event activity function, say $e(t)$, representing a "voiced stop" attribute. On one hand, some of the events in the ensemble provide positive reinforcement for $e(t)$. On the other hand,

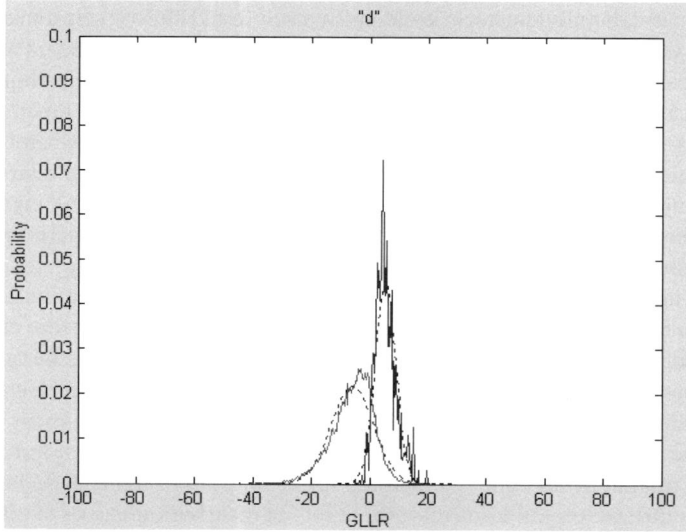

Figure 13. An example of verifying phone "d" using likelihood ratios of HMMs trained with TIMIT data.

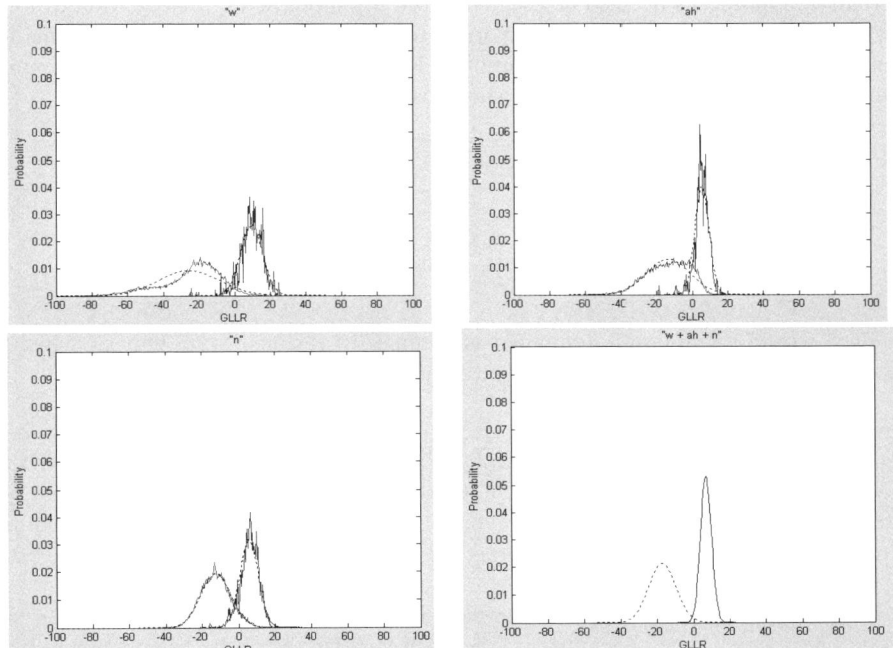

Figure 14. Verifying the word "one" (bottom right) based on evidences of verifying the 3 phones, "w" (top left), "ah" (bottom left) and "n" (top right) in it.

some lower-level evidences may interfere with the higher-level evidences. Evidence combination can be accomplished by designing a mapping function from some of the time series in the ensemble to *e(t)* such that *e(t)* serves as an evidence time series, for the next level of knowledge representation, such as phones, syllables, and words.

In addition, a stochastic combination theory to form strong event verifiers from a collection of weak event detectors, such as *boosting* (e.g. [89][98]), is a useful mathematical tool to combine low-level, redundant events. Parsing of event lattices, by extending the deterministic CYK algorithm (e.g. [4]) to probabilistic parsing with variable segment boundaries, is also an important set of tools to be developed in order to combine a set of multiple evidences in time with unknown gaps in-between.

To demonstrate phone detection, we estimate the two competing distributions in Figure 12 using HMM *generalized log likelihood ratio* (GLLR in Eq. (3)), computed as the log likelihood difference of a desired target phone model and a general speech filler model [96]. The phone models were built with the TIMIT [34] training utterances. One the right part in Figure 13, we plot the distribution for phone "d" and on the left we have the histogram for all the other "non-d" segments. A typical result is that the curve on the right is sharper (less variance) than the one on the left (larger variance due to the more variety of non-target speech data). The mean of the right Gaussian density is greater than zero, indicating a correct detection most of the time, while the mean of the left Gaussian density is less than zero, showing correct rejection for most "non-d" samples.

For detecting the word "one", shown in Figure 14 (bottom right), based on the LLR statistic in Eq. (3), we plot in Figure 14, three sets of distribution curves similar to those in Figure 13 for detecting the three corresponding phones, "w", "ah" and "n" in the

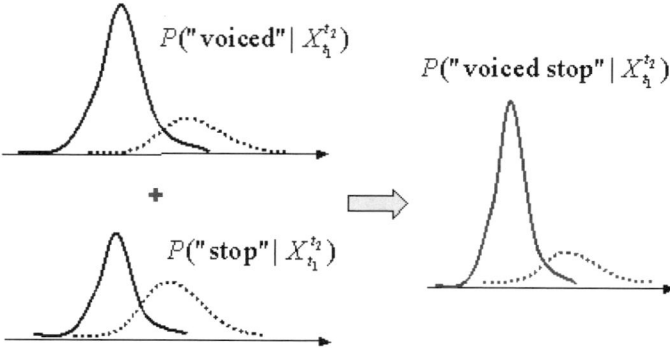

Figure 15. Verification of composite hypotheses.

word. By approximating the three sets of histograms with Gaussian densities, we can compose the Gaussian curves for detecting the word "one". It is noted that it is easier to detect words than phones, because the composed competing Gaussian curves show a better separation, or equivalently less overlapping nature. Theory in sequential hypothesis testing also provides many guidelines for designing sequential evidence mergers (e.g. [94]).

We can also perform evidence combination at the raw speech attribute level. So far, we don't have experimental results yet. They will look similar to the ones shown in Figure 14 for sequential evidence combination. One such example is to merge the "front vowel" and "nasal" attributes to form a higher level event, such as "a front vowel followed by a nasal". In addition, to verify composite hypotheses conceptually, like the event "voiced stop" shown in the right part of Figure 15, we need to come up with two set of curves as shown in the left part of Figure 15 for detecting the two corresponding speech attributes, "voiced" and "stop", respectively. If the two events on the left are not heavily correlated, we argue that the curves of the combined evidence will give a better separation than those for either of the two attributes, similar to what were demonstrated in Figure 14. Because of the redundancy in the overall set of detected speech attributes and evidences, a perfect detection of raw attributes, however small, is not required in the detection-based ASR framework.

4.4 Beyond Word Transcription

As described in Section 3, the data-driven approach to ASR is built upon the Bayes decision theory. The framework assumes that the recognition problem involves a (fixed) number of classes, say M, of observations, each of which is associated with a distribution function. Given such a probability space (with all the distributions known), the recognition system designer can construct a decision scheme based on the MAP policy expressed in Eq. (1) to determine the class identity of an observed pattern (out of the *close set* of M classes).

In contrast, the class of problems that involve the need to deal with observations of unassociated classes (i.e., not belonging to any of the M classes) is called an *open-set* pattern recognition problem. Since the observation whose class identity is to be determined may not fall into any of the established set, and thus no probability measure is

(a) Diagnostic evaluation of detectors (at speech event level):

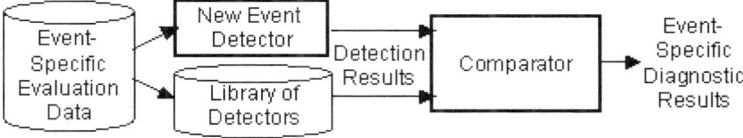

(b) Diagnostic evaluation of speech recognizers (at word level):

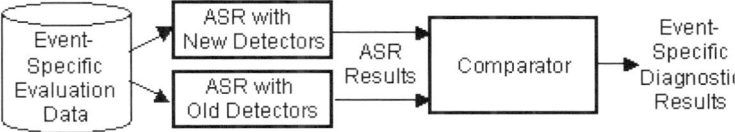

Figure 16. An objective platform evaluating: (a) detection modules; (b) ASR system performance.

available to describe it, the MAP rule becomes irrelevant. We need a formulation different from the Bayes theory.

Practical speech recognition applications, as expected, often involve open-set problems. These deviations appear in the form of out-of-vocabulary words or phrases, out-of-grammar phrases or sentences, and various forms of speech disfluencies, such as partial words, hesitation, and repairs. It seems clear that a complete specification of speech in order to facilitate close-set ASR is hard, even for simple tasks (e.g. [96]). As discussed in Section 4B, a partial understanding of ill-formed utterances is feasible through keyword detection and verification. The new event detection framework allows us to realize ASR capabilities beyond just word transcription in today's *speech-to-text* scenario. Instead we could anticipate a full description of speech attributes, encompassing all relevant human information embedded in speech utterances, even though we don't have a complete speech model.

5. An Open Platform for Collaborative ASR

Collection of language resources and objective evaluation on a large set of real-world sentences are two cornerstones in the advancement of ASR technologies [76]. In order to enjoy a fast progress with the new detection-based paradigm, a coordinated community effort is needed. In addition to evaluating the word error rate, which is commonly practiced in ASR benchmarking, we are interested in the performance of the detectors at both the low-level attribute and high-level evidence levels. To facilitate an objective evaluation at the detector level, two scenarios can be considered [60]. The first is a side-by-side, relative comparison between two detectors, old and new, shown in Figure 16(a). The other task is similar to the evaluation of speaker verification systems, by plotting target and competing distributions similar to Figure 13, and ROC curves, and reporting *equal error rates*. The key to the success of this evaluation methodology is a common test set of *event-specific evaluation data* that is designed to maximize the coverage of the target attributes being tested in different contexts. There will be plenty of "anti-attributes" in the test set to evaluate the false alarm rates also. A *library of attribute-specific detectors* is also essential. Since the tests are done at the attribute and evidence levels, they should offer plenty of diagnostic information to help with improving detector performances.

The other key component shown in Figure 16(b) is the ASR system evaluation at the word level. We can again design a set of event-specific evaluation utterances that is rich in the specific feature being tested. For example, we could collect sentences with plenty of nasal attributes to compare an ASR system, with a new nasal detector, with the same system configuration but with an old nasal detector. This meets the so called "*plug-'n'-play*" requirement that one can realize the whole system by only working at a module level. In doing so, the entry barriers to ASR research can be greatly lowered. It also facilitates remote collaboration that different groups can work on different modules of the same system and both contribute to developing the whole system. Or they can work on the same module and be able to compare notes in order to improve the technology.

6. Conclusion

We have reviewed the technology advances in automatic speech recognition in the last four decades of the 20th Century. Although we have witnessed a tremendous progress and seen many spoken language applications and services deployed and used in our everyday life, it is safe to conclude that the ASR problem is far from being solved. In order to surpass the current ASR capabilities and alleviate some of the limitations, it is time we take advantage of the vast body of knowledge available in speech science in order to advance ASR technology. We have shown that, knowledge sources, when properly utilized, greatly enhance the ASR accuracies over those achieved by the state-of-the-art systems. We have also introduced a detection-based ASR paradigm that is collectively solved by the speech community using a "divide and conquer" strategy. In this bottom-up framework, it requires building a bank of high performance speech event detectors and a collection of effective evidence merger and verifiers. Researchers in the speech science community are thus enabled to contribute to designing any part of the ASR systems, using existing and newly developed knowledge and techniques. An open platform for knowledge sharing and objective technology evaluation is also proposed to facilitate the establishment of a Collaborative ASR Community of the 21st Century. We expect this effort to greatly lower barrier entries to ASR system development, lead to a second wave of fast technology progress, and eventually close the performance gap between machine and human recognition of speech.

Acknowledgements

The author owes his sincere gratitude to his past colleagues at Bell Labs, Murray Hill, for endless and stimulating discussions. Such precious opportunities will be greatly missed. He also thanks his Georgia Tech students, Jinyu Li, for generating Figure 11, and Yu Tsao, for producing Figures 13 and 14.

References

[1] Acero, A. *Acoustical and Environmental Robustness in Automatic Speech Recognition*. Boston: Kluwer, 1992.

[2] Ali, A.M.A, Van der Spiegel, J. and Mueller, P. "Acoutic-phonetic features for the automatic classification of fricatives." *J. Acoust. Soc. Am*. 109: 2217-2235, 2001.

[3] Ali, A.M.A, Van der Spiegel, J. and Mueller, P. "Acoutic-phonetic features for the automatic classification of stop consonants." *IEEE Trans. Speech, Audio Proc*. 9(8):833-841, 2001.

[4] Aho, A.V. and Ullman, J.D. *The Theory of Parsing, Translation, and Compiling*, Vol. 1, Englewood Cliffs, NJ: Prentice Hall, 1972.

[5] Allen, J. "How do humans process and recognize speech." *IEEE Trans. Speech and Audio Proc*. 2(4): 567—577, 1994.

[6] Atlas, L. "Modulation spectral transforms - Aapplication to speech separation and modification." In *Dynamics by Ear, Eye, Mouth and Machine, An Interdisciplinary Workshop*, Kyoto, Japan, 2003.

[7] Bahl, L.R., Jelinek, F., and Mercer, R.L. "A maximum likelihood approach to continuous speech recognition." *IEEE Trans. Pattern Analysis, Machine Intelligence*, 5(2): 179-190, 1983.

[8] Bahl, L.R., Brown, P.F., De Souza, P.V., and Mercer, R.L. "Tree-based language model for natural language speech recognition." *IEEE Trans. Acoust., Speech, Signal Proc*.37(7): 1001-1008, 1989.

[9] Baker, J.K. "The DRAGON system: An overview." *IEEE Trans. Acous., Speech, Signal Proc*. 23: 24-29, 1975.

[10] Bellegarda, J.R. "Exploiting latent semantic information for statistical language modeling." *Proc. IEEE* 88(8): 1279-1296, 2000.

[11] Bilmes, J. and Zweig, G. "The graphical models toolkit: An open source software system for speech and time-series processing," *Proc. ICASSP*, 2002.

[12] Bourlard, H. and Morgan, N. *Connectionist Speech Recognition – A Hybrid Approach*. Boston: Kluwer, 1994.

[13] Bregman, A.S. *Auditory Scene Analysis: The Perceptual Organization of Sounds*. Cambridge, MA: MIT Press, 1990.

[14] Bridle, J., *et al*. "*An Investigation of Segmental Hidden Dynamic Models of Speech Coarticulation for Automatic Speech Recognition*," Final Report, 1998 JHU Workshop on Language Engineering, pp. 1-61, 1998.

[15] Brown, P.F., Cocke, J., Della Pietra, S.A., Della Pietra, V.J., Jelinek, F., Lafferty, J.D., Mercer, R.L., and Roossin, P.A. "A statistical approach to machine translation," *Computational Linguistics*, 16: 79-85, 1990.

[16] Chomsky, N. and Halle, M. *The Sound Pattern of English*. New York: Harper and Row, 1968.

[17] Church, K.W. *Phonological Parsing in Speech Recognition*. Boston: Kluwer, 1987.

[18] Cox, R.V., Camm, C.A., Rabiner, L.R., Schroeter, J. and Wilpon, J.G. "Speeech and language processing for next-millennium communication services." *Proc. IEEE* 88(8): 1273-1314, 2000.

[19] Davis, S.B. and Mermelstein, P. "Comparison of parametric representations of monosyllabic word recognition in continuously spoken sentences." *IEEE Trans. Acous., Speech, Signal Proc*. 28(4): 357-366, 1980.

[20] Dayan, P. and Abbott, L.F. *Theoretical Neuroscience: Computational and Mathematical Modeling of Neural Systems*. Cambridge, MA: MIT Press, 2001.

[21] DeGroot, M.H. *Optimal Statistical Decisions*. New York: McGraw-Hill, 1970.

[22] DeMori, R. (ed.), *Spoken Dialogues with Computers*. San Diego: Academic Press, 1998.

[23] Deng, L. "Computational models for speech production." In *Computational Models for Speech Pattern Processing*, R. Moore (ed.) Berlin: Springer-Verlag, pp. 199-214, 1997.

[24] Divenyi, P. (Chair), *Perspectives on Speech Separation – a Workshop*, http://www.ebire.org/speechseparation/, 2003

[25] Elman, J.L. "Finding Structures in time." *Cognitive Science* 14: 179-221, 1990.

[26] Fant, G. *Acoustic Theory of Speech Production*. the Hague: Mouton, 1970.

[27] Fant, G. *Speech Sounds and Features*. Cambridge, MA: MIT Press, 1973.

[28] Fiscus, J.G. "A post-processing system to yield reduced word error rates: Recognizer output voting error reduction (ROVER)." *Proc. 1997 ASRU Workshop*, pp. 347-352, 1997.

[29] Flanagan, J.L. *Speech Analysis, Synthesis and Perception*, 2nd edition. Berlin: Springer-Verlag, 1972.

[30] Fosler-Lussier, J.E. *Dynamic Pronunciation Models for Automatic Speech Recognition*, Ph.D. Dissertation, Department of Electrical Engineering and Computer Science, University of California, Berkeley, 1999.

[31] Furui, S. *Digital Speech Processing, Synthesis and Recognition.* Marcel Dekker, 2001.

[32] Gales, M.J.F. and Young, S. J. *"Parallel Model Combination for Speech Recognition in Noise."* Technical Report, CUED/ TR135, 1993.

[33] Gao, Y., Bakkis, R., Huang, J., and Zhang, B. "Multistage coarticulation model combining articulatory, formant and cepstral features." *Proc. Int. Conf. Spoken Lang. Proc.*, pp. 91-94, 2000.

[34] Garofolo, J.S., Lamel L.F., Fisher, W.M., Fiscus, J.G., Pallett, D.S., and Dahlgren, N.L. *"DARPA TIMIT Acoustic-Phonetic Continuous Speech Corpus."* U.S. Dept. of Commerce, NIST, Gaithersburg, MD, 1993.

[35] Gauvain, J.-L. and Lee, C.-H. "Maximum a posteriori estimation for multivariate gaussian mixture observations of Markov chains," *IEEE Trans. Speech Audio Proc.*, 2(2), 291-298, 1994.

[36] Gauvain, J.-L. and Lamel, L. "Large vocabulary continuous speech recognition: advances and applications." *Proc. IEEE*, 88(8): 1181-1200, 2000.

[37] Gersho, A. and Gray, R.M. *Vector Quantization and Signal Compression.* Boston: Kluwer, 1992.

[38] Ghitza, O. "Auditory nerve feedback as a basis for speech processing." *Proc. IEEE Int. Conf. Audio Speech Sig. Proc.*, pp. 91-94, 1988.

[39] Greenberg, S., Hollenback, J. and Ellis, D. "Insight into spoken language gleaned from phonetic transcription of the Switchboard corpus." *Proc. Int. Conf. Spoken Lang. Proc.*, 1996.

[40] Haykin, S. *Neural Networks: A Comprehensive Foundation.* Toronto: McMillan, 1994.

[41] Huo, Q. and Lee, C.-H. "On-line adaptive learning of the continuous density hidden Markov model based on approximate recursive Bayes estimate." *IEEE Trans. Speech Audio Proc.* 5(2): 161-172, 1997.

[42] Huo, Q. and Lee, C.-H. "Robust Speech recognition based on adaptive classification and decision strategies." *Speech Communication*, 34: 175-194, 2001.

[43] Jelinek, F. "The development of an experimental discrete dictation recognizer." *Proc. IEEE* 73(10): 1616-1624, 1985.

[44] Jelinek, F. *Statistical Method for Speech Recognition.* Cambridge, MA: MIT Press, 1997.

[45] Juang, B.-H., Levinson, S.E., and Sondhi, M.M. "Maximum likelihood estimation for multivariate mixture observations of markov chains." *IEEE Trans. Information Theory*, Vol. IT-32(2): 307-309, 1986.

[46] Juang, B.-H., Chou, W., and Lee, C.-H. "Discriminative Methods for speech recognition." *IEEE Trans. Speech Audio Proc.* 5(3): 257-265, 1997.

[47] Juang, B.-H. and Furui, S. "Automatic Speech recognition and understanding: A first step toward natural human-machine communication." *Proc. IEEE* 88(8): 1142-1165, 2000.

[48] Junqua, J.-C. and Haton, J.-P. *Robustness in Automatic Speech Recognition: Fundamentals and Applications.* Boston: Kluwer Academic Publishers, 1996.

[49] Katagiri, S., Juang, B.-H., and Lee, C.-H. "Pattern recognition using a generalized probabilistic descent method." *Proc. IEEE* 86 (11): 2345-2373, 1998.

[50] Katagiri, S. (ed.) *Handbook of Neural Networks for Speech Processing.* Artech House, 2000.

[51] Katz, S.M. "Estimation of probabilities from sparse data for the language model component of a speech recognizer." *IEEE Trans. Acoust., Speech, Signal Proc.* 35(3): 400-401, 1987.

[52] Kawahara, T., Lee, C.-H., and Juang, B.-H. "Key-Phrase detection and verification for flexible speech understanding." *IEEE Trans. Speech Audio Proc.* 6(6): 558-568, 1998.

[53] Klatt, D. "Review of the ARPA speech understanding project." *J. Acous. Soc. Am.* 62(6), 1977.

[54] Kohonen, T. *Self-Organizing Maps.* Berlin: Springer-Verlag, 1995.

[55] Launay, B., Siohan, O., Surendran, A.C., and Lee, C.-H. "Towards knowledge-based features for HMM based large vocabulary automatic speech recognition." *Proc. IEEE Int. Conf. Audio Speech Signal Proc.*, 2002.

[56] Lea, W. (ed.), *Trends in Speech Recognition.* Englewood Cliffs, NJ: Prentice Hall, 1980.

[57] Lee, C.-H. "A unified statistical hypothesis testing approach to speaker verification and verbal information verification." *Proc. COST Workshop on Speech Technology in the Public Telephone Network*, pp.62-73, 1997.

[58] Lee, C.-H. "On stochastic feature and model compensation approaches to robust speech recognition." *Speech Communication* 25: 29-47, 1998.

[59]   Lee, C.-H. "Statistical confidence measures and their applications." *Proc. ICSP-2001*, pp. 1021-1028, 2001.

[60]   Lee, C.-H. (Chair), *NSF Symposium on Next Generation Automatic Speech Recognition*, http://www.ece.gatech.edu/~chl/ngasr03, 2003.

[61]   Lee, C.-H., Rabiner, L.R., Pieraccini, R., and Wilpon, J.G. "Acoustic modeling for large vocabulary speech recognition." *Computer Speech and Language* 4(2): 127-165, 1990.

[62]   Lee, C.-H., Soong, K.F and Paliwal, K.K. (eds.) *Automatic Speech and Speaker Recognition: Advanced Topics*. Boston: Kluwer, 1996.

[63]   Lee, C.-H. and Huo, Q. "On adaptive decision rules and decision parameter adaptation for automatic speech recognition." *Proc. IEEE* 88(8): 1241-1269, 2000.

[64]   Lehmann, E.L. *Testing Statistical Hypotheses*. New York: John Wiley, 1959.

[65]   Leggetter, C.J. and Woodland, P.C. "Maximum likelihood linear regression for speaker adaptation of continuous density hidden Markov models." *Computer Speech and Language* 9: 171-185, 1995.

[66]   Levinson, S.E. "Structural methods in automatic speech recognition." *Proc. IEEE* 73: 1625-1650, 1985.

[67]   Lippmann, R. "Speech recognition by human and machines." *Speech Communication* 22: 1-14, 1997.

[68]   Ljolje, A. and Riley, M.D. "Optimal Speech recognition using phone recognition and lexical access." *Proc. Int. Conf. Spoken Lang. Proc.*, pp. 313-316, 1992.

[69]   Makhoul, J., Kubala, F., Leek, T., Liu, D., Nguyen, L., Schwartz, R., and Srivastava, A. "Speech and language technologies for audio indexing and retrieval." *Proc. IEEE* 88(8): 1338-1353, 2000.

[70]   Mozer, M. "Neural net architectures for temporal sequence processing." In *Predicting the Future and Understanding the Past*, A. Weigend and N. Gershenfeld (eds.), Addison-Wesley, 1993.

[71]   Ney, H. and Ortmanns, S. "Progresses in dynamic programming search for LVCSR." *Proc. IEEE* 88(8): 1224-1240, 2000.

[72]   Nilsson, N.J. *Problem-Solving Methods in Artificial Intelligence*, New York: McGraw Hill, 1971.

[73]   Niyogi, P. and Ramesh, P. "A detection framework for locating phonetic events." *Proc. Int. Conf. Spoken Lang. Proc.*, 1998.

[74]   Olive, J.P., Greenwood, A., Coleman, J., Greenwood, A., *Acoustics of American English Speech: A Dynamic Approach*. New York: Springer, 1993.

[75]   Ostendorf, M. and Roukos, S. "A Stochastic segment model for phoneme-based continuous speech recognition," *IEEE Trans. Acoust., Speech, Signal Proc.*, 37: 1857-1869, 1989.

[76]   Pallett, D.S. "A look at NIST's benchmark ASR test: past, present, and future." *Proc. IEEE ASRU Workshop*. pp. 483-488, 2003.

[77]   Parthasarathy, S. and Coker, C. "On Automatic estimation of articulatory parameters in a text-to-speech system." *Computer, Speech and Language* 6: 37-75, 1992.

[78]   Rabiner, L.R. "A tutorial on hidden Markov models and selected applications in speech recognition." *Proc. IEEE* 77(2): 257-286, 1989.

[79]   Rabiner, L.R. and Schafer, R.W. *Digital Processing of Speech Signals*. Englewood Cliffs: Prentice-Hall, 1978.

[80]   Rabiner, L.R. and Juang, B.-H. *Fundamentals of Speech Recognition*. Englewood Cliffs: Prentice-Hall, 1993.

[81]   Rahim, M., Lee, C.-H. and Juang, B.-H. "Discriminative utterance verification for connected digit recognition." *IEEE Trans. Speech Audio Proc.* 5(3): 266-277, 1997.

[82]   Ramesh, P. and Niyogi, P. "The voice feature for stop consonants: acoustic phonetic analysis and automatic speech recognition experiments." *Proc. Int. Conf. Spoken Lang. Proc.*, 1998.

[83]   Reddy, R. (ed.), *Speech Recognition, Invited Papers Presented at the 1974 IEEE Symposium*. New York: Academic Press, 1974.

[84]   Riley, M.D. "A statistical model for generating pronunciation networks." *Proc. IEEE Conf. Acoust. Speech Sig. Proc.*, pp. 737-740, 1991.

[85]   Rosenfeld, R. "Two decades of statistical language modeling: Where do we go from here?" *Proc. IEEE* 88(8), 1279-1296, 2000.

[86]   Sankar, A. and Lee, C.-H. "A maximum-likelihood approach to stochastic matching for robust speech recognition," *IEEE Trans. Speech Audio Proc.* 4(3): 190-202, 1996.

[87]   Seneff, S. "A Joint synchrony/mean-rate model of auditory speech processing." *J. Phonetics*, 16: 55-76, 1988.

[88] Shamma, S. "On the role of space and time in auditory processing." *Trends in Cognitive Sciences*, 5(8): 340-348, 2001.

[89] Shapire, R. "The strength of weak learnability," *Machine Learning*, 2, 197-227, 1990.

[90] Sukkar, R.A. and Lee, C.-H. "Vocabulary independent discriminative, utterance verification for non-keyword rejection in subword based speech recognition." *IEEE Trans. Audio Speech Proc.* 4(6): 420-429, 1996.

[91] Sumita, E., Yamada, S., Yamamoto, K., Paul, M., Kashioka, H., Ishikawa, K. and Shirai, S. "Solutions to problems inherent in spoken-language translation: The ATR-MATRIX approach." *Proc. MT Summit VII*, 1999.

[92] Stevens, K. *Acoustic Phonetics*. Cambridge, MA: MIT Press, 1998.

[93] Surendran, A.C., Lee, C.-H., and Rahim, M. "Non-linear compensation for stochastic matching." *IEEE Trans. Speech Audio Proc.*, 7(6): 643-655, 1999.

[94] Wald, A. *Sequential Analysis*. New York: John Wiley, 1947.

[95] Waibel, A., Geutner, P., Tomokiyo, L.M., Schultz, T., and Woszczyna, M. "Multiliguality in speech and spoken language systems." *Proc. IEEE* 88(8): 1166-1180, 2000.

[96] Wilpon, J.G., Rabiner, L.R., Lee, C.-H., and Goldman, E. "Automatic recognition of keywords in unconstrained speech using hidden Markov models." *IEEE Trans. Acous. Speech Signal Proc.*, 38(9): 1870-1878, 1990.

[97] Young, S., Odell, J., Ollason, D., Valtchev, V. and Woodland, P. *The HTK Book (for HTK Version 2.1)*. Cambridge: Cambridge University, 1997.

[98] Zitouni, I., Kuo, H.-K.J., and Lee, C.-H. "Boosting and combination of classifiers for natural language call routing systems." *Speech Communication*, 41: 647-661, 2003.

[99] Zue, V.W. "Acoustic-Phonetic knowledge representation: implications from spectrograms reading experiments." Tutorial paper presented at the 1981 *NATO ASI on Speech Recognition, Bonas, France*, 1981.

[100] Zue, V.W., Glass, J., Phillips, M. and Seneff, S. "The MIT Summit speech recognition system: A progress report." *Proc. DARPA Speech and Natural Language Workshop*, pp.179-189, 1989.

[101] Zue, V.W. and Glass, J.R. "Conversational interfaces: Advances and challenges," *Proc. IEEE* 88(8): 1166-1180, 2000.

Dynamics of Speech Production and Perception
P. Divenyi et al. (Eds.)
IOS Press, 2006

Automatic Phonetic Transcription and Its Application in Speech Recogniser Training – A Case Study for Hungarian

Péter MIHAJLIK, Péter TATAI and Géza GORDOS
Department of Telecommunications and Media Informatics
Budapest University of Technology and Economics
Budapest, Hungary

Abstract. Unlike English, many languages use phonetic writing style, e.g., the Slavic languages, Turkish, Hungarian, etc. For these languages the pronunciation modeling for an ASR (Automatic Speech Recognition) system is relatively easy, because merely some transcription rules have to be developed instead of huge dictionaries. Due to rule-based automatic transcriptions, such a solution can be much more flexible than dictionary-based ones since dynamically changing vocabularies can be transcribed without a-priori knowledge of the input words. This chapter discusses rule-based automatic phonetic transcriptions developed for Hungarian speech recognition. It first introduces the basic technologies of automatic speech recognition for the sake of readers not familiar with this scientific field; then it discusses the role of phonetic transcription in speech recogniser training. Next, our method is presented for transcribing Hungarian texts automatically. This technique is an extension of the traditional linear transcription approach; its output is called 'optioned' because it contains pronunciation options - including cross-word coarticulations - in parallel arcs. Comparing our 'optioned' transcription to other kinds of transcriptions, significant improvements in recogniser training efficiency can be experienced. The acoustic models trained with our automatically made phonetic transcriptions perform on independent test data practically at the same level as the acoustic models obtained using manual phonetic segmentation of the whole training database.

Keywords. Automatic speech recognition, pronunciation modeling, automatic phonetic transcription

Introduction

Automatic speech recognition (ASR) has been an extensively researched area in the past few decades, and now it has reached the level of practical applicability and is already in use, mainly in telephony applications. The current technology is phone-based, so the words to be recognised have to be transcribed into phone sequences; this process is called phonetic transcription, which has a significant role in ASR, as will be shown.

The operation of contemporary recognisers is based on statistical models, which is, perhaps, their most important feature. This means that the characteristics of the basic phone-units – which are often called acoustic models, i.e., the models of the speech-sounds – are estimated using a large speech database recorded from hundreds or thousands of speakers. In other words, the most successful ASR approach is somewhat similar to the human method: "First teach it, then use it!" A key point in teaching a speech recogniser – i.e. estimating the parameters of the acoustic models – is the need for the correct, or at least, consistent phonetic transcription of the recorded training speech.

Some training algorithms require not only the uttered phone sequence, i.e., the phonetic transcription, but also the time-boundaries of the speech sounds. Based on the transcription and some initial acoustic models, the approximate time-boundaries can be generated using a special technique called "forced alignment", which will be discussed later. Nevertheless, a great amount of spoken text has to be transcribed phonetically. This is time-consuming, tedious work for a human, so it is an expensive procedure. Since the Hungarian orthography and pronunciation are in relatively close correspondence, it seemed plausible to automate the process of phonetic transcription as well. However, as we have experienced, the development of a general transcription method for ASR purposes is not a straightforward task.

In this paper we give a very brief introduction to the basics of current mainstream speech recognition technology, and show the role of phonetic transcription in speech recogniser training. This is followed by a discussion of the main difficulties in automatic phonetic transcription (APT) for ASR, namely, alternative pronunciation options, and the different behaviour of adjacent consonants at morpheme or word boundary. Then we propose a method for individual words and extend it for longer training texts. After that, we present and analyse our experimental results obtained on speaker- and gender-independent isolated-word recognition tasks. In the experiments, the acoustic models were trained with various phonetic transcriptions; their qualities – in terms of recognition rates on an independent test database – are compared to each other. Our automatic phonetic transcription method outperforms the other transcription techniques, including the manual method, and performs nearly as well as the manual *segmentation*.

1.   A Few Words About Automatic Speech Recognition Technologies

As mentioned earlier, today's most successful ASR technology is based on a statistical approach, often referred to as the Hidden Markov-Model (HMM) technique. The core of this technology is that every speech sound is modelled by one or more simple HMMs and these phone-models are joined to each other, depending on the recognition task, resulting in a "big" HMM. This composite HMM is a directed graph, which always has a single starting and a single ending node, and is able to recognise any of the possible phone sequences, represented by a path between the start and the end node.

1.1 Recognition

First, the sound – the intensity change of the air-pressure – is converted to electromagnetic signal by a microphone, and then it is digitised. An acoustic pre-processing step follows, which transforms the waveform into a frequency-domain signal. Then further transformations are executed on the resulted short-time spectra, such as Mel-filtering, logarithm calculation, DCT, and addition of temporal derivatives. The result of the pro-

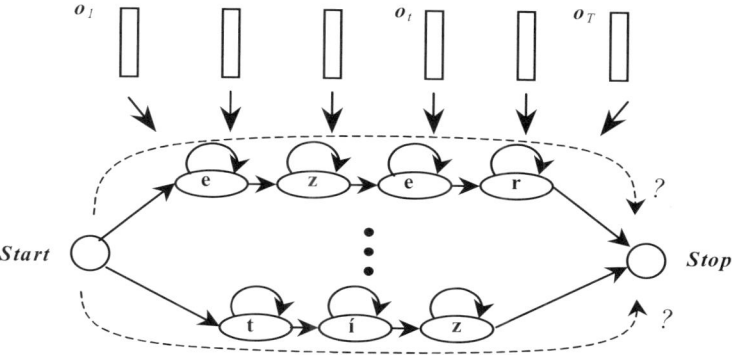

Figure 1. Illustration of HMM-based isolated-word number recognition (*ezer* "thousand", …, *tíz* "ten" are parallel branches representing recognition alternatives).

cess is a sequence of feature vectors (o_1, o_2, …, o_T) equally spaced in time, where each vector characterises the respective part of the speech signal. This pre-processing step is often called parameterisation or feature extraction.

The main task of the recogniser is to choose the best, i.e., most likely path between the start and end node according to the actual feature vector sequence. Each phone-model has its own "similarity" function, which provides the likelihood measure of an incoming feature vector, so the simplest means of operation is to measure the likelihood of each feature vector in each phone-model and then choose the most likely phone-sequence among all possible paths. An efficient implementation of this method is the Viterbi algorithm [3]. For the sake of simplicity, each phone model consists of one HMM state in this example, but typically three states with "left-to-right" topology are used for each model.

1.2 Training of acoustic models

In order to be able to compute the likelihood of a feature vector in a phone model, the likelihood function of the sound model must be estimated in some way. This estimation process is called "training of acoustic models". Generally the Maximum Likelihood (ML) criterion is used, which can be illustrated by the following example: if we would like to estimate the likelihood function of the phone-model [ɔ], then it is expected that on average the likelihood function responds with the maximum value in cases of feature vectors originated from an [ɔ] sound as compared to feature vectors originated from any other sound ([aː], [b], …).

There are two main approaches to perform such training: the initialisation training and the embedded training. Both require a great amount of recorded speech – the more the better – because the likelihood functions to be determined are estimated from statistics of feature vectors derived from a training speech database. It can be shown that the continuous density function of the distribution of training feature vectors corresponding to the given state fulfils the criterion mentioned above.

- **Initialisation training:** In this case the boundaries of the speech sounds are needed, so each feature vector can be unambiguously mapped to a phone-model. Then, the likelihood functions of the phone-models can be estimated one by one typically by a **K-means algorithm** as mixtures of Gaussian-functions [3]. To refine the estimation the Viterbi realignment is used [8]. The training within this approach is relatively effective in terms of quality of acoustic models and convergence speed; however, it requires not only the uttered phone sequence but also the exact boundaries of the speech sounds.

- *Embedded training:* The other, widely used training method is the embedded **Baum-Welch re-estimation** procedure [8]. If an acoustic model is given, its summarised likelihood on a speech sample can be increased by applying the Baum-Welch re-estimation formulae. In other words, if we have a trained recogniser and the uttered phone sequence is known, the recogniser can be refined further to fit better to the speech utterance. An important characteristic of this approach is that no information is needed about the boundaries of the speech sounds; it merely requires the phone sequence, i.e., the phonetic transcription of the recorded training speech. This is an advantage as compared to the previous approach; this embedded training, however, requires an initially trained acoustic model set which, if not present, can be substituted by so called "flat models", but then the convergence of training iterations can be unacceptably inferior. Often, the embedded training iterations are applied after a K-means and Viterbi initialisation training to further refine the acoustic models.

1.3 Forced alignment

Forced alignment is a commonly used technique that deserves to be described in some detail. In fact, the basic forced alignment method is an extremely simplified recognition procedure aiming only at the temporal segmentation of the input speech-signal, based on its phonetic transcription. The way of doing this is the following: according to the precise phonetic transcription of the input speech, the phone-models are sequentially joined to each other resulting in a *linear* hidden Markov-model. This HMM is used for recognising the input speech utterance. Actually, the recogniser has no other choice but to recognise the actual given phone-sequence; therefore it is called "forced" alignment. Thus, the result of the recognition is trivial, since there is only one path between the start and end node, so we utilise only the side-effect of the recognition process, namely, the mapping of every feature vector to a phone-model whereby the input speech is segmented at the phone-level.

This simple recognition procedure is able to determine the approximate boundaries of the sounds in the speech sample based only on the phonetic transcription. Of course, some trained acoustic models are needed for the recognition, too.

This method allows one to choose freely among training techniques requiring either segmentation or not, assuming that an initial acoustic model set is available, which always can be prepared by a small amount of manual work (i.e., manual phonetic segmentation and initialisation training).

2. Phonetic Transcriptions Techniques for Recogniser Training

As mentioned earlier, the recorded words and sentences have to be accompanied by their correct phonetic transcription at the training phase. There are many possible ways to produce phonetic transcriptions.

- ***Manual method****:* Perhaps one of the highest quality solutions is to listen to all recordings and do each and every phonetic transcription "by ear". This approach has a great advantage: independently of the written text, the actual, *uttered* phone sequence is recorded which otherwise might not be the case due to misreading. But as usual, the "human-factor" causes failures, too. This kind of transcription technique, however, requires a qualified employee with excellent hearing abilities, also the work is very monotonous and tiresome. So, considering the quite large amount of speech data (typically some 10 hours or more) this is a really expensive method. If the time boundaries of the phones are also determined during this process, it is called manual segmentation.

- ***Computer-aided manual method****:* In a variant of the previous system, an automatic phonetic transcription based on the known read text is made first, and the human task is merely to modify the automatic transcription where necessary after listening to the recorded speech. It could be noted that currently for Hungarian, as well as for other languages, the majority of training materials are read speech, so the source text is generally available. This transcription method is faster than the previous one, but the automatically generated phone transcriptions might bias the listener and the technique still needs a huge amount of human work, especially if segmentation is also performed simultaneously.

- ***Automatic-method****:* Another approach is to do the phonetic transcriptions completely automatically based on the source read text. Undoubtedly, once an APT technique is readily available, this is the fastest and the most inexpensive way, but of course, where the "printed" and "spoken" text differ, the automatically made phonetic transcription will contain errors.

- ***Human-aided automatic method****:* In a variant of the previous system a manual checking of the source text is made first after a quick listening of the recordings. The aim of this step is to correct or indicate if evident errors are made during the reading (such as misreading, stopping in the middle of the word, hesitation…). This step is frequently called annotation and requires much less human work than the correction of APT errors in the computer-aided manual case. The automatic phonetic transcription of an annotated text may be very close to the result of the manual method.

Generally, the last mentioned approach is preferred on the basis of price/quality ratio. However, there is a theoretical difficulty with the automatic generation of the (guessed) uttered phone sequence, i.e., the actual utterance realization of a read text cannot be predicted in advance, because very often variations in the pronunciation can occur. While in the case of isolated words the number of alternative phonetic realisations is generally one or two, the number of possible pronunciations of a complete sentence is much higher. The source of the variations is not only that a sentence includes more words and so, trivially, the product of word variations can be high; additional phenomena arise due to the optional pauses between words and the phonological interactions at word boundaries. In the case of training sentences, however, the real difficulty is that the pronunciation options cannot be directly represented, because the training algorithms by default need an *actual* linear phone sequence, as opposed e.g. to the isolated-word vocabulary transcription.

We have elaborated a special technique to solve the problem described above. Our method is the following: first a special – we call it "optioned" – phonetic transcription is generated automatically from the annotated source text for every sentence. This kind of transcription contains parallel phone-sequence options allowing alternative pronunciations.

Illustration:

> Original source text:
>
> > *Mit csinálsz, Bandi?*   "What are you doing, Andrew?"
>
> Annotated source text:
>
> > *mit csinálsz Bandi*
>
> Possible phonetic transcriptions:
>
> > m i t t͡ʃ i n a: l s sil b ɔ n d i
> > m i t͡ʃ i n a: l s sil b ɔ n d i
> > m i t t ʃ i n a: l z b ɔ n d i
> > m i t ʃ i n a: l z b ɔ n d i
>
> Optioned phonetic transcription:
>
> > m i < t | > t͡ʃ i n a: l < s sil | z > b ɔ n d i

In this example the optioned transcription includes four possible phonetic transcriptions. A pronunciation option begins with "<", the alternative phonetic realization are separated by "|", and the return from an option is denoted by ">". "sil" denotes speech silence.

In the next step these optioned transcriptions are used in the forced alignment. For this procedure the basic forced alignment method has been extended to handle parallel alternatives. The forced alignment chooses a uniquely estimated phone-sequence among all possible pronunciations allowed by the optioned transcription. In this step the time boundaries of the speech sounds are determined, too, but they can be discarded if not needed. So, essentially the computer is used for "listening" to the recordings, instead of humans.

Though representing alternative pronunciations of *words* in forced alignment is a commonly used technique, taking into account the optional cross-word coarticulations, i.e., assimilations at word boundaries is not a typical approach.

The question is how well this method performs, and how the "optioned" phonetic transcriptions can be generated automatically. For the answer we had to work in the reverse direction: first we generated the transcriptions automatically and then conducted some experiments to evaluate the effect of optioned phonetic transcriptions applied in speech recogniser training. The rest of the article is devoted to this issue.

3. Automatic Phonetic Transcription of Hungarian Texts

In the following we discuss the problems related to automatic phonetic transcription of Hungarian, give a method for isolated words, and then extend it for training sentences.

3.1 Introduction

The Hungarian alphabet is based on the Latin alphabet but it is extended by special accents like *ó, é, ű, ö* etc. (vowels only). Similarly to other languages, some phonemes are denoted by two or more characters (consonants only); these will be called multi-character letters, e.g., '*sz*' pronounced as [s], or its long counterpart '*ssz*' pronounced as [s:].

Though the Hungarian writing has about a thousand year tradition, the language – including the writing system – was renewed in the XIX. century. As a result, we still have a phonetic writing system: generally the pronunciation of a word can be predicted from its orthography. The difficulties arise merely on morpheme boundaries. As Hungarian is a heavily agglutinating language consonant congestion in the suffixation and similar dynamic events influencing the pronunciation occur quite frequently.

3.2 Problems

The process of phonetic transcription can be divided into two main steps. The first one is to identify the letters in the input text, with a special care to the multi-character letters, which abound in Hungarian, and then to convert them into phonemes; the result is the canonical phonemic transcription. At the second step, the interactions of adjacent speech sounds or phonemes are taken into account, and so we get the phone-sequence(s) of the input word according to its actual pronunciation(s) as an output phonotypical transcription.

3.2.1 First step: Segmentation of orthographic words to letters

With respect to automating the segmentation of Hungarian words into letters, one has to deal with the following problems:

1. The identification of multi-character letters in the input word can be ambiguous if higher-level linguistic knowledge is not applied in the source text.

   An example of the decoding ambiguity of the *csz* string:

   láncszem → *l á n cs z e m* or *l á n c sz e m* ?   "chain-loop"
   kulcszörgés → *k u l c sz ö r g é s* or *k u l cs z ö r g é s* ?   "jingle of a key"

2. Further difficulties arise when dealing with traditionally spelt or foreign words and acronyms, (like *Batthyány*, *e-mail*, *ABC*...). In these cases it makes no sense to segment the words into letters; obviously they should be handled as exceptions.

So, the first problem is to identify the letters in the text, and then they can be converted one by one into phonemes.

3.2.2 Second step: Handling phonological processes

Once the canonic phonemic transcription is arrived at, there is often no need for further processing. However, in many cases the pronounced sequence of phones is different from the canonical form because of the interaction of neighbouring phonemes or speech sounds. Particularly, the consonants may change, due to assimilations, mergers etc. These phenomena are widely known and often described as pronunciation rules [2].

A difficulty that prevents the direct application of these rules in a computer-based system is that they utilize higher-level linguistic information, which is not available by default. Moreover, the rules sometimes allow more correct pronunciation options and it is not trivial how to handle them.

Let us see some examples for the pronunciation ambiguity of phoneme-pairs or triplets:

– [t j]:

[l a: t j ɔ] → [l a: c: ɔ] "somebody can see it"

[a: t j a: r o:] → [a: t j a: r o:] "passageway"

In the first case, only the pronunciation involving [c:] is correct, while in the second case only the [t j].

– [t ʃ]:

[ɔ p a: t ʃ a: g] → [ɔ p a: tʃ: a: g] or [ɔ p a: t ʃ a: g] "abbey" [1]

Both pronunciations are correct.

– [ʃ t]:

[ɛ z y ʃ t] → [ɛ z y ʃ t] "silver"

[ɛ z y ʃ t b a: ɲ ɔ] → [ɛ z y ʒ d b a: ɲ ɔ] "silvermine" [1]

The sound [b] voices not only the adjacent sound [t], but the more distant [ʃ], too.

– [s t g]

[e: b r ɛ s t g ɛ t]→ [e: b r ɛ z d g ɛ t] or [e: b r ɛ z g ɛ t] "somebody is waking up somebody"

The [d] can optionally be dropped.

Therefore the traditional linear phone sequence output approach that is adequate in speech synthesis cannot be kept in speech recognition. Here, all correct pronunciation options should be represented in some way in the phonetic transcription.

3.3 Our automatic phonetic transcription method

In the following we introduce a method to transcribe individual (orthographic) words into phonotypical phone sequences including pronunciation options. Also, the majority of the previously outlined problems can be handled within this framework. The main steps of the method are as follows:

3.3.1 Morpheme analysis

Most of the problems described above can be handled by taking the morphological structure of words into account. Therefore, the first step of our method is to perform morphological segmentation. The words are passed to a morphological analyser that inserts special symbols at morpheme boundaries. This method was originally proposed in Wothke [7] and our system uses similar symbols to theirs:

= before a stem

+ before a derivational affix

% before an inflectional affix

Example:

     kulcszörgés → =kulcs=zörg+és   "jingle of a key"

3.3.2 Identification of letter boundaries

After the boundaries of the morphemes have been determined, the input word can be segmented into letters on a morpheme-by-morpheme basis. This turns out to be a much easier task than segmenting the original word because ambiguous combinations of the letters almost never occur inside morphemes.

Utilising that observation, Hungarian morphemes can be segmented unambiguously into letters with the following method. The alphabet, including long consonants, is stored in a table. The first letter of the morpheme is the longest (containing the most characters) letter of the table that matches the beginning of the morpheme. This letter is detached and the process is continued on the remaining part of the morpheme.

Example:

     =dzsessz=szín=ház → = dzs e ssz = sz í n = h á z   "jazz-theatre"

3.3.3 Letter to phoneme conversion

Due to the close correspondence, the mapping of letters to phonemes can be considered unambiguous and can be done letter by letter. As a result we get a phoneme sequence, the canonical phonemic transcription of the input word extended with morpheme boundary symbols.

Examples:

     = t a x i → = t ɔ k s i

     = ly u k → = j u k

In the next step, we will switch from phonology to the phonetic level. Therefore, the segmental units will be referred to as "phones" or "speech sounds" rather than "phonemes". Also, the brackets surrounding phonetic transcriptions will be omitted from now on.

3.3.4 Application of phonological rules

The pronunciation variants of the input word are generated with the appropriate application of Hungarian phonological rules. For treating the problems described in the previous section, we use the formalism below, after Wothke [7] which permits generation of alternative outputs at each rule and is able to utilise morpheme boundary information.

$$\mathbf{X\{Y\}Z} \;\to\; \langle \mathbf{W1}|\ldots|\mathbf{Wn}\rangle$$

This rule changes the extended phone string Y to the alternative phone strings W1, …, Wn if it occurs in the phonetic transcription of the input word with X left and Z right context. Both X and Z are extended phone string sets as string elements permitted. The use of phone sets is described later in this section.

Examples of the simple use of this formalism:

     Rules (merger of consonants)

  1. {t = j} →   <t j>

    2. {t % j} →   <c:>

    3. {t + ʃ} → <t ʃ| tʃ:>

Application:

    1. = aː t = j aː r oː → = aː t j aː r oː: "passage"

    2. = l aː t % j ɔ → = l aː c: ɔ   "somebody can see it"

    3. = ɔ p aː t + ʃ aː g → = ɔ p aː <t ʃ| tʃ:> aː g   "abbey"

There are two types of rules, depending on their direction of application: "forward rules" and "backward rules". In the case of forward rules, the best matching rule is sought from the beginning of the extended input phone string and applied if it exists. The search then continues with the next phoneme until the word ends. In the case of backward rules, the evaluation sequence is the opposite. Backward rules provide a convenient way to formulate rules of assimilation:

    Pronunciation rules (backward rules):

$$\text{VOICING} = \{\text{b} \quad \text{d} \quad \text{ɟ} \quad \text{g} \quad \text{z} \quad \text{ʒ} \quad \widehat{\text{dz}} \quad \widehat{\text{dʒ}} \}$$

    //comment: consonants, which can change the preceding consonant from voiceless to

    //voiced

    {t} VOICING   → d

    {t=} VOICING → d

    {s} VOICING   → ʒ

    ...

and their application:

    = ɛ z y ʃ t = b aː ɲ ɔ → = ɛ z y ʒ d b aː ɲ ɔ   "silver-mine"

In this example, the variable "VOICING" defines a phone set. When it occurs in a rule, it matches any of the phones on the right hand side of its definition, in this example it matches [b], [d], [ɟ], ... Starting with the second rule, [t] is changed into [d]. In the next step, this [d] changes the preceding [s] into [ʒ], using the third rule.

The rules are structured into groups. The evaluation direction is the same within each group, so that a group of rules is evaluated at one time as described. The phonotypical phonetic transcription of the input word, including the pronunciation alternatives, is generated by the sequential application of rule groups.

The rule groups may have illustrative linguistic meanings. With the organization of groups illustrated in Figure 2, words that are the subject of more than one pronunciation rule can also be transcribed.

The shortening/lengthening/insertion/dropping of vowels and consonants can hardly be algorithmically described, and therefore they are handled as exception-like rules. (Examples: *szőlő* → [s ø lː ø:] "grapes", *lesz* → [l ɛ sː] "it will be", *juh* → [j u] "sheep" etc.)

Actually, in Figure 2 – excluding the dashed line block – the pronunciation is modelled in the phonological level. Of course, the scope of this pronunciation modelling is limited, but many "problematic" words can be transcribed in this way as shown in the right side of the figure. The morpheme boundary symbols are not shown.

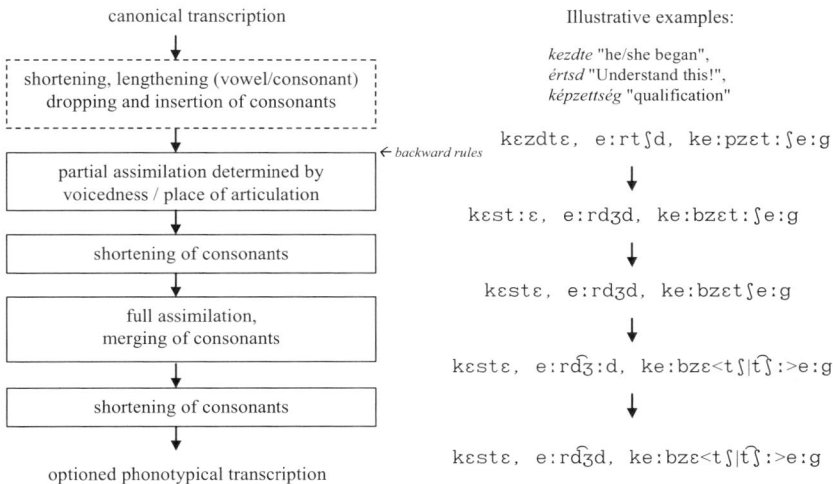

Figure 2. The generation of phonotypical transcription including alternatives by means of formalized pronunciation rules.

3.3.5 Text to graph conversion

Finally, the phonotypical transcription containing the pronunciation options – which we call optioned phonetic transcription – is converted to graph representation. The result is a pronunciation phone-network, which can be effectively stored and used in the computer. Of course, this last step is not a subtask of the phonetic transcription, it is a wholly separate procedure but, as it nearly always follows the transcription process, we include it in the description here.

Example: a z o < n m | mm > ó d → 0 1 a;

1 2 z;
2 3 o;
3 4 n;
4 5 m;
3 5 mm;
5 6 ó;
6 7 d;

3.4 Extension of the algorithm for training sentences

The previously presented method generates the optioned phonetic transcription of an input word. The question is: how can it be enhanced to transcribe whole sentences? Fortunately, the answer is quite simple: only the introduction of word boundary symbols and the corresponding rules are necessary, otherwise the entire process described is applicable.

An example rule:

{t \\ = s} → <t sil s | t s | t͡s :>

//comment: symbol "\" denotes the beginning and ending of a word

Application: *Mit szólsz?* "What do you say?"

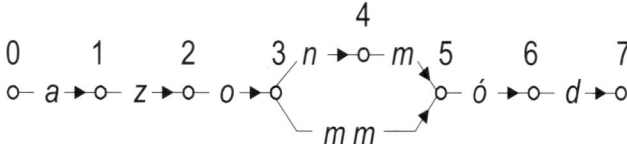

Figure 3. The pronunciation graph representation of the Hungarian word *azonmód* [ɔ z o n m oː d] or [ɔ z o mː oː d] "right away".

$$\backslash = m \ i \ \% \ t \ \backslash \backslash = s \ o: \ l \ \%s \ \backslash \qquad \rightarrow$$
$$\backslash = \ m \ i \ \% <t \ sil \ s \ | \ t \ s \ | \ \widehat{ts} :> o: \ l \ \%s \ \backslash$$

Due to optional pauses between words and possible consonant clusters across word boundaries, it is not a straightforward job to construct a compact set of rules for sentences. But our aim is to perform well the optioned phonetic transcriptions for the large majority of the sentences; the elaboration of a perfectly precise technology would be unrealistic.

Since the training algorithms are statistical, they are relatively insensitive to transcription or other errors. The only important thing is that there should be many more correct forms than erroneous. But if this is true, do we really need the optioned transcriptions? Would it not be enough or better to use some simple – automatically or manually made - linear phone-sequences for training? To answer these questions we carried out some experiments, which will be described in the following section.

4. Experimental Comparison of Speech Recognisers Trained with Different Phonetic Transcriptions

We conducted two different experiments to evaluate the efficiency of our method developed for transcribing training sentences. Three different kinds of phonetic transcription were used for training, and the recognition efficiencies of the resulting acoustic models were compared to each other in a series of tests.

The experimentation was based on the HTSD (Hungarian Telephony Speech Database) [6]. It consists of various utterances of 500 speakers, primarily read speech recorded in normal environment through fixed or mobile network. A part of the database – comprising phonetically rich sentences and words – is particularly elaborated; we utilised this fraction to do the comparison mentioned above. This particular part (12 sentences and 4 words per speaker) is manually segmented at the phone level, and it further includes the original automatic segmentation as well. To be precise, the developers of the database performed some forced alignment with automatic linear transcription of the annotated source texts and then corrected the phonetic segmentation manually. So, by leaving the time boundaries out from the segmentations, we get the "opponents" of our "optioned" phonetic transcription, namely, the "computer-aided manual" and the "human-aided automatic" transcriptions.

Our fundamental aim was to investigate the significance of phonetic transcription in recogniser training. Investigation effectively meant training the speech recognisers with differently made transcriptions and testing them on independent speech data. Among the four basic transcription methods discussed in Section III we excluded the fully manual and automatic ones because of their impracticality. Hence, our examinations were focused on the other two types of transcription methods, and to our advanced technique.

During the experimentation the standard Mel-frequency Cepstral Coefficients (MFCCs) were used as feature vectors [8]. The logarithmic energy was appended to the first ten cepstral coefficients and then the first and second temporal derivates were calculated and appended to the original vector resulting in a 33 dimensional feature vector. No cepstral mean subtraction or energy normalisation was performed at the parameterisation of the utterances.

Before using the whole training database, initial investigations were done. The aim of these experimentations was to see if a moderate amount of data is sufficient to evaluate the transcription methods, or not. There was a practical reason, too: at the beginning of the work only the first 100 speakers' data was available.

4.1 Initial experiments

Because of the limited training data, context independent (monophone) models were used with three states per model. As a pre-processing step, training utterances, which had a noise marker in the annotation, were excluded. Then we made a comparative analysis of phonetic transcription methods in the following way:

- First we split the speech data of the 100 speakers into two parts. The acoustic models used later for forced alignment were trained on the first 50 speakers' data utilising manual segmentation, and only the other 50 speakers' data was used for further experimentations.

- The mentioned three types of phonetic transcriptions were collected for every sentence. For simplicity the "computer-aided manual" and "human-aided automatic" transcriptions will be referred in the followings to as "manual" and "automatic", respectively. The optioned phonetic transcription was generated by our transcription method from the annotated source text. (The morpheme analysis step was not implemented yet in the algorithm.)

- Forced alignment – using the acoustic models trained on the other half of the material – was performed with all three transcriptions for all sentences. As a result we got three segmentations for all training utterances.

- Initiated with these three segmentations, three training procedures were performed in exactly the same way using the Cambridge Hidden Markov-Model Tool Kit (HTK) functions [8]. All training consisted of 26 stages. The first step was the k-means and Viterbi training (Hinit) with 1 Gauss function per phonemodel, and it was followed by the embedded Baum-Welch re-estimations (HERest) with mixture increments through mixture splitting. (Mixture number: the number of Gauss-functions at a phone-model)

- After each training step a Hungarian city name recognition test was carried out on an independent telephony speech database with a vocabulary size of 500. The test data comprised of the city name part of the SpeechDat-Hungarian database [5]. The non-noisy marked utterances of the first 500 speakers were used (413 recordings altogether). The recognition rates are shown in Figure 4.

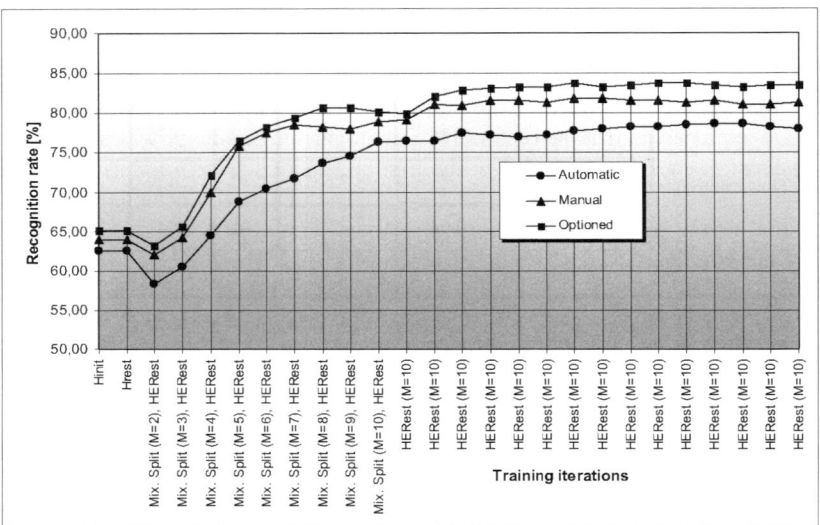

Figure 4. City name recognition error rates referring to the acoustic models of speakers 50-99, trained using different phonetic transcriptions.

In order to control our results, we repeated the whole series of experiments by swapping the first and second half of the hundred speakers available.

As it can be seen, our automatic optioned phonetic transcription method outperformed in both cases not only the traditional automatic but the manual method, as well.

However, it is important to mention that the acoustic models used for the forced alignments were measured as significantly better than the acoustic models trained based on *transcriptions*. We measured 10.4% and 11.1% WERs when the acoustic models were trained with the first and the second half of the training data based on *manual segmentation*, correspondingly. In these cases, the acoustic models were taught applying initialisation training (k-means algorithm and Viterbi realignment) utilising directly the manually checked phone boundary information.

We conclude that in this case – where only a few training data are present – the application of optioned transcriptions results in considerably better acoustic models than the application of manual or automatic linear *transcriptions*, but it provides significantly worse results than the application of precise manual *segmentations*.

Though these results were promising, further investigations were necessary to reduce the uncertainty caused by data insufficiency.

4.2 Experiments utilising the entire training database

In order to draw valid conclusions the investigations were extended to all 500 speakers' data in the HTSD. In this case there was an adequate amount of data to train context dependent (cross-word triphone) acoustic models. Similar to the previous experiment noisy recordings were removed from the database (about 15%); the total length of training material was about 5 hours.

Our aim was to build and compare the best recognisers available; therefore we conducted several experiments based on the training part of the HTSD to find an optimum

		Initial ER	Best ER	N	#	Relative ER
Manual Segmentation		6.85%	6.85%	0	415	—
Transcriptions	Optioned	7.26%	7.02%	2	425	+2.4%
	Manual	7.71%	7.58%	2	459	+10.6%
	Automatic	9.06%	8.93%	1	541	+30.4%
Monophone case*		19.4%		—	1280	+191%

Table 1. A summary of experimental results obtained on the whole training database. Initial ER: Recognition error rate after the initialisation training. Best ER: The lowest recognition error rate after N embedded training iterations. N: Number of the embedded training iterations required for the best result. #: Number of recognition errors. Relative ER: Relative increasing of the error rates (reference: manual segmentation) * The recognition results of the acoustic model set used for forced alignment.

training strategy. The optimal technique found was the following: using the Flexi-Train tool [4] developed at our Laboratory, an initialisation training was performed first. Initialisation meant not only k-means and Viterbi training with 10 mixtures, but monophone to triphone conversion, and rule-based clustering of the triphones, too. Then the acoustic models were refined by embedded training iterations until the recognition rates on independent test data decreased. With the application of this training strategy a recognition error rate of 2.67% was achieved on the SpeechDat City name task when using manual segmentation.

However, because of the low number of test utterances, the City name task is not adequate to test recognition efficiencies if good estimates of these statistical quantities are needed. Besides, SpeechDat Hungarian consists of only fixed network telephone speech. Therefore in the new tests a novel database was used, the twin database of HTSD, the HTSD-II (in Hungarian it is called "BeszTel") developed at our department. The structure of this material is equivalent to the HTSD, except that in HTSD-II there is no transcription or segmentation at all. (Of course, separate talkers acted in the two databases.) This database is currently not publicly available.

The test set was constructed as follows: 14 utterances of each speaker were collected, targeting short and middle length words (e.g. "yes/no" answers, numbers < 10, command words, surnames, family names, city names, etc.) – there was no overlap between the types of utterances in the training and test databases. Then the recordings marked as noisy were filtered out, since the aim of the experiments was not noise robustness evaluation. At the end altogether 6057 test utterances remained.

The test dictionary was created in such a way that the source texts of the test set were merged and the duplicates were removed. As a result we got a vocabulary with a size of 934. The transcription of the vocabulary elements was performed with our transcription tool, but this time only one typical pronunciation per item was allowed. In other words, for the dictionary transcription a traditional linear human-aided automatic method was applied. The average utterance length in the dictionary was 7.2 phones, or 3.1 syllables (calculation was based on the phonetic transcription).

In this way we obtained a sophisticated isolated-word recognition task applicable to

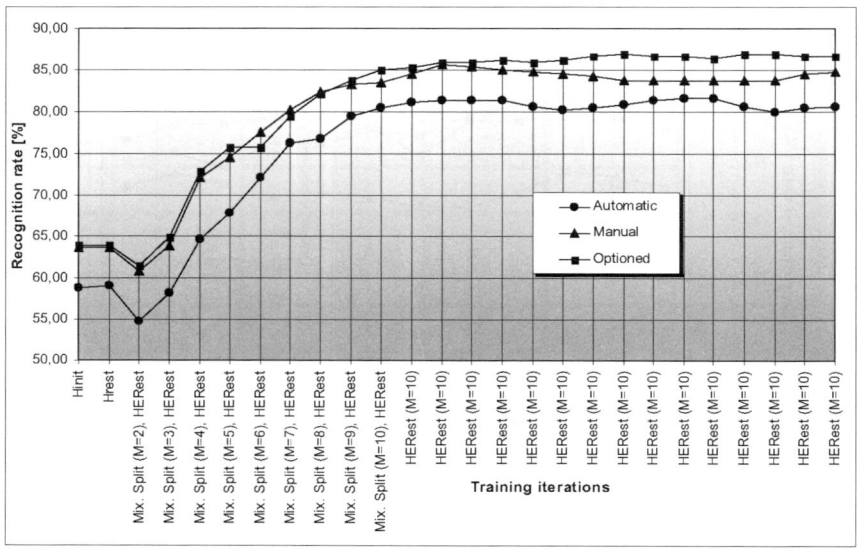

Figure 5. City name recognition error rates referring to the acoustic models of speakers 0-49, trained using different phonetic transcriptions.

measure the quality of any acoustic model set with high confidence. In the experiments we always used this practical task – referred to as "HTSD-II task" – to test the accuracy and to compare the differently trained recognisers.

The comparative analysis was carried out as follows:

- First the transcriptions ("automatic", "manual", and "optioned") and the manual segmentations were collected or generated for the entire training database.

- Then all three transcriptions were converted to segmentations by forced alignment with the acoustic models used for the same purpose in the initialisation experiments. (Those monophone models were used, which were trained on the first 50 speakers' data.)

- The previously described training procedure was applied for all the four cases of segmentations. Each training step was followed by a test on the HTSD-II task. The manual segmentation acted as a reference to the transcriptions.

- Finally we evaluated the recognition results. A summary of the experiments is shown in Table 1.

4.3 Evaluation of recognition results

The results are convincing: the "optioned" transcription performed significantly better than the "manual" transcription, which was definitely superior to the "automatic" one as measured by recognition rates. The validity of experimental results is supported by the observable stability of recognition error rates; the embedded training iterations could hardly refine the thoroughly estimated acoustic models of the initialisation training.

There are two explanations of these results. First the "optioned" method does not have "human-factor" errors. Second, it must be mentioned here that the term "manual"

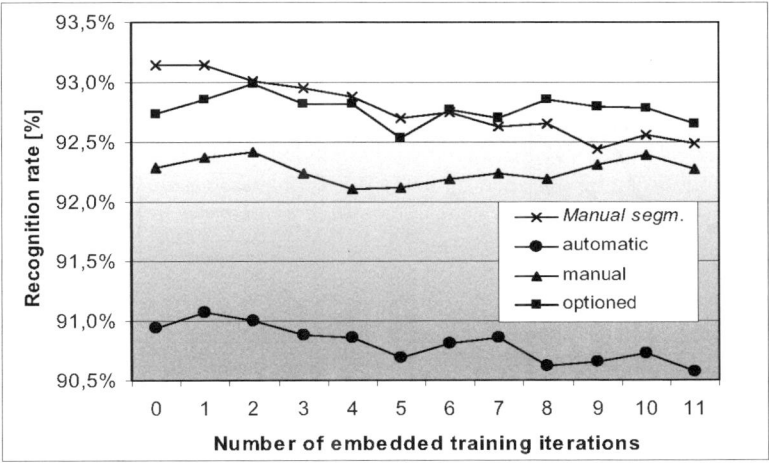

Figure 6. Recognition rates referring to the acoustic models trained using various phonetic transcriptions and to the acoustic model set trained on manual segmentation. The initialisation training is followed by several embedded training iterations.

was used in the experiments as a shortened form of the term "computer-aided manual"; accordingly, these transcriptions were made by *manual corrections of automatically made transcriptions*. Therefore, the manually corrected phonetic transcription can be biased, as discussed in Section III, especially if the quality of the automatically made transcriptions is inferior, e.g., because the pronunciation rules do not take deeper phonological processes into account. Probably both assumptions are applicable considering the relatively high error rates of the original "automatic" transcriptions. Though the superiority of an automatic transcription method amongst transcription techniques containing manual method, as well, was somewhat unexpected, we found it more interesting than the slight difference between the results of the optioned *transcription* and of the manually made *segmentation*.

In what follows we make an attempt to explain the possible cause of this phenomenon. First of all, as it is generally accepted, training a speech recogniser requires only a few manually segmented "bootstrap" data, and increasing the amount of hand-labelled data has only a little effect on the acoustic model quality [8]. So, the small difference in recognition rates is not surprising when the results of the manual segmentation based training and the phonetic transcription based training are compared to each other. Note that in the first case manual segmentations for the entire training database was used directly while in the second case only the first 50 speakers' manual segmentation was used indirectly. What is unexpected, it is the small ratio of the error rates (2.4% relative!). A possible explanation is the following: the "manual" transcription is less accurate than the "optioned" one, therefore the adjusting of segment boundaries by hand cannot improve the training beyond a limit (which was in our case 10.6%, relative). When considering the results of the transcriptions (see Table 1) the previous finding seems reasonable.

Now we have come to the point where conclusions can be drawn. From the *theoretical* point of view, it would be very interesting to do the following comparisons in order to complete the investigation of phonetic transcription and segmentation methods: first do the transcriptions fully manually to avoid the influence of automatic method (this would be the "manual" method using the terminology of Section III), and compare it to the "optioned" one. Then correct the *segmentations* resulted by forced alignment of these transcriptions *by hand*, and observe if an achievement in the error rates similarly to the "computer-aided manual" method's 10.6% appears.

From practical point of view, it can be is concluded that effectively the same quality of acoustic models can be obtained by using our sophisticated *automatic transcription* method or by applying the highly expensive *manual phonetic segmentation*.

5. Summary

In this article we summarized our work and experiences with Hungarian phonetic transcription in speech recognition training. We also gave a short introduction on speech recognition principles for people not familiar with this scientific field.

We have developed a method for transcribing Hungarian texts automatically, which is an extension of the traditional linear transcription approach. Its output is called "optioned" because it contains pronunciation options in parallel arcs. Cross-word phonological processes are modelled in the transcription, as well. We presented our experiences with promising improvements in training efficiency. The achievements were due to the application of deeper linguistic (phonological) knowledge. With the training technique developed not only the quality of the acoustic models can be enhanced, and the amount of the required manual work can effectively be reduced, but also, practically, the efficiency of recognisers trained on the full manual segmentation can be attained.

Acknowledgements

The authors wish to thank Dr. Klára Vicsi, and László Tóth for the HTSD phonetically segmented database, and a special thank is due to Máté Szarvas for his kind support in terms of scripts, tools, and advice.

References

[1] Fekete, L. *Magyar Kiejtési Szótár (Hungarian Pronunciation Dictionary)*. Budapest: Gondolat, 1992.
[2] Hedvig, O. and Puster, J. (eds.) *A Magyar Helyesírás Szabályai (The Spelling Rules of Hungarian)*. Budapest: MTA, Akadémiai kiadó, 1994.
[3] Rabiner, L. and Juang, B.H. *Fundamentals of Speech Recognition*. Englewood Cliffs, NJ: Prentice Hall, 1993.
[4] Szarvas, M., Fegyó, T., Mihajlik, P. and Tatai, P. "Automatic recognition of Hungarian: Theory and practice." *Int. J. Speech Technology*. 3: 237-251, 2000.
[5] Vicsi, K. and Virág, A. "Speechdat-Hungarian (Technical Report)." *http://www.fee.vutbr.cz/SPEECH-DAT-E/sample/fixed3hu/doc/ED1_12_5_v12.doc*, 1999.
[6] Vicsi, K., Valyon, Z., Teleki, Cs., Gordos, G., Tóth, L., Kocsor, A., and Csirik, J. "MTBA – Magyar nyelv, telefon beszéd adatbázis" (Hungarian Telephony Speech Database). *http://luna.ttt.bme.hu/speech/MTBA.htm*, 2002.
[7] Wothke, K. *Automatic Phonetic Transcription Taking into Account the Morphological Structure of Words*. IBM Scientific Center Technical Report, Heidelberg, 1991.
[8] Young, S., Kershaw, D., Odell, J., Ollason, D., Valtchev, V., and Woodland, P. *The HTK Book*. Cambridge: Microsoft, 2000.

Dynamics of Speech Production and Perception
P. Divenyi et al. (Eds.)
IOS Press, 2006

263

Speech Inversion: Problems and Solutions

Victor N. SOROKIN

Institute for Information Transmission Problems
Russian Academy of Sciences
Moscow, Russia

Abstract. Inverse problems with respect to vocal tract shape, area function, articulatory parameters or control commands appear both in the theory of speech production and perception, and in technical applications like speech recognition, synthesis and compression. The inverse problems are ill-posed because of non-unique mapping from acoustical parameters to area function, to articulatory parameters, to control commands. The observation of speech pathology, especially laryngectomy and glossectomy, and artificial disturbance of speech production and perception have lead to the hypothesis of the so-called internal model used by the articulatory control system to transform motor commands in order to achieve desired acoustic or articulatory patterns. This hypothesis is supported by the theory of ill-posed inverse problems. One of the most powerful methods of ill-posed problems solving is the variational one where a mathematical model of speech production is used together with some criteria of optimality and constraints to obtain a stable solution. The measured acoustical parameters of the speech signal serve as external constraints while the geometry of the vocal tract, the mechanics of the articulation, the aerodynamics, and the phonetic properties of the language play the role of internal constraints. Optimality criteria, such as the work of articulation and the muscle force, provide good accuracy for both static and dynamic tasks, and reproduce the effects of the bite-block and motor control reorganization for different articulation rates.

Keywords. Speech inverse problems, ambiguity, constraints

Introduction

The observation of speech pathology, especially natural disturbance following laryngectomy or glossectomy, and artificial disturbance of speech production and perception have led to the hypothesis that there is an internal model used by the articulatory control system for transforming motor commands to achieve desired acoustic or articulatory patterns [39]. The internal model is considered as a module (rather, a resident program) that is aware of the anatomy of a particular speaker and of the mechanics, aerodynamics, and acoustics of speech production processes together with phonetic properties of language [33][34]. It is assumed that the internal model uses this information for current control and to predict and compensate for perturbations. The parameters and even the structure of the internal model may change in the course of vocal tract growth, after surgery on articulators, or as an adaptation to a permanent dental prosthesis. Many compensating processes occur in real time, i.e., dynamically. It happens, for example, when listening to one's own speech with transformed formant frequencies or fundamental tone. Compensatory response latency for the electrical stimulation of the lower lip depressor muscle [10], or for a sudden jerk applied to the jaw or lip, fell within the range 25–80 ms [1]. This does not leave time for tentative movements and implies some feed-forward mechanisms [13]. The mechanisms of internal model action must be based on solving inverse problems at such levels as "acoustics: articulatory control", "acoustics: articulatory parameters", "acoustics: place of articulation", "articulatory parameters: articulatory controls", and so on. The inverse problem can be defined as a problem of identifying parameters for a process generator from parameters of the observed process.

Chistovich [8] and Liberman and Mattingly [19] have speculated about the possibility of speech perception not only at the acoustical level but also at the articulatory level. Electrical activity was found in the auditory cortex for a listener observing articulatory movements of a speaker, while non-speech mimics does not evoke such an activity [24][6]. It is well known from everyday speech practice that visual information enhances speech perception, especially in adverse conditions or for foreign language. It may imply that speech perception refers to motor components in addition to acoustical parameters of speech.

At the level of description by discrete symbols, speech is similar to error–correcting codes. Compensation for noise and distortion is achieved by the use of a hierarchical structure (code structure) formed by differential cues for phonemes, morphemes, syllables, words and sentences. From the analysis of speech code structure it follows that gross acoustical cues are sufficient for reliable speech recognition if there is no acoustic noise or signal distortion, and there are strong syntactic and semantic constraints [41]. Information on the place of articulation is required for adverse acoustical environment and linguistic uncertainty. The determination of this cue is difficult at the acoustical level, and vocal tract shape identification would be helpful. Experiments with functional MRI have revealed that speech motor areas of the brain are more active under conditions in which speech is degraded by noise [5][30]. This strongly supports the hypothesis on the reality of motor component analysis in speech perception.

Speech learning during childhood and foreign language acquisition for adults is governed by listening to other people, and transforming acoustic patterns perceived in motor controls of the speaker. We know the speech inverse problems are solvable, because humans do learn to speak and sometimes successfully compensate for pathology.

Inverse problems are known for the considerable mathematical difficulties associated with them. It is therefore necessary to positively show how speech inversion problems can be solved. A mathematical analysis of the problem is required to understand the conditions of speech inverse problem solving. However, a purely mathematical approach to speech inverse problem solving is unproductive because it requires information unavailable at the physiological or acoustical level. Properties of speech production and perception must play the dominating role. In particular, one may suppose that articulatory control and speech perception for static and dynamic segments of a speech are provided by different means. In the experiments with functional MRI and acoustic stimulation by gradient sound, the experimenters found that the transient response and sustained response are localized in different areas of the brain [29]. This may imply that the internal model receives feedback signals labeled according to the type of a segment - static or dynamic.

A mechanism of bite–block compensation for steady–state isolated vowels should differ from a mechanism of compensation for a sudden jerk applied to the jaw or lip. In the first case, the inverse problem must be solved only with respect to the position of articulators. In the latter case, the velocity and timing of articulators must be corrected. The reorganization of EMG and articulatory movements for different speaking rates also points to the existence of mechanisms sensitive to speech production dynamics. It will be shown below that these mechanisms are the result of specific properties of inverse problem solving at different levels.

1. Ambiguity

The plasticity of speech control system and its ability to maintain acoustic parameters of speech in spite of various kinds of perturbation is based on the non-isomorphic mapping from one level of speech production to another one. However, it makes the inverse mapping from acoustical parameters to vocal tract shape, articulatory parameters or controls kinematically non-unique. This notion of non-unique mapping in the acoustical space in the space of vocal tract shapes is generally accepted. However, the mathematical properties of the mapping are not widely known.

A simple example of acoustics–to–area function non-uniqueness can be shown by means of the Schroedinger method of small perturbations. Let

$$\frac{1}{S}\frac{\partial}{\partial x}\left(S\frac{\partial P}{\partial x}\right) - \frac{1}{c_0^2}\frac{\partial^2 P}{\partial t^2} = 0 \tag{1}$$

be the wave (Webster) equation of the vocal tract with the corresponding set of eigenvalues $\{\lambda^{(0)}\}$ and eigenfunctions $\{\varphi^{(0)}(x,\lambda^{(0)})\}$. $P(x,t)$ is acoustical pressure, $S(x)$ is area function, c_0 is sound velocity, and x is the coordinate along the vocal tract midline. If the perturbed area function is

$$S(x) = S_0(x) + S_1(x) \tag{2}$$

where $S_1(x) \ll S_0(x)$ for any x, then the perturbed eigenvalues are λ_i, and

$$\lambda_i^2 = \lambda_i^{(0)2}(1 + \eta_i) \tag{3}$$

where

$$\eta_i = \frac{a_i}{\lambda_i^{(0)2}} - b_i - c_i \tag{4}$$

$$a_i = \int_0^l S_1(x)[\varphi_i^{(0)'}(x)]^2 dx \tag{5}$$

$$b_i = \int_0^l S_1(x)[\varphi_i^{(0)}(x)]^2 dx \tag{6}$$

and

$$c_i = S_1(l)\varphi_i^{(0)}(l)\varphi_i^{(0)'}(l) - S_1(0)\varphi_i^{(0)}(0)\varphi_i^{(0)'}(0) \tag{7}$$

where l is vocal tract length. The prime is a derivative for x. It is seen that parameters a_i and b_i can be the same for different perturbation functions $S_1(x)$ if the integrals in (5) and (6) remain the same. Therefore there are an infinite number of area functions consistent with a given set of resonance frequencies. This means that a unique solution to static inverse problems with respect to the area function is impossible unless information on speech production is used.

Equation (4) suggests a way to restrict the number of variants in vocal tract deformation when matching formant frequencies measured in the speech signal with resonance frequencies calculated by an acoustical model. The smaller the area function is in a given part of the vocal tract, the more some resonance frequencies may be affected. We know that the perturbation of the uniform tube's area function affects an eigenvalue if it is applied around the extremum or on the node of the corresponding eigenfunction. This property can be illustrated by a simple example with area perturbation concentrated in one point, with the coordinate $x = x_0$, $S_1(x) = \varepsilon\delta(x-x_0)$, where δ is a delta–function. Then, assuming that there is free radiation from the vocal tract at the point $x = l$ (i.e., $\varphi_i^{(0)}(l) = 0$), and the wall at the point $x = 0$ is absolutely rigid (i.e., $\varphi_i^{(0)'}(0) = 0$), we obtain $c_i = 0$, and

$$\eta_i = \frac{\varepsilon\{[\varphi_i^{(0)'}(x_0)]^2 - [\lambda_i^{(0)}\varphi_i^{(0)}(x_0)]^2\}}{\lambda_i^{(0)2}} \tag{8}$$

It is seen that the perturbation most affects the ith eigenvalue when $\varphi_i^{(0)}(x_0) = 0$ (the node of the ith eigenfunction) or $\varphi_i^{(0)'}(x_0) = 0$ (the extremum or the inflection of ith eigenfunction). The frequency of the ith resonance will not change if $\varphi_i^{(0)'}(x_0)^2 = [\lambda_i^{(0)}\varphi_i^{(0)}(x_0)]^2$, or $\varphi_i^{(0)}(x_0) = 0$ and $\varphi_i^{(0)'}(x_0) = 0$ simultaneously (the inflection of the ith eigenfunction at the node). This perturbation property of acoustic systems was first described by Rayleigh [23]. Carré uses it for determination of sensitive areas in the vocal tract [7]. These areas may serve as constraints in the process of solving the inverse problem with respect to vocal tract shape if a specific codebook is constructed for the representative number of target areas.

It follows from Equation (8) that controllability for the resonance frequencies is limited. It is very difficult to achieve independent control for more than three resonances due to the continuity of area function along the vocal tract [33].

Considerations of the speech inverse problem's non-uniqueness is usually confined by "acoustics: area function" conversions. However, the same area in the acoustically sensitive places can be obtained with different displacement of articulators. For example, the distance between the lips depends on lip and jaw displacement; the distance between the tongue tip and the alveolar ridge depends on tongue and jaw displacement. Due to the activity of pharyngeal muscle constrictors, the same area may correspond to different displacements of vocal tract walls in the frontal and midsagittal planes. These are examples of non-unique mappings from area function to articulatory displacements.

The same displacement of an articulator can be achieved with different muscle activation. For example, the vertical position of the tongue tip is determined by the activity of muscles *longitudinalis superior, longitudinalis inferior, styloglossus, palatoglossus* and *genioglossus*. Jaw raising may be executed with different combinations of *masseter* and *temporalis* muscles contraction. The *masseter* muscles are mainly intended for mastication, but we also found muscle activity was found during rapid articulation [33]. Therefore, "displacement–muscle activity" mapping is not just non-unique but also depends on the style of speech. Furthermore, the same muscle contraction may be produced by the excitation of different motor units [9].

This consistent non-uniqueness at all levels of speech production is beneficial for the flexibility of the articulatory control system. Differences in the dimension and shape of the fixed surfaces in the vocal tract for different people does not prevent the generation of sounds with phonetically conditioned acoustic parameters. The influence of muscle paralysis, food in the mouth, dental prostheses, cigarettes or pipes is also compensated for, at least partially. However, due to their non-unique mapping properties, from an abstract mathematical point of view speech inverse problems fall into the class of "ill–posed" problems. According to Hadamard's definition, a problem is well posed if (1) the solution exists for any admissibly exact data; (2) the solution is unique; and (3) the solution is stable with respect to admissible data perturbations. Not all inverse problems are ill–posed, only those in which at least one condition is not satisfied. For speech inversion, condition (2) is not satisfied due to the ambiguity in speech production. Condition (3) is also often not satisfied. This makes speech inversion an ill–posed problem.

Kinematically, any instantaneous solution consistent with the structure of speech production as discussed above considered is good. However, there is no guarantee that a sequence of solutions will be consistent in dynamics. Usually, it demonstrates improbable jumps in vocal tract shape that require muscle forces outside of the physiological range. A neuromotor command cannot follow the previous one before a certain period of time [28]. This discontinuity of commands, together with the inertiality of the articulators, limits the velocity of change of vocal tract shape. Clearly, articulatory dynamics is the most powerful factor in stabilizing inverse problem solving for continuous speech.

2. Regularization

For a long time, ill–posed problems were considered intractable (i.e., "Can you hear the shape of a drum?"). However, a growing corpus of data on the compensation ability of the articulatory control system made us reconsider mathematical approaches. See Schroeter and Sondhi [27], and Sorokin *et al.* [40] for a review of and references to the history of speech inversion. The modern approach to speech inversion is based on the general theory of ill–posed problems developed in Tikhonov and Arsenin [42], and Tikhonov *et al.* [44]. They found that some approximate solution to ill–posed problems might be obtained by means of "regularization." In this method, a special term is added in the inverted equation, making the process of solving stable and unique with respect to the solution. This term depends on a particular task.

The most effective regularization is the variational one. This method consists of varying the parameters of a mathematical model describing the process to be inverted, in order to minimize a discrepancy between the observed and calculated parameters of an input signal, together with some criterion of optimality. Thus, the hypothesis of the internal model is supported by the theory of ill–posed inverse problems—if we believe that inverse problem solving is involved in the activity of articulatory control system of a speaker, then a model of speech production for the speaker must be present in the system. If, in the perception of speech of other speakers, motor components are somehow used, then a set of parameters for the transformation of the listener's internal model should be learned.

A general model of speech production is the transformation of articulatory parameters z to acoustical parameters u using a continuous operator of speech production A, such that $Az = u$, $z \in Z$, and $u \in U$. Z is the set of admissible articulatory parameters, and U is the set of admissible acoustical parameters. This is the forward problem which is solvable in opposite to the inverse problem where z must be found for the given u. In practice, the exact operator A and the value of u is unknown, but we have an approximate model A_h and measurements u_δ, where h and δ are the accuracy of the estimates. Therefore, instead of solution z, only quasi-solutions $z_{h\delta}$ may be obtained from the conditional minimum of the functional that includes an optimality criterion and a discrepancy between observed and computed parameters. In particular, the functional may be presented as follows:

$$M(z_{h\delta}) = a\Omega(z) + \rho^2(A_h z, u_\delta)/\beta \tag{9}$$

the regularization parameter $a = a(h,\delta)$. $\rho(A_h z, u_\delta) = \|A_h z - u_\delta\|$ is the discrepancy for the approximate data, the functional $\Omega(z)$ is a criterion of optimality, and β is the penalty parameter. This functional is applicable both to static and dynamic inverse problems. Technically, the solution to problem (9) can be obtained by the method of penalty functions with iterative changes of the penalty parameter $\beta_k = \beta_k \gamma_\gamma^k$, $\gamma_\gamma \ll 1$, $k = 1, 2, ...K$. Given appropriate choices of parameters β_0 and K, the vector $z^{(K)}$ is a good approximation to $z_{h\delta}$.

The accuracy of an approximate solution can be estimated in relation to the theoretically best attainable accuracy [44]. In this way, various methods can be compared, but the best attainable accuracy itself remains unknown. The method described in Equation (9) provides a relative error not worse than double the least attainable error. This "method of calibrating curves" was used by Sorokin, Leonov, and Trushkin [40] to estimate the stability and accuracy of inverse problem solutions for randomly and independently disturbed formant frequencies, with the amount of disturbance ranging up to 20%. We found that the solution errors were actually independent of the degree of disturbances, and that the range of articulatory parameter disturbance for vowels was less than 5%.

Equation (9) shows that a solution to the ill–posed problem may be found if (1) a mathematical model A_h of the process to be inverted is known, (2) the optimality criterion $\Omega(z)$ is determined, (3) the discrepancy r is defined, and (4) there is a set of appropriate constraints. Not every solution to speech inversion is acceptable in a particular application. In order to obtain plausible solutions, the optimality criterion and constraints must be physiologically and acoustically justified.

3. Mathematical Models of Speech Production

The mathematical model of speech production A_h in Equation (9) includes a model of vocal tract anatomy (describing fixed surfaces of the vocal tract), an articulatory model (describing the kinematics and dynamics of articulators), an algorithm converting articulatory parameters into a vocal tract area function, a model of aerodynamics, and an acoustical model. A model of articulatory controls is also required for the dynamic inverse problem.

Vocal tract anatomy is described by vocal tract length for phonetically neutral vocal tract shape; the geometry of the nasal cavity, jaw, lips, velum; and the 3–dimensional shape of the hard palate, the back wall of the vocal tract, pharynx, and the side cavities in the pharyngeal region (the *sinuses piriformis*). The shape and geometric dimensions of the vocal folds are also needed in the inverse problems for the vocal source. In the articulatory control system, the data for inverse problem solution may be obtained during speech learning. In the mathematical modeling of inverse problem solving, some of the data may be obtained from magnetic resonance imaging [42][45][2] or X-ray measurements [46], or another electromagnetic system. However, there is a lack of important information on the distribution of the geometric parameters among speakers due to the expense and complexity of experiments required to obtain this type of data. Thus the identification of geometric parameters must be included in the process of inversion. Fortunately, such a complex inverse problem must be solved only one time (or a few times) for a particular speaker simulating a kind of speaker adaptation.

Articulatory models with a small number of parameters cannot reproduce vocal tract shapes with high accuracy. The number of articulatory parameters is determined by the articulatory structure and direction of muscle forces. A kinematic model with 17 articulatory parameters was proposed by Sorokin [33], and used in inverse problems for vowels and fricatives. These parameters should include the following:

- *Vocal slit width* determines voiced or voiceless closure and parameters of turbulent noise excitation for fricatives.
- *Larynx height* is independent parameter although often it is correlated with the vertical displacement of the tongue root.
- *Velum height*, which may be interpreted as an *angle of velum rotation*. The velum arises due to the contraction of *levator palatini* muscle, and moves down usually because of passive elastic deformation of soft tissues.
- The lips are elastic bodies. Theoretically, an infinite number of eigenfunctions describes their elastic deformations. However, in practice, only the first eigenfunction is observed in lip movements [33]. The contractions of *orbicularis oris* (the circular muscle in the lips) change the distance between lip ends thus

providing lips *protrusion*. The upper and lower lip can move in the vertical direction independently though in articulation their movements are correlated, so instead of two parameters only *distance between lips* may be used.

- The jaw has two parameters employed in articulation—*the angle of jaw rotation* about the tempomandibular joint and *the horizontal displacement of jaw pivot* along the articular surface of the temporal bone. The latter parameter is often used in sounds with the alveolar place of articulation, especially for the fast rate of articulation [33].

- Extrinsic muscles, *styloglossus, hyoglossus, palatoglossus, mylohyoid,* and the lower part of the *genioglossus* control *horizontal and vertical coordinates of the tongue root.*

- The *styloglossus, palatoglossus* and certain part of *genioglossus* muscle can rotate the tongue about its root as a solid body. The *angle of rotation* is the parameter controlled in the articulatory model.

- The tongue is an elastic body as well. Its elastic deformations are usually described by means of the finite–element method. This method is computationally cumbersome. There is another method that provides both the shape and temporal characteristics of the tongue: the tongue can be considered as an elastic bent plate, and its elastic deformations are found as a solution to the equation in partial derivatives. Four eigenfunctions for the tongue body and one eigenfunction for the tongue tip approximate tongue shapes with good accuracy [33]. The tongue tip sometime appears as an independent articulator controlled by anterior parts of the *longitudinalis superior* and *longitudinalis inferior* muscles. *One coefficient* for the tongue tip is sufficient for the description of its shape and movements. Coefficients for four eigenfunctions of the tongue body are not independent. They are computed as the response to extrinsic muscles contraction with *the geniouglossus* divided by three intersected parts [15]. Hence, there are *three controls* for tongue body shape.

- The upper and lower fibers of the *transversalis* muscle can make the tongue convex or concave.

- The contraction of the middle part of *the geniouglossus* often forms a groove in the tongue. All these effects can be modeled by *one coefficient* of the transverse eigenfunction for the tongue. According to the recent MRI and X-ray studies, the pharynx width must be included in the articulatory model. *Two coefficients* for two eigenfunctions found from the statistical analysis describe the transversal shape of the pharynx.

In total, there are 17 physiologically adequate articulatory parameters.

The dynamic inverse problem requires a physiologically–justified mathematical model of articulation complete with a model of controls. All articulators except the tongue can be considered as lumped systems subject to the ordinary differential equation:

$$m_j z_j'' + r_j z_j' + c_j\left(z_j - z_j^{(0)}\right) = f_j(t), \qquad j = 1, \ldots, n \qquad (10)$$

Here z_j is the articulatory position at time t, $z_j^{(0)}$ is the articulatory parameter for the neutral position, z'_j is the velocity, z_j'' is acceleration of the jth articulator, m_j is mass, r_j is resistance, c_j is an elasticity associated with the articulator, and $f_j(t)$ is a function of control provided by muscle force. According to the modal control theory, the dynamics of the tongue's elastic deformations can also be described by a composition of the second order ordinary differential equations.

Equation (10) may be rewritten in the form

$$z_j'' + 2g_j z_j' + \omega_j^2 \left(z_j - z_j^{(0)} \right) = f_j(t)/m_j, \qquad j = 1, \ldots, n \qquad (11)$$

In the mathematical modeling below presented, the parameters $g_j = r_j/m_j$ and $\omega_j^2 = c_j/m_j$ were identified in separate experiments and described in [38].

On the basis of X-ray measurements taken simultaneously with EMG recording of articulatory muscles, Leonov and Sorokin [16] have found that the controls, in the form of piecewise linear discontinuous functions, provide an error in articulatory movements approximation comparable with the accuracy of measurements while muscle forces were in the physiologically plausible range. The computed controls for velum movements were correlated with the EMG of the *levator palatini* muscle, the only muscle lifting the velum. Also, the computed controls for the tip of the tongue movements were correlated with the EMG of the *longitunalis superior* muscle. Therefore, the dynamic articulatory model controls $2n$ temporal parameters, where n is the number articulatory parameters.

A model of the cross-sectional area function is a part of the speech production model. Usually, mathematical models of articulation describe vocal tract shape in the midsagittal plane. It is implied that the vocal tract area function S is a rather simple function of vocal tract width w and distance d between the surface of the articulatory organs and the surface of the fixed parts of the vocal tract. Simultaneous MRI measurements of vocal tract shape and its area function have revealed the necessity of accounting for the vocal tract's width in order to achieve a computation error in the range of measurement accuracy. Pharynx width actively changes during articulation [42][2]. Principal component analysis shows that 2 eigenvectors describe 94% of pharyngeal width variability, and 2 parameters are needed to describe the neutral shape of the pharynx in the frontal plane. Average values for the wall mass and elasticity per unit of vocal tract length are necessary for the accurate computation of resonance frequencies.

The resonance frequencies of the vocal tract are calculated by solving Equation (1). Computing the acoustical parameters of fricatives is done by an aerodynamic model that calculates the Reynolds number along the vocal tract and determines the characteristics of turbulent noise. The model includes a cumbersome system of non-linear differential equations [22][35], here omitted. It was used both for vowel and fricative inverse problems. The solution for vowels requires no turbulent noise, while the computation of the spectrum of fricatives requires turbulent noise excitation [37][38].

4. Articulatory Codebook

Like any optimization problem, the variational approach to speech inverse problems doesn't guarantee the finding of the global optimum. The usual remedy is to start the optimization process from different initial positions. For this purpose, a codebook can

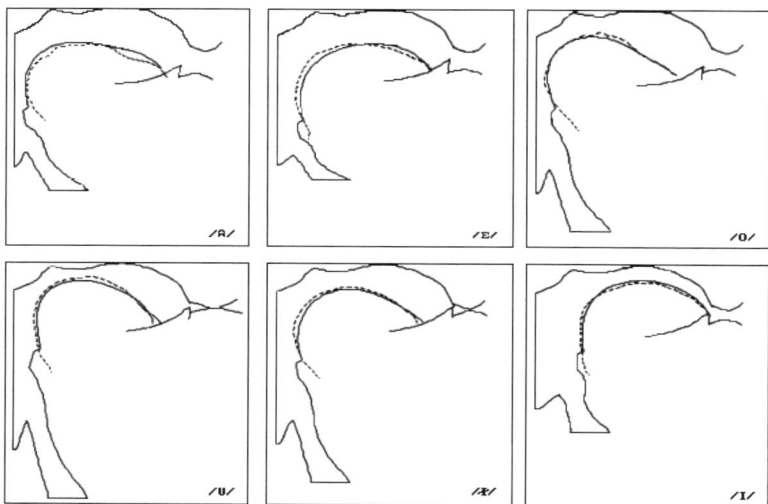

Figure 1. Outlines of the X-ray images of vocal tract shape (dashed lines); the inverse solution (solid lines).

be used. A codebook comprises a number of articulatory parameters and corresponding acoustic parameters found by means of forward problem solving for a mathematical model of speech production. In certain circumstances, the codebook may provide good solutions to the inverse problem even without evoking an optimization process, thus making almost instantaneous decisions.

A static codebook, shaped by means of an abstract articulatory–acoustic model with the fixed anatomic parameters, may contain too many cells. For example, Schroeter and Sondhi [26] used a static codebook with over 200,000 cells. Still, such a codebook can be deficient if the inverse problem is considered for many speakers. If the inverse problem is stated, like the speech recognition problem, for an unknown speaker, then the codebook must include geometric parameters of the vocal tract and vocal tract walls (the distribution of mass, elasticity and losses along the vocal tract) for a variety of speakers. In addition, the dynamic inverse problem requires a codebook with information on the dynamic parameters of the articulators, depending on their sizes. The number of necessary cells in a codebook can be much reduced if it is constructed only from samples taken along the trajectories of articulators recorded by means of an X-ray or electromagnetic system and, if necessary, complemented by simulation with an articulatory synthesizer [38].

All the information necessary for codebook shaping exists in the articulatory control system of the speaker, because the system has complete access to control commands, articulatory positions, and acoustic parameters for phonetic elements of speech. During speech production, the human codebook may be used for mapping from perceived acoustical parameters to controls just as it is used in mapping from articulatory positions to neuromotor controls. Hence, the concept of the codebook does not contradict to the potential capability of the control system.

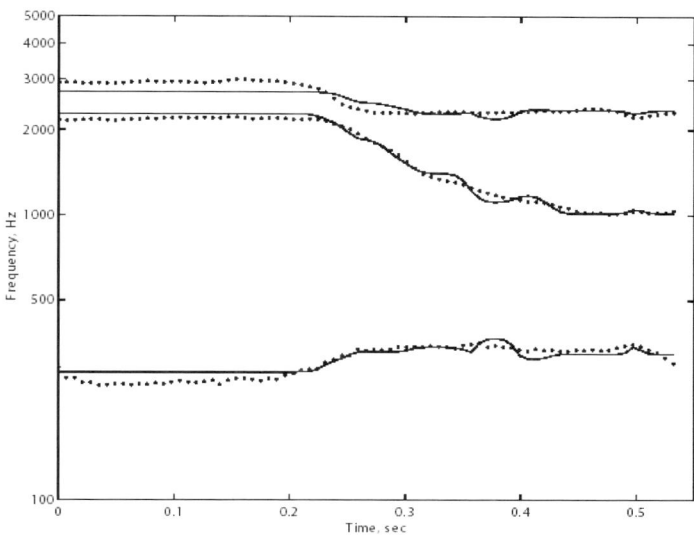

Figure 2. Formant tracks for the dipthong /iu/. The measured formats are shown by the solid lines; the inverse solutions are shown by dotted lines

5. Constraints

An ill–posed problem may even become well posed if a sufficient number of proper constraints are used. For example, the inverse problem with respect to the unconstrained function $S(x)$ in Equation (1) has a unique solution if very specific information is available, such as the infinite number of eigenvalues for at least two different boundary conditions [4]. With this respect, vocal tract anatomy determines kinematic and dynamic constraints, which substantially facilitate inversion even with the above–mentioned non-uniqueness of inverse mapping.

There are external and internal constraints involved in solving the inverse problem. The external constraints are related to acoustic and language properties whereas the internal constraints are related to anatomy and muscle power limitations. Six kinds of constraints are conceivable at present:

1. Limitations on the contractive force f_n of the nth muscle $0 \leq f_n \leq f_{n\ max}$. This kind of constraint determines the maximum velocity and acceleration of articulators.

2. Constraints related to the anatomy of the vocal tract. The articulatory parameters are confined to a certain range of values due to physical and language limits $z_{j\ min} \leq z_j \leq z_{j\ max}$. Parameters of articulatory dynamics, i.e., mass, elastic resistance, and damping for each articulator are constrained as well.

3. The functional class of transformations connecting a set of articulatory parameters to the area function of the vocal tract, $S(x,z)$. Here x is the coordinate along the vocal tract's axis and z is the vector of articulatory parameters $\mathbf{z} = z(z_1, z_2, ..., z_N)$, where N is the number of articulatory parameters.

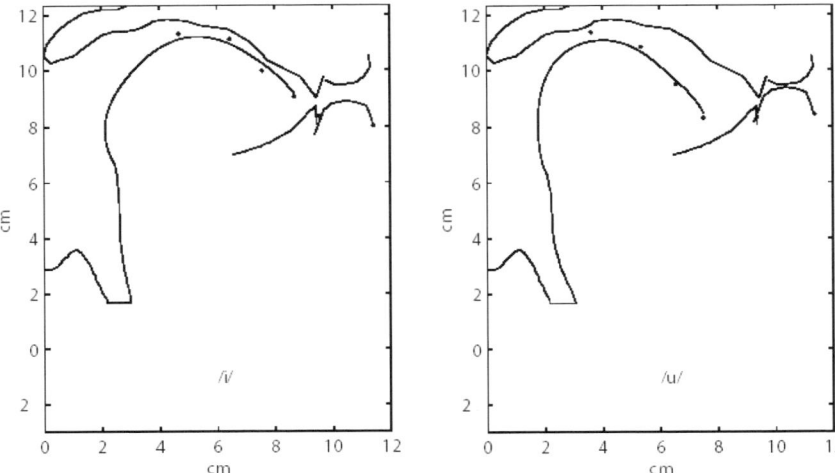

Figure 3. Vocal tract shapes reconstructed for dipthong /iu/.

4. Constraints on the shape of the vocal tract. For example, the controlled value may be a cross-sectional area function in certain regions of the vocal tract. Area function constraints for vowels are one-sided: $S(x, z) \geq S_{min}$, $x = x_{min}$, and $x = 0$ on the vocal slit. S_{min} is determined by the condition of non-turbulent airflow, when the Reynolds number Re is less than a threshold, $Re < Re_{critical}$. The constraints for fricatives are two sided: $S_{min} \leq S(x, z) \leq S_{max}$, where S_{min} and S_{max} determine the condition of air-flow turbulence, that is, $Re \geq Re_{critical}$. For stops, $S_{min} = 0$ when complete closure must be achieved. The area of the velum port is $S_{vp} > 0$ only for nasals (including nasal vowels). For the remaining sounds, $S_{vp} = 0$. Obviously, this kind of constraint may be correctly applied only in cases when a speech segment is previously recognized as vowel, fricative, closure or nasal.

5. Acoustical constraints. These constraints have the form $0 \leq \rho(u, u_\delta) \leq \Delta\rho$, where $\rho(u, u_\delta) = \|u - u_\delta\|$ is a discrepancy of the measured acoustical data u_δ and the output u is calculated by using the mathematical model. It is known that for different styles and rates of speech, or for different positions of a speech segment with respect to a stressed vowel, the acoustical characteristics of the same sound are different. This implies that while solving the inverse problem, acoustic goals may be achieved with different accuracy, and therefore the limit $\Delta\rho$ may depend on linguistic factors.

6. Finally, the complexity of motor commands planning and programming may also serve as a constraint for the optimization process. This follows from Mandelbrot's law for the frequency of word appearance, which is derived from the principle of information maximization under conditions of limited expense for code generation [21]. The Mandelbrot law explains why short words are more frequent than long words and why the sounds with the smallest number of features should be more frequent than sounds more features [41]. Apparently, the

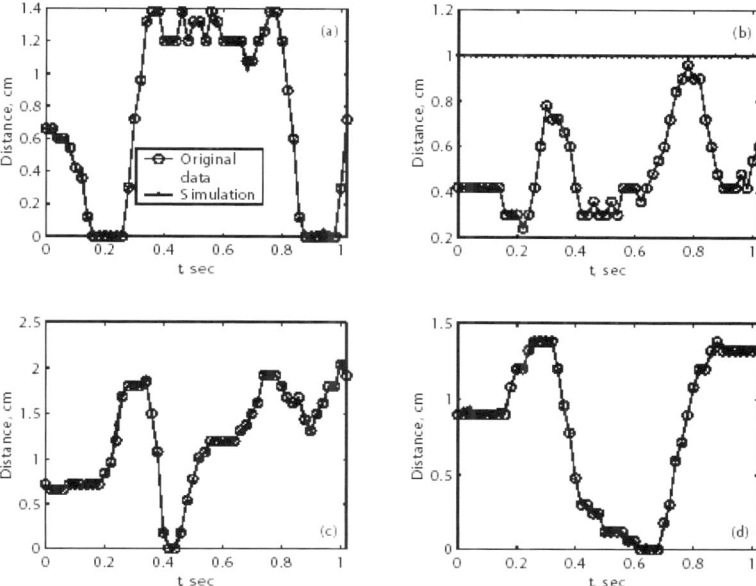

Figure 4. Utterance *panikapa*. Distances between (a) lips; (b) upper and lower incisors; (c) tongue tip and hard palate; and (d) tongue and velum.

factor of complexity should have the most influence at the level of continuous speech and may be somehow correlated with the principle of synergy [3].

6. Discrepancy

The discrepancy measure ρ in (9) plays an important role in the process of inversion. It describes the difference between the acoustical parameters, computed and measured. Levinson and Schmidt [18] and Sondhi and Schroeter [32] used the difference between the amplitude spectrum of the speech signal and the calculated spectrum to analyze vowel inversion. This approach is susceptible to vocal source differences and to the amplitude–frequency distortions imposed by a communication channel. Discrepancy in the cepstrum space may be used to suppress the influence of vocal source variability using the compensation of spectrum tilt, although Hogden *et al.* [14] did not find any advantage in using the cepstrum discrepancy over the spectrum one for inverse problem solving. The comparison of formant frequencies F_k measured in the speech signal and computed resonance frequencies F_k^* is adequate for vowels. The discrepancy $\rho = \max \left| 1 - F_k^*/F_k \right|, k = 1, 2, 3$ was found to be optimal [36]. In real environments, the speech signal is usually accompanied by background noise and distorted by chamber reverberation and communication channels. Errors in estimating formant frequencies can degrade the accuracy of speech inversion. Robust models of speech analysis are needed to provide sufficiently accurate acoustic parameters as input to speech inversion procedures. Some approaches to speech analysis models are considered in the present book.

Formant frequencies are not informative for fricatives. Instead, the discrepancy based on the Cauchy–Bounjakovsky inequality may be used [37]. It is invariant to the gain of each spectrum:

$$\rho = 1 - \frac{\displaystyle\int_{0}^{l} S(\omega)S^*(\omega)\,d\omega}{\left[\displaystyle\int_{0}^{l} S^2(\omega)\,d\omega \int_{0}^{l} S^{*2}(\omega)\,d\omega\right]^{1/2}} \tag{12}$$

This measure is conveniently normalized to 1, $0 \le \rho \le 1$, and $\rho = 0$, only if both measured $S(\omega)$ and computed $S^*(\omega)$ spectra are equal, such that $S(\omega) = S^*(\omega)$, where ω is circular frequency (in radian/sec).

There is widespread agreement among physiologists that the motor control system uses some energy criterion of optimality. However, it seems, that there are different sets of optimality criteria regulating different styles of speech and regulating the production of different phonetic elements. My 1987 paper describes a case involving steady–state positions of an articulator [34]. In statics, the velocity z'_j and acceleration z''_j both equal zero, and Equation (10) reduces to $c_j \Delta z_j = f_j(t)$. The displacement Δz from the neutral position $z_j^{(0)}$ of the jth articulator, $\Delta z_j = z_j - z_j^{(0)}$, and the coefficient of elastic resistance c_j , are the only parameters which affect the possible criterion of optimality. The criterion of force minimum, $\sum_j f_j = \min$, provides $\Omega_F(z) = \sum c_j |\Delta z_j| = \min$. The criterion of energy minimum, $\sum f_j^2 = \min$ corresponds to $\Omega_W(z) = \sum c_j^2 \Delta z_j^2 = \min$, which is proportional to the work minimum. Both criteria require the maximum displacement for the articulator with the minimal elastic resistance, but the latter one also depends upon the displacement. The criterion Ω_W was used for the inverse problem with respect to vocal tract shape in the midsagittal plane for vowels recorded by an X-ray microbeam system (at the University of Wisconsin) with a chain of gold pellets superimposed on the tongue of the male and female speaker. The computed and measured tongue shape was very similar, and the average absolute error between the computed and measured frequency for the first four formants were $\varepsilon_1 = 4.6\%$, $\varepsilon_2 = 6.8\%$, $\varepsilon_3 = 2.4\%$, and $\varepsilon_4 = 9.5\%$, for the male speaker, and $\varepsilon_1 = 17.2\%$, $\varepsilon_2 = 14.3\%$, $\varepsilon_3 = 15.1\%$, and $\varepsilon_4 = 12.3\%$ for the female speaker [36]. The accuracy obtained is comparable with the measurement accuracy. The same criterion was applied to measurements with cineradiography for the same male speaker [40]. The errors for formant frequency computation were $\varepsilon_1 = 8.4\%$, $\varepsilon_2 = 29.7\%$, and $\varepsilon_3 = 12.8\%$, which is somewhat higher than in the previous experiments due to the acoustic noise of the X-ray apparatus. Nevertheless, the measured and computed tongue shapes are very similar (as shown in Figure 1), which demonstrates the stability of the solution discussed in section 3.

The criterion Ω_W has also provided good accuracy in spectrum and vocal tract shape computation for the steady–state fricatives generated by an articulatory synthesizer [37]. In addition, this criterion is appropriate for relatively slow movements, such as diphthongs. Figure 2 shows formant tracks, measured and computed for diphthong / *iu*/ from the X-ray microbeam data base [46]. Figure 3 shows vocal tract shapes reconstructed for the first and last moment of /*iu*/ articulation. Inversion was found for three formant frequencies measured from the speech signal and synchronously recorded coordinates of 6 pellets inside of the mouth.

The criterion Ω_W may also be involved in the mechanism of articulatory compensation for the bite–block. In the simulation experiments, data for articulatory movements were obtained from a cineradiographic film for the utterance *panikapa*, which was cut from continuous speech. The inverse problem was solved with respect to control commands when the input data were the distances between the lips and the upper and lower incisors, and between the tongue and the hard palate, the velum, and the back wall. Then the jaw position was fixed to simulate the bite–block effect (dots in the Figure 4b), and the inverse problem was solved again with the original (undisturbed) input data as target trajectories. Figure 4 shows that, in spite of the bite–block, the original data were accurately reproduced, and the necessary lip and alveolar closures were achieved. This was due to a reorganization of lip and tongue movements, which is not shown in Figure 4. The zero distance in Figure 4a corresponds to the lip closure (the initial and final /p/ in *panikapa*), the zero distance in Figure 4c corresponds to the alveolar closure (*n* in *panikapa*), and the zero distance in Figure 4d corresponds to the velar closure (*k* in *panikapa*).

It is interesting that the inverse problem with the bite–block was solved faster than the problem using the original data. The optimizer found that the jaw was fixed, and did not try to move it, thus reducing task dimension. This accounts for the observation of immediate compensation for the bite–block in the first pulse of the vocal source [20][11]. It also implies the use of proprioceptive, not acoustic, information in the process of bite–block compensation.

The criterion Ω_W controls only articulatory positions. It does not use information on velocity or acceleration. Nevertheless, as it is clearly shown in the experiments modeling the bite–block for continuous speech, this criterion affects the articulatory dynamics of articulatory movements reorganization.

For continuous speech, even at a normal speaking rate, the first and the second term in (10) may prevail over the third one. Thus the energy criterion for the dynamic inverse problem requires a criterion related to the velocity or acceleration of articulators. Shirai and Kobayashi [31] and Schoentgen and Ciocea [25] used the criterion $\Omega_V(z) = \sum_j (dz_j/dt)^2$, which is analogous to kinetic energy. The criterion $\Omega_A(z) = \sum_j m_j (d^2z_j/dt^2)^2$, used in [17], directly refers to accelerations, in which m_j is the mass of the jth articulator.

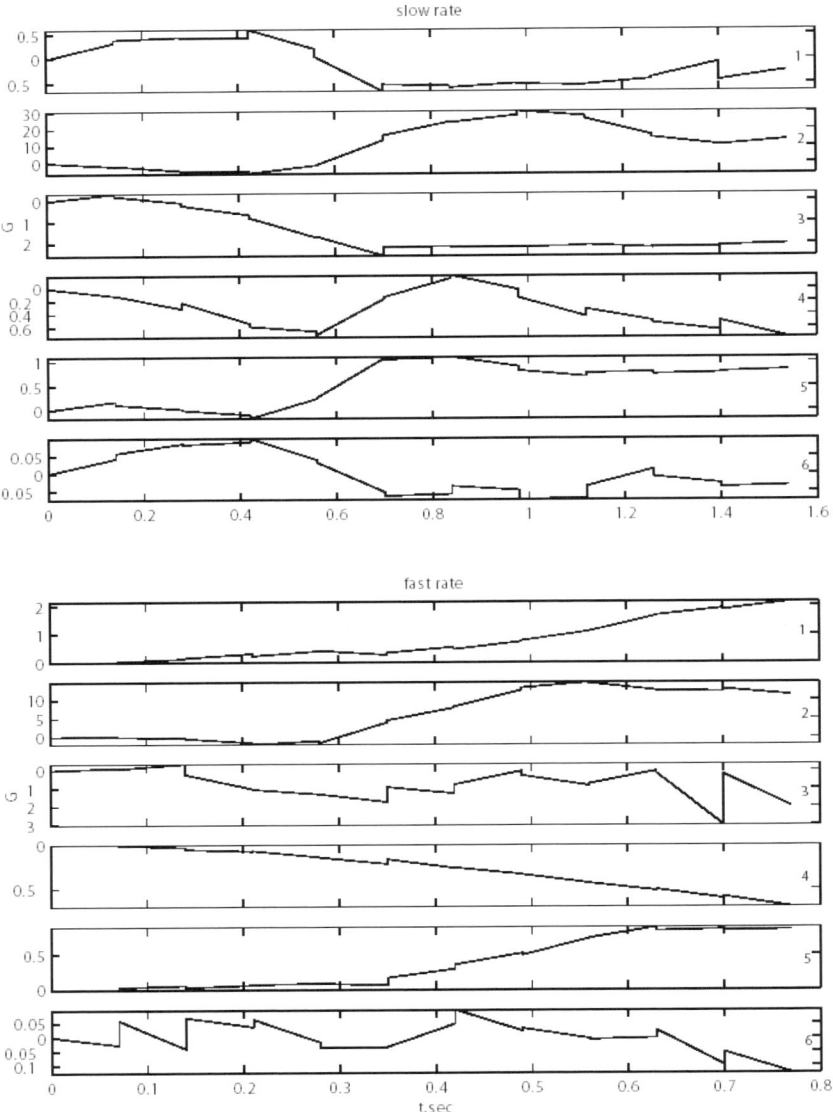

Figure 5. Control forces (in grams) for diphthong /ai/: (1) lower lip; (2) tongue tip; (3) angle of jaw rotation; (4) horizontal displacement of tongue root; (5) vertical displacement of tongue root; and (6) angle of tongue rotation.

Controls and articulatory movements reorganization is observed for the same speaker speaking with different articulation rates. Changes occur not only in duration, but in amplitudes and relative timing of EMG potentials and articulatory movements as well. Gay *et al.* [12] were the first to find such a reorganization. The criterion $\Omega_W(z)$ does not (and obviously cannot) initiate controls reorganization for different rates of articulation since it takes into account only the final position of articulators, not their dynamics. Criteria $\Omega_A(z)$ and $\Omega_V(z)$ both reproduce the effect of control commands reorganization in the experiments simulating different articulation rates by the articulation model. Figure 5 shows reorganization of control commands for the diphthong /ai/ spoken by the speaker JW11 from the database [46]. The inverse problem with respect to control commands for 15 articulatory parameters was solved with the use of 3 formant frequencies and the tracks of several pellets placed on the lips, jaw, and the anterior part of the tongue. The upper panel in Figure 5 shows the "slow rate," corresponding to inversion from the original data to controls. The lower panel corresponds to inversion from the "acceleration" of the original data provided by halving the sampling period. One can see that the shape and timing of controls is changed for all articulatory parameters with the exception of the tongue tip.

The criteria $\Omega_A(z)$ and $\Omega_V(z)$ also demonstrate bite–block compensation in continuous speech in experiments with a "fixed jaw."

Jointly, the criteria $\Omega_W(z)$ and $\Omega_A(z)$ allow the accurate reproduction of articulatory movements and acoustic parameters on a level comparable to the accuracy of the measurements. These criteria, simultaneously applied, provide an accurate reproduction of speech signals from inverse problem solutions. Figures 6 and 7 show the sonograms of the syllable /asha/ and the phrase /the other/ computed for the original utterance (left side of the sonograms) and the utterance re-synthesized after inverse problem solving (right side of the sonograms). Not only do the sonograms look very similar, but the original and re-synthesized speech signals are perceptually almost identical. These are examples of solutions to dynamic inverse problems with the use of energy criteria.

The muscles controlling articulators are striated. These muscles must consume energy to maintain any steady–state position different from the neutral state. This property indicates that the optimality criteria may be presented in a form integrated over some time period. This assumption was examined in experiments which recorded joint movements of the jaw and tongue–tip by an X-ray microbeam system for two modes: speech mode, for the sequence /tatatata/ with different speaking rates; and non-speech mode, with the instructions "slowly elevate and lower the tongue–tip, without touching the hard palate." It was found that the individual movements of the jaw and tip of the tongue in speech and non-speech modes are controlled by different criteria of optimality: in the speech mode, only energy criteria integrated over time periods of about 100 ms or more provide good approximation of the movements, while in the non-speech mode the displacements of the tongue tip and jaw are well reproduced by the instant cri-

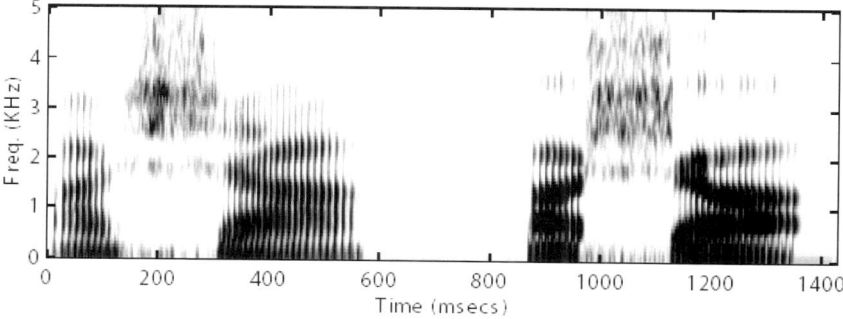

Figure 6. Sonograms for the original utterance /asha/ (left) and the re-synthesized one after inverse problem solving (right).

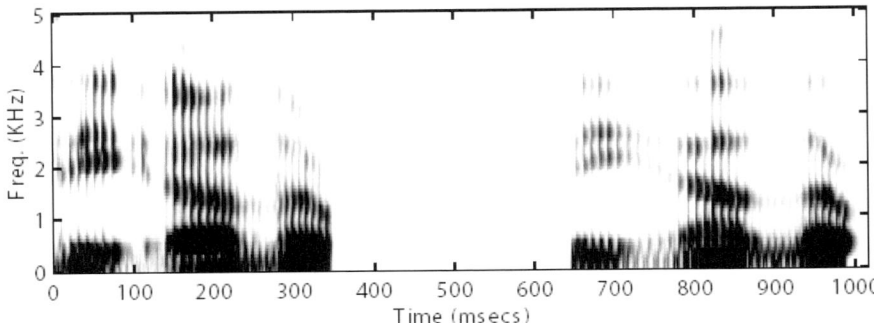

Figure 7. Sonograms for the original phrase /*the other*/ (left) and the re-synthesized one after inverse problem solving (right).

teria $\Omega_W(z)$ or $\Omega_A(z)$ [17]. This is consistent with the notion that speech and non-speech movements are controlled by different centers in the cerebral cortex.

7. Conclusion

The theory of an internal model in the speech production system is supported by the results of the mathematical modeling of dynamic reorganization of articulatory controls. The main mechanism of internal model activity relies upon solutions to various inverse problems, by means of which feedback signals from the hearing system and proprioceptors are transformed to neuromotor commands. Controls, articulatory parameters, and vocal tract shape can be computed from acoustic parameters not only for steady–state speech segments but for continuous speech as well. The energy criteria of optimality play an important role in inverse problem solving. Reorganization of control commands in compensating for a bite–block or sudden disturbance to articulatory movements, and for different speaking rates, may be affected by the criteria.

References

[1] Abbs, H., Gracco, L. and Cole, K.J. "Control of multi-movement coordination: Sensorimotor mechanisms in speech motor programming." *J. Motor Behav.*,16: 195–231, 1984.
[2] Badin P. and Engwall O. "An MRI study of Swedish fricatives: Coarticulatory effects." *Proc. 5th Seminar on Speech Production*, pp. 297-300, 2000.
[3] Bernstein, M.A. *The Coordination and Regulation of Movements*. Oxford: Pergamon, 1967.
[4] Borg, G. "Eine Umkehrung der Sturm—Liouvilleschen Eigenwertaufgabe." *Acta Math.* 78: 1-96, 1946.
[5] Callan, D. E., Callan, A. M., Kroos, Ch. and Vatikiotis-Bateson, E. "Neural processes underlying perception of audiovisual speech production." *Proc. 5th Seminar on Speech Production*, pp. 273-276, 2000.
[6] Calvert, G., Brammer, M., Bullmore, E., Campbell, R., Williams, S., McGuire, P., Woodruff, P., Iversen, S. and David, A. "Activation of auditory cortex during silent lip-reading." *Science* 276: 593-596, 1997.
[7] Carré, R. "Speech gestures by deduction, gesture production and gesture perception." *In this volume, 2006.*

[8] Chistovich, L. A., Ventsov, A. V., Granstrem, M. P., Zhukov, S. Ja., Zhukova, M. G., Karnickaja, E. G., Kozhevnikov, V. A., Lisenko, D. M., Fiodorova, N. A., Haavel, P. H., Chistovich, I. A. and Shupljakov, V. S. *Fisiologija rechi. Vosprijatie rechi chelovekom (Speech Physiology. Speech Perception).* Leningrad: Nauka, 1976. [Russian]

[9] Cooper, D.S. and Folkins, J.W. "The temporal sampling problem in electromyographic studies of speech musculature." *J. Acoust. Soc. Am.* 71: S33, 1982.

[10] Folkins, J. and Zimmerman, G. "Lip and jaw interaction during speech: Responses to perturbation of lower-lip movement prior to bilabial closure." *J. Acoust. Soc. Am.* 71: 1225-1233, 1982.

[11] Fowler, C.A. and Turvey, M.T. "Immediate compensation in bite–block speech." *Phonetica* 37: 306-326, 1980.

[12] Gay, T., Ushijima, T., Hirose, H. and Cooper, F. "Effect of speaking rate on labial and consonant–vowel articulation." *J. Phonetics* 2: 47-63, 1974.

[13] Gracco, V.L. and Abbs, J.H. "Programming and execution processes of speech movement control: Potential neural correlates." In *Motor and Sensory Processes of Language*, E. Keller and M. Gopnik (eds.), Hillsdale, NJ: Lawrence Erlbaum, pp. 163-201, 1987.

[14] Hogden, J., Lofqvist, A., Gracco, V., Zlokarnik, I., Rubin, P. and Saltzman, E. "Accurate recovery of articulator positions from acoustics: New conclusions based on human data." *J. Acoust. Soc. Am.* 100: 1819-1834, 1996.

[15] Leonov, A.S. and Sorokin, V.N. "Inversion from articulatory movements to control forces", *Proc. 5th Seminar on Speech Production*, pp. 17-20, 2000.

[16] Leonov, A.S. and Sorokin, V.N. "Inverse problem for the vocal tract: Identification of control forces from articulatory movements." *Pattern Recognition and Image Analysis* 10: 110-126, 2000.

[17] Leonov, A.S. and Sorokin, V.N. "Optimality criteria in inverse problems for tongue–jaw interaction." *Proc. Eurospeech,* pp. 2353-2356, 2003.

[18] Levinson, S.E. and Schmidt, C.E. "Adaptive computation of articulatory parameters from the speech signal." *J. Acoust. Soc. Am.* 74: 1145-1154, 1983.

[19] Liberman, A. and Mattingly, I. "The motor theory of speech perception revised." *Cognition* 21: 1-36, 1985.

[20] Lindblom, B.E.F., Lubker, J. and Gay, T. "Formant frequencies of some fixed mandible vowels and a model of speech motor programming by predictive simulations." *J. Phonetics* 7: 147-161, 1979.

[21] Mandelbrot B. "Contribution à la Théorie Mathématique des Jeux de Communication." *Ph.D. Thesis*, Publ. De l'Inst.de Statistique de l'Univ. de Paris, 2, 1953.

[22] Muller, E.M. and Brown, W.S. "Variations in the supraglottal air pressure wave form and their articulatory interpretation." In *Speech and Language*. New York: Academic Press, pp. 317-389, 1980.

[23] Rayleigh, Lord (J.W. Strutt). *The Theory of Sound.* London, 1894.

[24] Sams, M., Aulanko, R., Hamalainen, H., Lounasmaa, O., Lu, S. and Simola, J. "Visual information from lip movements modifies activity in the human auditory cortex." *Neurosci. Lett.* 127: 141-145, 1991.

[25] Schoentgen, J. and Ciocea, S., "Kinematic formant–to–area mapping." *Speech Communication* 21: 227-244, 1997.

[26] Schroeter, J. and Sondhi, M.M. "Speech coding based on physiological models of speech production." In *Advances in Speech Signal Processing*, S. Furui and M.M. Sondhi (eds.), New York: Marcel Dekker, pp. 231-268, 1992.

[27] Schroeter, J. and Sondhi, M.M. "Techniques for estimating vocal tract shapes from the speech signal." *IEEE Trans. Speech Audio Proc.* 2, N1, Part 2: 133-150, 1994.

[28] Schmidt, R.A. "More on motor programs." In *Human Motor Behavior*, S. Kelso (ed.), Hillsdale, NJ: Lawrence Erlbaum, pp. 189-218, 1982.

[29] Seifritz, E., Esposito, F., Hennel, F., Mustofic, H., Neuhoff, J.G., Bilecen, D., Tedeschi, G., Scheffler, K. and Di Salle, F. "Spatiotemporal pattern of neural processing in the human auditory cortex." *Science* 297: 1706-1708, 2002.

[30] Sekiyama, K. and Sugita, Y. "Auditory–visual speech perception examined by brain imaging and reaction time." *Proc. 7th Int. Conf. Spoken Lang. Proc.*, pp. 1693-1696, 2002.

[31] Shirai, K. and Kobayashi, T. "Estimating articulatory motion from speech wave." *Speech Communication* 5: 159-170, 1986.

[32] Sondhi, M.M. and Schroeter, J. "A hybrid time–frequency domain articulatory speech synthesizer." *IEEE Trans. Acoust., Speech, Signal Proc.* ASSP-35: 955-967, 1987.

[33] Sorokin, V.N. *Theory of Speech Production.* Radio and Telecommunication, Moscow, 1985. [Russian]

[34] Sorokin, V.N. "Coordination of muscles and articulators." *Proc. XIth Int. Cong. Phon. Sci.*, Vol. 3, pp. 382-384, 1987.

[35] Sorokin, V.N. *Speech Synthesis.* Science, Moscow, 1992. [Russian]

[36] Sorokin, V.N. "Determination of vocal tract shape for vowels." *Speech Communication* 11: 71-85, 1992.

[37] Sorokin, V.N. "Inverse problem for fricatives." *Speech Communication* 14: 249-262, 1994.

[38] Sorokin, V.N. and Trushkin, A.V. "Articulatory–to–acoustic mapping for inverse problem." *Speech Communication* 19: 105-118, 1996.

[39] Sorokin, V.N, Olshansky, V., and Kozhanov, L. "Internal model in articulatory control: Evidence from speaking without larynx." *Speech Communication* 25: 249-268, 1998.

[40] Sorokin, V.N., Leonov, A.S. and Trushkin, A.V. "Estimation of stability and accuracy of inverse problem solution for the vocal tract." *Speech Communication* 30: 55-74, 2000.

[41] Sorokin, V.N. "Some coding properties of speech." *Speech Communication* 40: 409-423, 2003.

[42] Story, B., Titze, I. and Hoffman, E. "Vocal tract area functions from magnetic resonance." *J. Acoust. Soc. Am.* 100: 537-554, 1996.

[43] Tikhonov, A.N. and Arsenin, V.Ya. *Solution of Ill–Posed Problems.* New York: Wiley, 1977.

[44] Tikhonov, A.N., Leonov, A.S. and Yagola, A.G. *Nonlinear Ill–Posed Problems.* New York: Chapman and Hall, 1998.

[45] Titze, I., Story, B. and Hoffman, E. "Vocal tract area functions for an adult female speaker based on volumetric imaging." *J. Acoust. Soc. Am.* 104: 471-487, 1998.

[46] Westbury, J. *X-ray Microbeam Speech Production Database: User's Handbook.* Madison, WI: University of Wisconsin, 1994.

Dynamics of Speech Production and Perception
P. Divenyi et al. (Eds.)
IOS Press, 2006

Computer-Assisted Pronunciation Teaching and Training Methods Based on the Dynamic Spectro-Temporal Characteristics of Speech

Klára VICSI
Department of Telecommunication and Mediainformatics
Budapest University of Technology and Economics
Budapest, Hungary

Abstract. This chapter provides a general overview of computer based speech learning and training methods, which are used for teaching speech handicapped persons or for pronunciation teaching in the field of language learning(CALL: Computer Assisted Language Learning). It will discuss how these systems can present the dynamic spectro-temporal characteristics of speech for students, and how these have been used with success in such tasks like training basic speech abilities, improving pronunciation, practicing intonation, gaining speaking fluency and evaluating the pronunciation. The technology includes speech recognition, synthesis, analysis, manipulation and visualisation. Among these systems a newly developed process-oriented, multi-modal speech correction method is described in detail, developed in the frame of the European SPECO project (Contract no.977126). The system has been developed for teaching and training 5-10 year-old speech handicapped children and it has been developed for four languages: English, Swedish, Slovenian and Hungarian. Correction of disordered aspects of speech is done by real time visual presentation of the speech parameters, in a way that is understandable and interesting for young children, while remaining correct from the acoustic-phonetic point of view.

Keywords. Speech pronunciation teaching and training, computer-assisted language learning (CALL), speech recognition, speech visualization, speech handicapped, hearing impaired, speech therapy

Introduction

The latest results in computer technology and digital speech processing make possible the construction of systems that improve the quality of speech learning and training. Speech training using these technologies is useful for speech-handicapped persons, especially hard-of-hearing and deaf children, but recently it has appeared in second language learning (CALL: Computer Assisted Language Learning) too. As more advanced speech technology emerges, its usefulness will increase. The capabilities of the technology include measuring and displaying the dynamic characteristics of speech parameters,

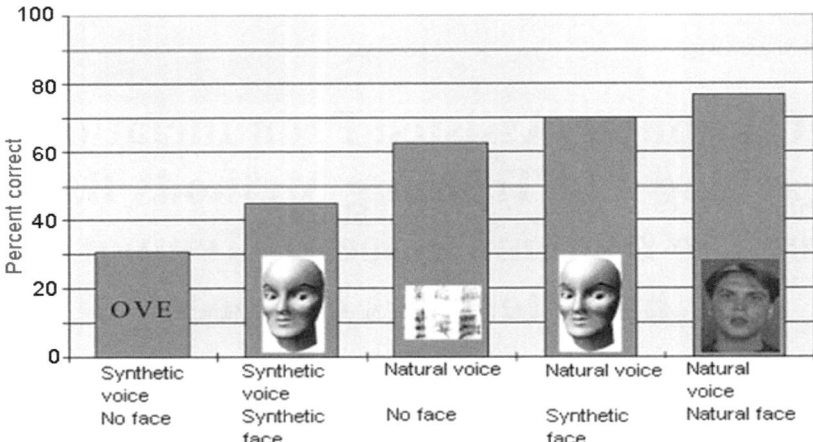

Figure 1. The importance of speech reading and body gesture in speech intelligibility when speech is supplemented by a synthesized face [5].

speech recognition, synthesis, manipulation and visualisation.

In this chapter, different feedback methods are discussed which are generally used in speech training systems. This description is not a detailed list of the existing systems, only a general overview, to give an average impression about this field of speech technology.

1. Types of Feedback

The aim of the computer assisted speech training systems is to provide an appropriate level of auditory and visual feedback to the student in order to point out possible direction for the improvement of the pronunciation. There are several possible training methods, which differ from each other mainly in the feedback.

1.1 Audio and visual feedback

The researchers in KTH (Royal Institute of Technology, in Stockholm) developed a speech intelligibility test to examine the role of visual information in speech intelligibility —in particular, speech reading and body gestures. Noisy synthetic and natural speech was supplemented by a visible synthesized or natural face and the intelligibility of the speech was examined [5].

The results obtained are presented in Figure 1. The results of the experiment show the improvement of intelligibility, when visual information is also given to the subjects.

1.2 Synthetic Face

A visual representation of the behaviour of the trainees' articulator is a direct and helpful method. These are the process-oriented systems [12].

The animated artificial agents, for example, model visual gestures in speech, utilis-

lip tracking

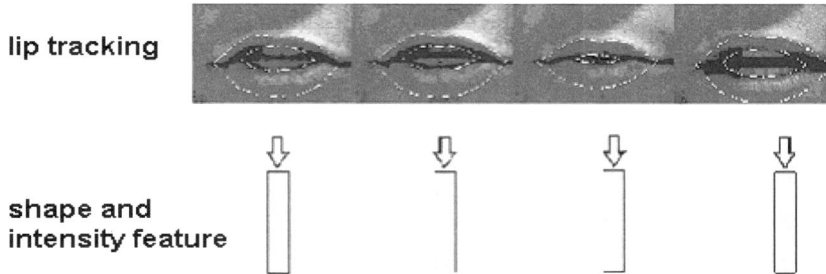

**shape and
intensity feature**

Figure 2. Extraction of visual speech features: Speech reading using probabilistic models [21].

ing a parametrically controlled visual speech synthesis based on a 3D polygonal model
of a face [8][23].

At IDIAP (Dalle Molle Institute for Perceptual Artificial Intelligence in Marrtingny,
Switzerland), a speech reading system locates and tracks the lips of a speaker over an
image sequence to extract visual speech information.

The extracted features describe the shape of the lips and the intensity of the mouth
area as presented in Figure 2. The main modes of intensity variation mainly account for
illumination and speaker differences rather than for speech information. Smaller modes
of intensity variation account for speech information and describe the visibility of teeth
and tongue. IDIAP models these features by Gaussian distribution and their temporal
dependencies by Hidden Markov Models.

The animated agents can improve learning and language training. Human faces
enrich interpersonal communication because they are informative, emotional and per-
sonal. We often communicate better in face-to-face situations because we are able to
combine many sources of information to perceive and understand, even when some of
the information is ambiguous or fuzzy. When producing speech, faces are informative
linguistically and the auditory and visual features of speech are often complementary. In
fact, animated faces such as "Baldi" can provide feedback that humans cannot by turning semi-transparent to show the movements of the tongue within the mouth from different angles, or by presenting visual patterns that represent acoustic phonetic features
of sounds [8][9].

1.3 Visualized Acoustic Properties

Another way to help students learn speech is to visualize the acoustic properties. These
systems record speech signals, play them back and eventually visualise them in order to
provide the user with feedback information. These systems work well if the measured
acoustic-phonetic parameters correspond adequately to the articulation movement. The
parameters can be visualized as sound pictures. Thus if the visualization process is correct, then there is a correspondence between the articulation and the sound pictures (Figure 3).

Visualized data can be diagrams and spectrograms, generally in comparative methods. The effectiveness of a system depends on the type of the acoustic processing giving
the acoustical parameters, and on the method of the visualisation. The visualised sound
parameters — the sound pictures — must be interesting and phonetically correct, pro-

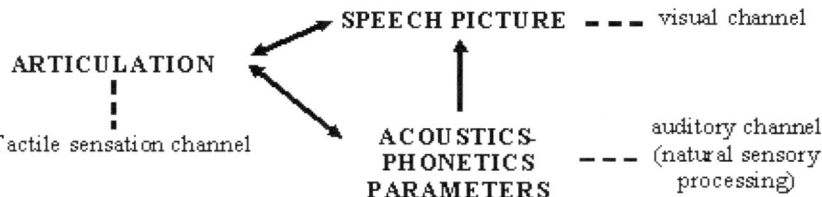

Figure 3. Correspondence between the articulation and the sound pictures.

viding feedback on whether and why the actual pronunciation is good or not.

Visualized data are often speech waveforms as in Figure 4. This kind of presentation is cheap, but hardly can give any useful and understandable help for students, however Bernstein and Christian wrote in their paper that experiments have shown in such cases a visual display of the talker not only improves the word identification accuracy [4], but also the speech rhythm and timing [22]. A large number of commercial pronunciation tutors on the market today offer this kind of feedback.

Experiences with spectral information on the displays suggest their potential use as pronunciation feedback. It is important to emphasize that the results depend first on the interpretation of the parameters, secondly on the method of visual presentation and thirdly on the instructions on how to interpret the displays. For example the spectrum interpretation by the IBM "Speech Viewer" of the /u/ sound in Figure 5(a) is dry and hardly understandable for young children, but the other type of its visualisation, presented in Figure 5(b), is clear and more age-appropriate: an apple falling off a tree, when the pronunciation is correct.

Others have experimented with using a real-time spectrogram display of speech to provide pronunciation feedback. Generally they use comparative methods, but these pictures are too complicated for 5-year-old children.

The SPECO System illustrated in Figure 6 belongs to the group using diagrams, spectrograms, and prosodic information, but a new interpretation technique was designed which is correct from an acoustic phonetic point of view, but easy to understand and interesting for children [34]. Auditory spectrograms are used by comparing the reference speech, (upper part in the Figures 6 and 7.) with the actual one (lower part in Figures 6 and 7.)

The important parts of the spectrogram of the practiced sound are emphasised by background pictures as you see it in the auditory spectrogram in Figure 7. In the correct pronunciation of the /s/ sound, the energy in the higher part of the spectrum is character-

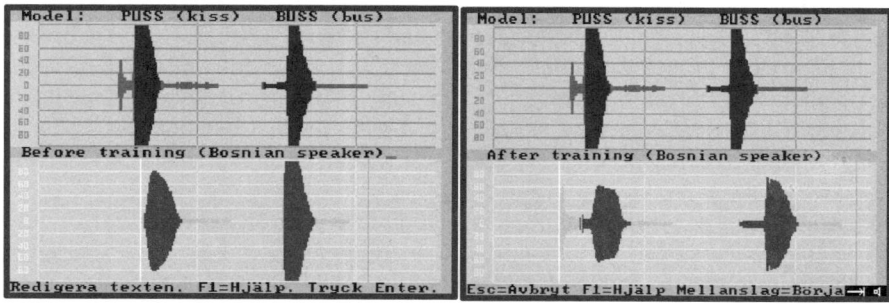

Figure 4. Wave form display in the IBM Speech Viewer.

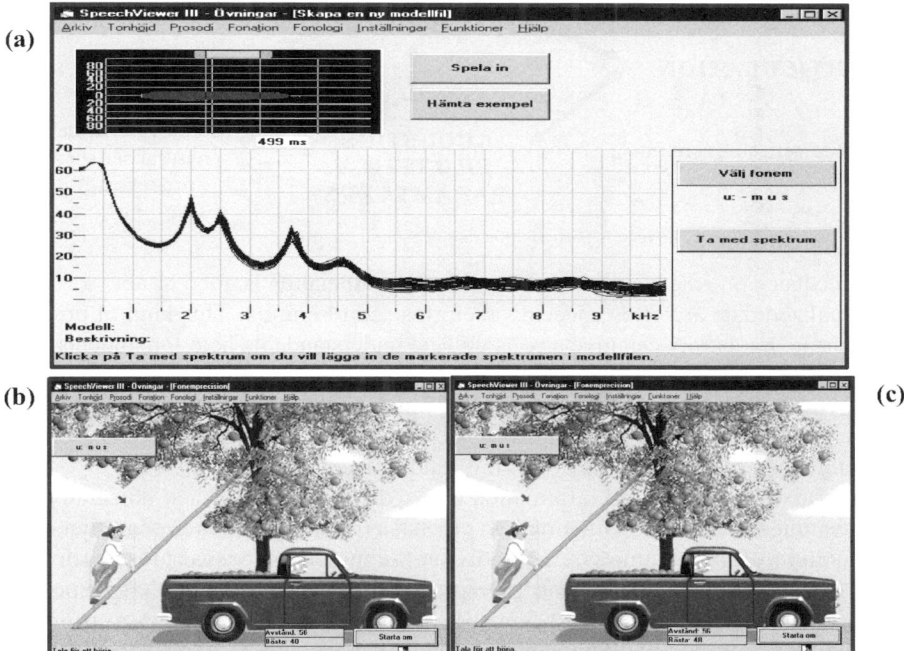

Figure 5. The spectrum display of the u sound in IBM Speech Viewer. a) Spectrum interpretation of the /u/ sound; b) Correctly pronounced /u/ sound; c) Incorrectly pronounced /u/ sound.

istic (the grey clouds must be covered by the spectral points, but the sheep must not have any).

Other systems focus on the supra-segmental feedback. Correct usage of supra-segmental features such as intonation and stress has been shown to improve the syntactic and semantic intelligibility of spoken language [10]. In spoken conversation, intonation and stress information not only help listeners to locate phrase boundaries and word emphasis, but also to identify the pragmatic thrust of the utterance (e.g., interrogative vs. declarative). One of the main acoustical correlates of stress and intonation is funda-

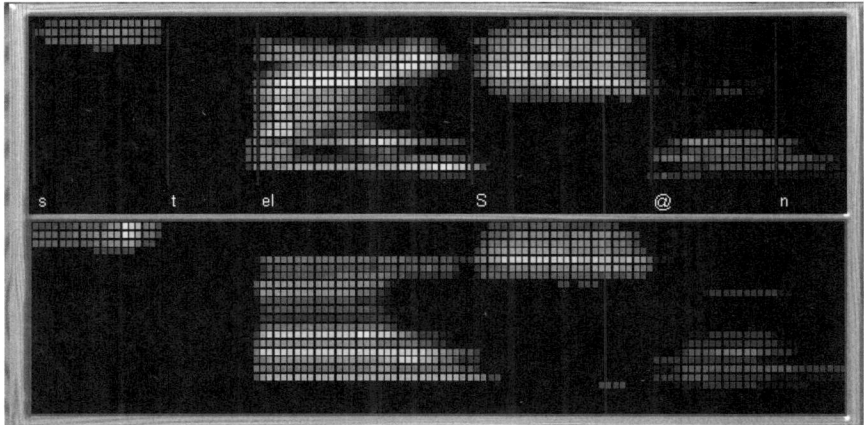

Figure 6. Auditory spectrogram of the word "station" in SPECO speech training system.

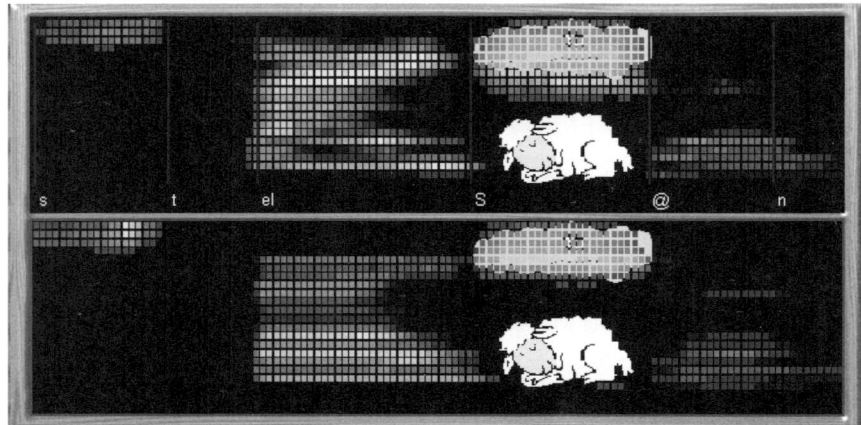

Figure 7. Auditory spectrogram of the word "station" in SPECO speech training system with a background picture.

mental frequency (F0); other acoustical characteristics include loudness, dynamics, duration and tempo. The presentation of dynamics in SPECO System are presented in Figure 8. Such displays can and have been used to provide valuable pronunciation feedback to students.

Experiments have shown that a visual F0 display of supra-segmental features combined with audio feedback is more effective than audio feedback alone [6][18], especially if the student's F0 contour is displayed along with a native model as in the Figure 9.

The feasibility of this type of visual feedback has been demonstrated by a number of simple prototypes [1][2][14][27][28]. We believe that this technology has good potential for being incorporated into commercial CALL systems.

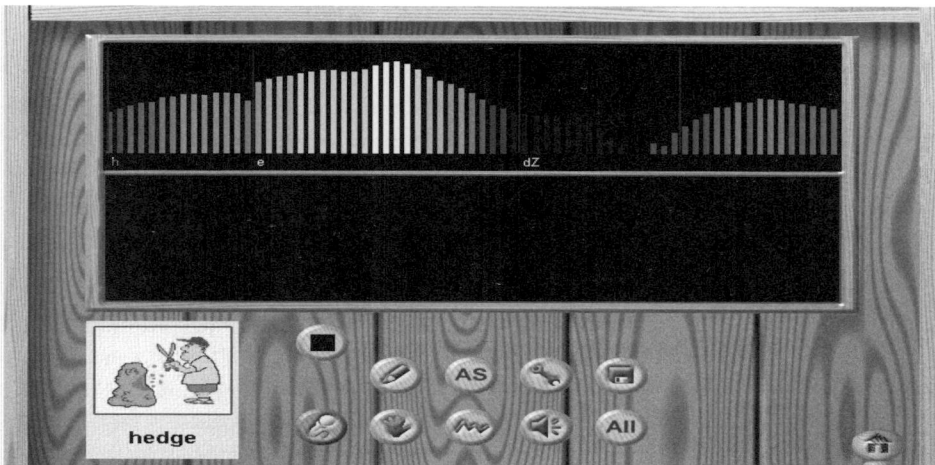

Figure 8. The presentation of dynamics of the energy in SPECO System. Light colours and longer columns represent higher volumes

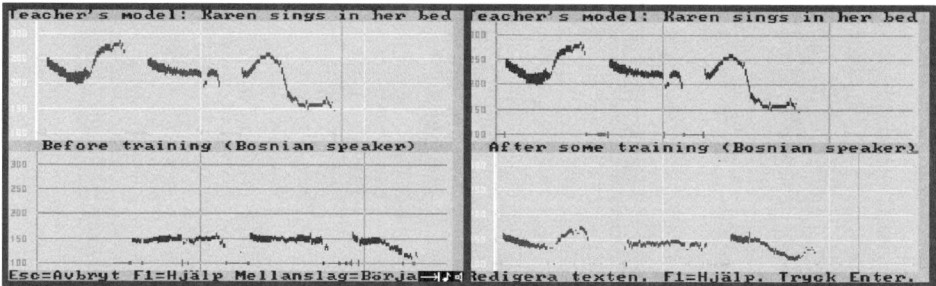

Figure 9. f_0 display in the IBM Speech Viewer.

1.4 Automatic Feedback

In the speech pronunciation learning process, the right feedback, either audio or visual, is very important and contributes to the speech development of the trainees. Moreover, many speech-training tools have some kind of automatic feedback too, based on the acoustic similarity between the trainee's production and a template. In the SPECO [33] and in the ISTRA (Indiana Speech Training Aid, [16]) systems for hearing impaired children, the acoustic similarity metric was estimated by measuring the similarity between a metric of each new utterance and a stored template, which represented the best recent utterances of the trainee.

In the other group of speech training systems, the phoneme-based Hidden Markov Models from the automatic speech recognition technology (ASR) are generally applied to the evaluation of pronunciation [19][24][15]. The teachers' opinions of the automatic efficiency of this last method are equivocal [36]. Sometimes these automatic judgements do not work perfectly on the basis of the automatic speech recognition technology or are not sensitive enough to make slight differences, leading the trainees astray so that they may get worse results than without using any automatic feedback.

From the perspective of speech technology, the key question is whether today's ASR techniques can be used to distinguish between good and poor pronunciations of a known word spoken by a child. By contrast, the normal goal of the ASR is to classify all utterances correctly, even if they are not pronounced accurately.

The systems can use either one type of feedback or all; it depends on the actual purpose of the tool.

2. General Method of the SPECO

In the following paragraphs a newly developed multi-modal, multi-lingual speech correction method is described in detail, developed in the frame of the European SPECO project (Contract no. 977126), directed by the author [32][31][35]. The SPECO system has been developed for speech handicapped persons; it uses the product-oriented teaching method that utilises visually displayed acoustic properties of speech. Children see and listen to the speech examples and compare them by auditory and visual feedback. An automatic feedback has been developed to help comparison, based on distance calculation between the spectral components of the typical auditory spectrums or spectro-

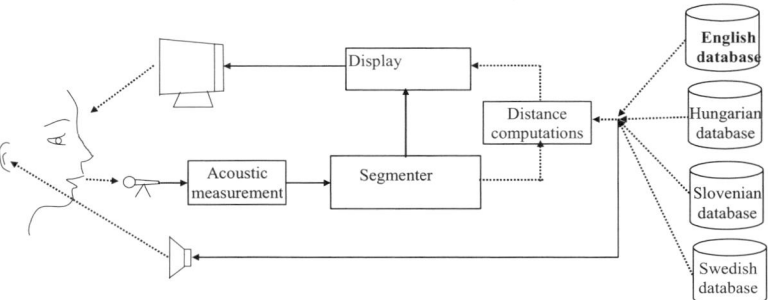

Figure 10. SPECO system structure.

grams and the child's speech.

This automatic feedback based differs in concept from those articulation teaching systems that have been developed on the basis of current speech recognizers (ASR). Nevertheless, the system uses many results and algorithms of ASR [17][20]. Moreover, we have developed a special training method that shifts from an initial focus on a simple sound production to the production of fluent speech on the basis of a big reference vocabulary. Systems are designed to provide training not only for speech production but for speech perception (discrimination and identification), too.

The first version of this multi-modal system was developed for Hungarian [32][31], and then the system was extended and developed further for English, Swedish, Slovenian, and more fluent Hungarian [35]. The project for the multilingual version was funded by the EU through the INCO-COPERNICUS program (Contract no. 977126), and it was called SPECO.

The system structure of this SPECO system is presented in Figure 10.

The system has two parts: one is a general language independent frame program, the Language Independent Database Editor and Measuring System; the other is the Language Dependent Database. This system contains many exercises and provides a teaching facility for developing fluent and intelligible speech using a large reference speech vocabulary. The editor measures the different acoustic-phonetic parameters of the speech signal, and helps the users to build a language-specific vocabulary, and to construct the appropriate sound support.

2.1 The Acoustic Measurement

The acoustic speech processor in our system is a simple auditory model that imitates only the low-level processing of the human hearing system, which is reasonably well-understood [37][38]. The model analyzes the speech signal with time, frequency and intensity resolutions that are similar to those of the human peripheral auditory system during speech perception. The data are valid for average speaking rates and the average speech intensity level (65 dB) [29][30].

Dividing the complex sounds into their frequency components is accomplished by 20 critical filter bands, from 80 Hz to 8 kHz. The filters have asymptotic slopes reflecting the filter characteristics of the human ear. The slopes of these filters are steeper towards high frequencies (25 dB/critical band) and flatter towards lower frequencies (10 dB/critical band) corresponding to masking curves.

In the present realisation, 20 IIR type (Infinite Impulse Response) digital filters are used. The parameters of the filters are calculated according to the following equations:

$$z = 13\arctg(0.76f) + 3.5\arctg(f/7.5)^2 \tag{1}$$

where z is the sound height in Bark, and f is the frequency. The width of the critical band is:

$$\left(\Delta f_{kr} = 25 + 75(1 + 1.4f^2)^{0.69}\right). \tag{2}$$

The transfer characteristic of the filter in logarithmic steps is the following:

$$10\log F(x) = 15.8 + 7.5(x + 0.5) - 17.5[1 + (x + 0.5)^2]^{0.5} \tag{3}$$

where the maximum of $F(x)$ is at $x=0$.

The time resolution is 10 ms, which represents one frame. The Sampling rate is 20 kHz, 16 bit. The measured speech parameters described below.

2.2 Dynamics of the Energy Changing in Time

The sound energy is measured in a 50-dB dynamic range, the integration time is 10 ms. A curve follows the change of the logarithmic energy level of the speech in the full band. (See Figure 8)

2.3 Pitch, Voiced-Unvoiced Detection

For pitch measurement the AMDF method is used [20], instead of a technique that would be better suited for the auditory model but would need much more computing capacities. A curve follows the change of the pitch from 80 Hz to 800 Hz. (See Figure 11.)

2.4 Intonation

Several types of normalization were compared to determine which one emphasizes the essence of the prosodic phenomena best. It was found that the most characteristic pitch contours were obtained using a logarithmic frequency scale with the frequency values normalized to the fundamental frequency of the vowel in the first syllable. So changes in the fundamental frequency were analysed by comparing it to the fundamental frequency in the first syllable. (See Figure 11.)

2.5 Auditory Spectrum

On the computer screen the energy of the spectral components is presented. The horizontal axis shows the frequencies in critical bands, from 1 to 20; the vertical axis shows the logarithmic energy level in dB in the bands. A curve is fit to the energy output of the

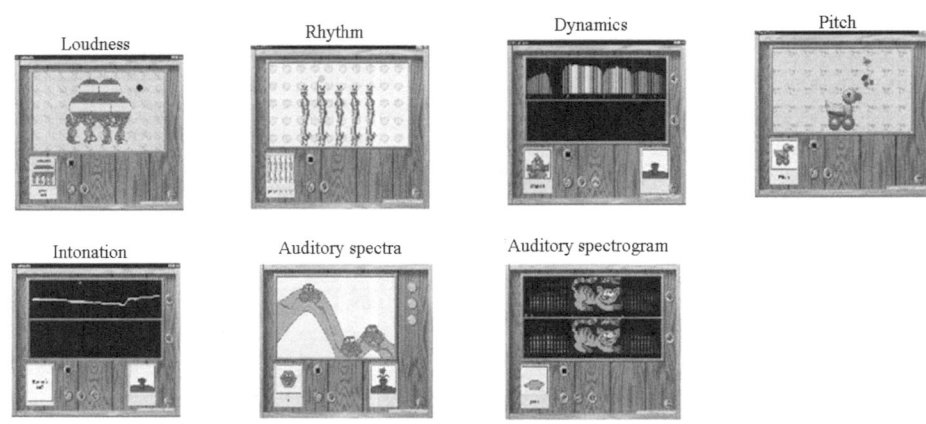

Figure 11. Speech pictures. **Loudness:** the position of a ball in the picture shows the value of the loudness over time. **Rhythm:** the position of a ball in the picture shows the value of the loudness over time; rhythm exercises are directed by different background pictures. **Dynamics:** The height and the brightness of the columns shows the value of the energy in every 10 ms; a diagram of the reference speaker is shown above a diagram of the student (which is empty at the recorded moment). **Pitch:** the pitch value is represented by the perpendicular movement of the duck's head. **Intonation:** this diagram presents the relative change of the fundamental frequency to the fundamental frequency of the middle of the vowel in the first syllable; a diagram of the reference speaker is shown above a diagram of the student (which is empty at the recorded moment). **Auditory spectrum:** a diagram shows the energy of the spectral component at a given moment. The background picture, the road, represents the spread of the energy value. **Auditory spectrogram:** a change in the energy of the spectral components in time (a diagram of the reference speaker is shown above a diagram of the student). Cats are on the background pictures at the position of the practised "ts" in the Hungarian word "patsa".

filter. Every 10 ms a new spectrum is measured and shown together with 9 earlier ones on the screen. (see Figure 14)

2.6 Auditory Spectrogram

On the computer screen the change of the energy of the spectral components in time (change of the auditory spectrum in time) is presented. The horizontal axis shows the time (the frame duration is 10 ms); the vertical axis shows critical bands, from 1 to 20. The logarithmic energy level output of the filters (in dB) are presented by colors. Light colours present high energy levels, while dark colours present low energy levels. (See Figures 7, 11 and 12.)

2.7 Spectrogram Differences

Spectrogram differences are given by comparing the auditory spectrogram of the reference example (upper picture) with the auditory spectrogram of the test item (lower picture). The reference and the test examples are warped to each other [26]. In the case of the best fitting outcome the two spectrograms are compared. At those spectral points where the difference in the corresponding spectral components of the corresponding frame is bigger than the threshold value (6dB), small rectangles are drawn. White rect-

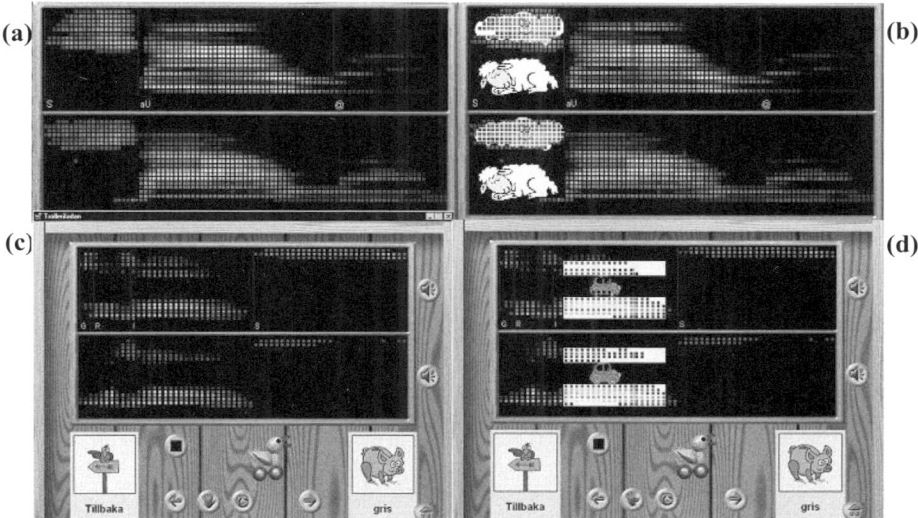

Figure 12. (a) Auditory spectrogram of the word "shower" in the SPECO speech training system in an example of practising the linguopalatal fricative consonant /S/. (b) Auditory spectrogram of the word "shower" in the SPECO speech training system with background pictures in an example of practising the linguopalatal fricative consonant /S/. (c) Auditory spectrogram of the Swedish word "gris" in the SPECO speech training system in an example of practising the vowel /i/ (the duck indicates the result of the automatic evaluation for the child). (d) Auditory spectrogram of the Swedish word "gris" in the SPECO speech training system with background picture in an example of practising the vowel /i/.

angles are drawn when the difference is negative, and green ones when the difference is positive.

2.8 The Visual Presentation

The aim of this method is to teach children how they can obtain information from visual speech pictures [7]. We undertook a detailed exploration to decide which numerical scale of loudness, pitch contour, spectral distribution, and so on, gives the most informative visual presentation (speech pictures) of these parameters. For example, how is it possible to draw a child's attention to the areas of maximum energy in the spectrogram?

Automatic begin/end processing is employed to detect the beginning and the end of the phrases. With the help of different time-warping algorithms [26][25], the corresponding sounds in the reference speech and in the imitation are shown with one immediately below the other, even though the durations of the reference speech and imitation may be different. In this way, the sounds in the reference speech and in the imitation may be easily compared. For example, the maximum energy parts of the auditory spectrogram of the practiced sound are emphasized by using cartoons as background pictures in the auditory spectrograms in Figures 12(a) and 12(b), which show an example of practising the linguopalatal fricative consonant /S/ (here the background picture is the ship with cloud) and in Figures 12(c) and 12(d), which show an example of practising the vowel /i/ (here the background picture is the two rectangles with the small car).

2.9 Vocabularies

Two types of vocabularies have been collected. One is the vocabulary of the reference examples in the program, presented to the child through the training. The other vocabulary is necessary to build up a statistical model of correct speech for automatic feedback.

2.9.1 Reference Speech Vocabulary

The reference speech vocabulary contains the prerecorded reference items. The speech pictures of the reference speech examples are clear and easy to read. The patient's goal during the therapy is to produce sound pictures similar to the reference examples in the vocabulary. In the vocabulary, all trained phonemes must be present in an isolated form, in carefully selected sound sequences, in words, in sentences and minimal pairs, in different sound positions and systematic sound sequences. The samples of the vocabularies are used as references. Although the acoustic speech processing and visual presentation are language-independent, the training method must be adapted to the language. Thus different vocabularies must be constructed for all the languages involved. The language-specific characteristics were taken into consideration in the construction of all the vocabularies.

The reference speech examples are produced by carefully selected persons who speak clearly. Their speech pictures must be clear and easy to read. The patients' goal during therapy is to produce sound pictures similar to the reference speech.

2.9.2 Children's speech database

It was necessary to build up databases for the construction of the statistical model of correct speech, to make the distance score evaluation of speech parameters between correct speech and speech of speech handicapped children. The text material contains all fricatives, affricates and vowels in sequences, in words and in sentences. Four different databases were collected for the four languages. The number of speakers (5- to 10-year-old children) changed according to the language.

It is very difficult to construct a database of correct children's speech. Two aspects had to be considered. On the one hand the text material had to be large enough to represent the language as much as possible. On the other hand the age of our speakers had to be chosen carefully. The length of the materials was limited, especially in the collection of children's speech. For example we had to take into consideration that the spoken utterances could not be longer than 10-15 minutes, especially in case of five-year-old speakers. It is also a very important aspect that the active vocabulary of five-year-old children is much smaller than the vocabulary of adults.

2.10 Statistical models of phonemes

2.10.1 Typical Auditory Spectra of Phonemes

Typical auditory spectrum patterns of vowels and sibilants were calculated from good examples of the Hungarian, Swedish, English and Slovenian children's speech databases, of isolated pronunciations and words. A typical auditory spectrum pattern is calculated as follows:

The spectrum pattern of a phoneme is calculated between $i=3$ and $I-2$. That means 2 frames at the beginning and at the end of the phonemes are left out of the calculation.

$$\bar{A}_n[phoneme] = \frac{1}{I-4} \sum_{i-3}^{I-2} A_i[phoneme] \qquad (4)$$

The spectrum pattern of a phoneme is calculated between i=3 and I-2. That means 2 frames at the beginning and the end of the phonemes are left out out of the calculation.

$$\bar{A}[phoneme] = \frac{1}{N} \sum_{n-1}^{N} \bar{A}_n[phoneme] \qquad (5)$$

where

$A_i = \{a_1, a_2, ..., a_f\}$

$f = 20$, the number of the critical band filters,
$I =$ the total number of frames in the phoneme, and
$N =$ the number of speakers in the children's speech database.

The calculated typical average spectrum patterns of sibilants are presented in Figure 13. All of the spectrum patterns are presented for the children, using one type of speech picture, shown as it is presented in case of the vowel /u/ in Figure 14. During training the child's spectrum lines must fall within the two spectrum lines on the speech picture.

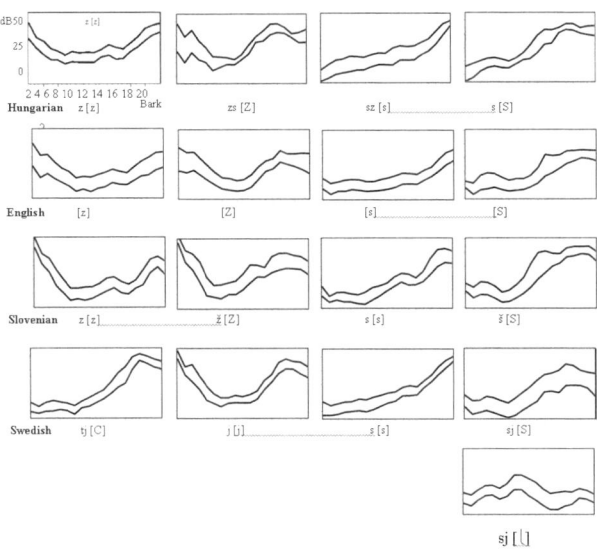

Figure 13. Typical auditory spectra of fricatives of four languages (fricatives are signed by their orthographic character [SAMPA]).

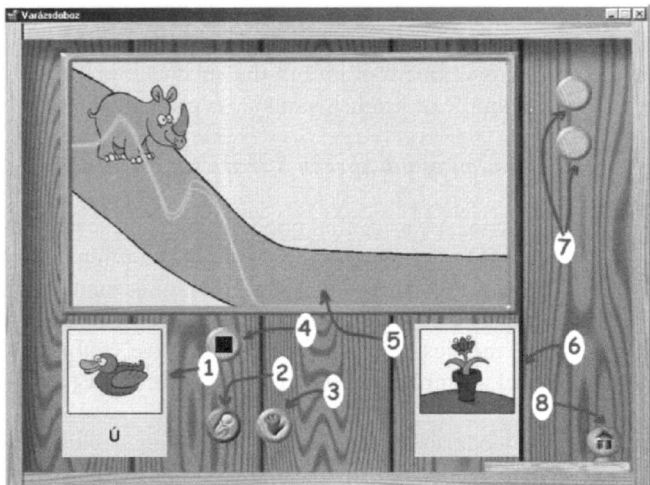

Figure 14. An example of the spectrum typed speech picture of vowel sound /u/ (5). Calling card (1). Func-
        tion-buttons (2, 3, 4, 7, 8). Card to show the result of automatic feedback with the flower, which
        blooms when a sound is pronounced correctly (6).

2.10.2 Typical Averaging Auditory Spectrogram and the Positioning of the background Pictures

One part of the training uses the auditory spectrogram. The spectrogram of the stored
speech of the reference speaker (the reference auditory spectrogram) is presented in the
upper part of the screen and the spectrogram of the child's pronunciation on the lower
part of the screen. Background pictures are presented with the reference auditory spectrogram to emphasize its important parts.

The average spectrograms (upper part of Figure 15) help the construction and the
positioning of the background pictures of each sound (lower part of Figure 15). The typical average auditory spectrograms have been calculated by averaging the energy values

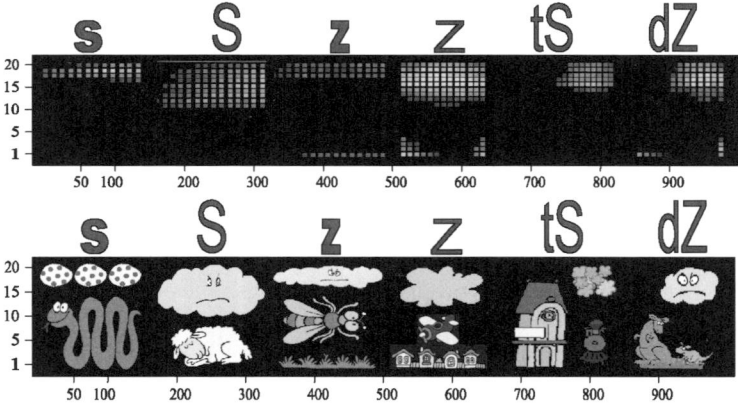

Figure 15. The typical average auditory spectrograms (upper) and the position of the background pictures
        (lower) for English sibilants.

of the spectrograms of the phoneme examples in words from the good and acceptable examples in the child speech database. This average auditory spectrogram is not identical with the reference auditory spectrogram but the spectrogram of a good reference speaker is close to it. An example of English sibilants is presented in Figure 15.

2.11 Distance Score Evaluation of the Speech Spectra for the Automatic Feedback

One important goal of this system was to find good distance measures that could facilitate the comparisons between the spectral components of the reference and the child's speech. This distance measure must mirror the judgement of listeners and the judgement of most of the people in the child's educational, public and cultural life.

The obtained distance metrics help with the quantitative evaluation of defective speech (automatic feedback) and are in good agreement with the displayed speech spectra [33].

The role of automatic feedback is very important in the teaching of severely hearing- impaired children. This feedback provides a good opportunity for practicing with no teacher other than the system alone.

2.12 Different Steps in the Therapy

Beside the exercises of basic speech elements as speech breathing, phonation of natural voices, speech rhythm, dynamics, and tones, detailed exercises were constructed from the voicing to the automation in the cases of sibilants and vowels. The system is based on an up-to-date technology, but the steps of traditional speech therapy were followed in both modules. These are the following: (1) sound preparation, (2) sound development, (3) training on words and (4) automation (meaning the achievement of a reliable production not requiring further instruction). Specific tasks have been constructed in a specific order involving the teaching experiences of the teachers of a given language. For example, in the case of sound development (2) of the linguopalatal fricative consonant / S/, we start to practice this sound together with a back vowel /u/, because pronunciation of this sound sequence is easier than, for example, one with a front vowel such as /i/. Thus one of the most important tasks was to construct a well-defined text.

In sound preparation (1) we can adjust different general speech parameters: loudness, rhythm, spectrum, pitch and so on. For example, it is possible to practice and develop the correct loudness of the child's speech, or to practice speech rhythm, or to develop the phonation of natural voices, and so on.

In the sound development exercises (2), the child can choose a phoneme and start to develop it. The vocabulary contains sound sequences constructed so that the phonemes being practiced occur in different positions and contexts in the syllable-sized units. For example, fricatives and affricates are presented in CV, VCV, VC and VC-VC-VC position and are sequenced with all the vowels and diphthongs. The order of the presentation of the sound sequences is important, so they are graded from the easier pronunciations to the more difficult ones.

In word training(3) the grouping of words is different in fricative support and vowel support. In fricatives and affricates support all phonemes are presented in initial, medial and final position in words. In vowel support all phonemes occur in one-syllable words

Name:
Job:
How long have you been using the program?
How good do you find this method from pedagogical point of view?
Does the user manual give orientation enough?
Is special skill necessary to the usage of the program?
Is training a pleasure for the children?
Do children understand the feedback in the program?
Are pictures understandable in the exercises "isolated sound"?
Are the speech pictures understandable for children in the exercises of syllables, words and sentences?
Is more training possibility necessary during the exercises?
Is less training possibility enough during the exercises?
Would any other kind of training possibilities be useful?
If yes, which ones?
What is your opinion about the exercises?
Have exercises developed the speech of the children? In what?
Preparation:
Sound development:
Practice in sentences:
Intonation:
Was it difficult to work with the program? If yes, please explain.
How long did it take for a phoneme in isolation to form perfectly?
How long did it take for a phoneme in continuous speech to form perfectly?
What is the difference with traditional therapy?
Did you like this method?
Any other ideas?

Table 1. A questionaire for the evaluation of SPECO project.

and in words of two or several syllables.

The contrast pairs are presented to the child to show the differences between the visual pictures of two phonemes in similar words.

Our aim of the therapy is to reach the speech level at which the patient speaks correctly without having to concentrate on the articulation. In this system the children can practice the sounds in sentences (4), too. Specially designed sentences, first simple, then complex, have been collected in the vocabulary of all participant languages.

Demo version of the SPECO system for the four different languages is presented on our webpage: http://alpha.ttt.bme.hu/speech/research.php.

2.13 Evaluation

During the development of the SPECO System we kept contact with therapists. They used the system for teaching during three or six months (it was changed according to the countries), and at the end of the training they filled in a special questionnaire that is presented in Table 1. On the base of their opinion we have developed the system further. This method helped us to construct a good program, but at the end of the development we wanted to know the effectiveness of the system.

A quantitative evaluation was based on a comparison of the intelligibility development of the children trained by the SPECO program, and by the traditional method (control groups). Different speech handicapped groups were examined.

40 6- to 8-year-old children were selected from 240 in the Hard of Hearing School in Budapest. Those 240 students represent the population of hearing handicapped children in Budapest. 40 children were grouped according to the degree of impairment. The

Type of the Groups	Pairs for listening	Decisions in the listening test		
		The FIRST word in the pairs is better [%]	The SECOND word in the pair is better [%]	Uncertain decision [%]
all groups together	1-2	18	55	26
	1-3	14	66	20
	2-3	22	40	39
control group	1-2	24	45	31
	1-3	14	58	28
	2-3	20	35	44
SPECO group	1-2	17	57	26
	1-3	14	67	19
	2-3	22	40	38
normal hearing (H)	1-2	15	74	11
	1-3	16	73	12
	2-3	24	22	54
small hearing impairment (SMH)	1-2	25	46	29
	1-3	21	64	14
	2-3	24	48	28
middle hearing impairment (MH)	1-2	16	62	22
	1-3	9	78	13
	2-3	20	52	27
severely hearing impairment (SH)	1-2	12	53	35
	1-3	12	57	31
	2-3	22	35	44

Table 2. The results of the listening test for the examination of the effectiveness.

groups (audiometric pre-examination was made without using a hearing aids) were the following:

8 children with normal hearing (H),

8 children with a small hearing impairment (SMH),

8 children with a medium hearing impairment (MH),

8 children with severe hearing impairments (SH),

8 children in the control group, trained only by the traditional method (2-2 children with H, SMH, MH, and SH).

Training in the control group was going on without SPECO program, with traditional methods, for the other four groups we made development on the basis of SPECO.

18 well-selected words were produced by the pupils in 3 phases:

1st phase before the training --- marked by 1.

2nd phase after the training --- marked by 2.

3rd phase after the summer holiday --- marked by 3.

Produced examples were recorded. After the first records there was an intensive speech development in the groups. Children participated individually in trainings, during 25 minutes, and 2-3 times per week. It became clear early during the development, that the planned therapy steps must be handed flexibly and modified how a given child can develop. There are plenty of possibilities because of the flexibility of program.

The main tasks were to arrange the following:

- appropriate speech breathing,
- phonation of natural voices,
- appropriate speech rhythm,

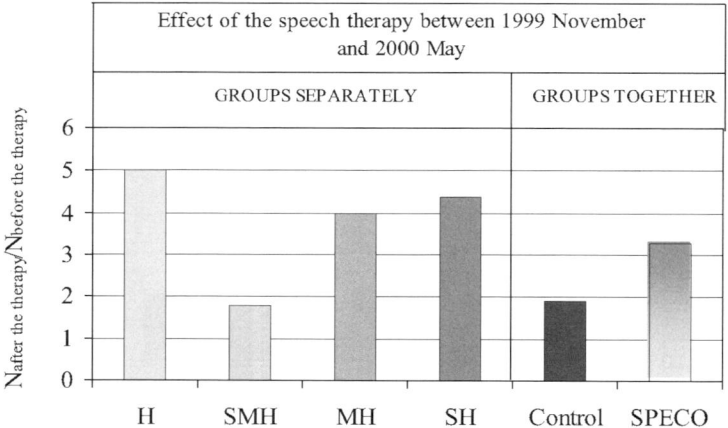

Figure 16. The effect of the speech therapy in the word pairs 1-2.

- appropriate dynamics,
- appropriate tone,
- appropriate pronunciation.

During the training users of the SPECO system were practicing continuously with the help of dictionary and the rich material of sentences of it, while the control group used the traditional memory cards, picture-books, and other exercise material.

Comparing the intelligibility of the recorded material of the 1st and the 2nd phases (marked: 1-2), the result provides information about the effectiveness of the SPECO method and about the quality of speech. A comparison of the speech of pupils in phases 2 and 3 (marked:2-3) shows whether the pupils could stay or not at the level they had reached during the training.

Words produced by each child were saved to separated files and marked with the child's monogram. The same words from two different phases of one child's training were concatenated to form a test word pair. The pairs of 1-2, 1-3 and 2-3 utterances were heard in random order resulted a rearrangement of the order of pairs and word order within the pairs, too. We have made 2160 (18x3x40) word pairs from the three records of the forty children, containing 18 words per record. We concatenated the mixed voice files in one big voice file, where there was a three second pause between words. After listening to the whole material we have made sure that as a result of mixing, a listener cannot identify, which child's record he/she hears and what time the record had been made.

30 non-expert young people (listeners) took part in the listening test. Listeners were asked to decide, which words were more understandable in the word pairs. They were allowed to note, too, if they could not make a decision. The listening test gave clear results presented in Table 2., where the decisions of the listeners are given according to the groups.

The SPECO group in the Table 2. gives the averaged result of the 4 groups, where the teacher used the SPECO system during training.In general the listeners found the words after the training much more understandable in all the groups. More listeners

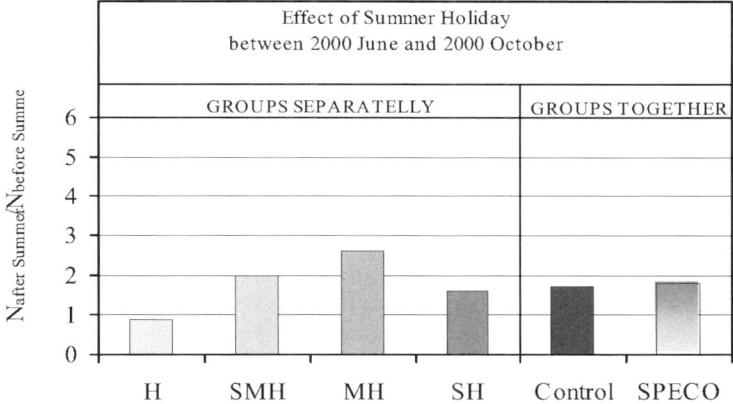

Figure 17. The effect of the summer holiday in the word pairs 2-3.

found the intelligibility better in those groups in which the SPECO system was used.

To see the effect of the speech therapy more precisely the 1-2 word pairs were examined separately. The number of the decisions in favor of the word recorded after therapy (N after the therapy) and before therapy (N before the therapy) were compared. See Figure 16.

The effect of the speech therapy is evident.The biggest improvement was found in the speech handicapped group with normal hearing. Perhaps in the case of children with severe hearing impairment positive changes are more hidden because they had problems not only with the pronunciation, but also with the power of voice, rhythm, etc., so with the suprasegmental elements, too. In spite of the intensive development there are remained some segments to be improved, that the intelligibility of speech does not improve for listeners so much. As it can be seen in Table 2., while in the case of speech handicapped children with normal hearing 11 percent of listeners could not decide, which word is more understandable, then in the case of severely hard of hearing children 35 percent of listeners could not decide it!

To see the effect of the summer holiday the 2-3 word pairs were examined separately, and compared the number of decisions in favor of the word recorded after the summer (N after summer) with the number of the decisions for the word recorded before the summer (N before summer) in word pairs. See Figure 17.

During summer holiday results do not deteriorate, listeners found development positive in every group. It shows in one hand, that the biologically determined spontaneous linguistic development was effective either in the case of the SPECO group, or in the case of the control group, and on the other hand, that the improvement in the quality of pronunciation was not only successful, but permanent as well.

The results show, that the effectiveness of SPECO depends on the type of hearing or speech handicap, but has given better results in every group than in the control groups, where a traditional speech therapy was applied.

3.   Conclusion

Research results written in this study hopefully can contribute to better realization of multi-sensored speech training processes.

On the basis of the evaluation of the SPECO System and on the basis of the opinion of the therapists we can tell the followings:

The intelligibility test is appropriate for examining of the development of articulation among the children, and can give good information about the effectiveness of a multimedia pronunciation training system.

The therapists were very satisfied with the SPECO method of learning. The summarised opinions of the teachers across four languages were very good. This tool is a good aid. It helps the therapist and gives a variety of learning experiences. Of course, especially for young children the visual tool itself does not substitute for the work of the speech therapist. On the other hand, in the case of older children, the system itself provides a good opportunity to practice alone.

Children can use this multimodal system by themselves very easily and they use it with pleasure, which is a very important factor from the point of view of efficiency. The visual feedback helps children to see whether their pronunciation is correct or not, and how far it is from the correct one. They are do not need to rely only on the teacher's opinion. In particular, this is very important in the case of speech handicapped children with hearing loss.

It was found that a consistently shorter time was required for improving a speech sound than was the case with corresponding children of similar mental ability and impairment level who had been instructed by traditional methods.

In those cases when sounds were very resistant to the traditional therapy, the new method helped to improve these sounds.

Naturally, this new method cannot be a substitute of the work of expert speech therapists, but it can help effectively with education, and it facilitates expert speech therapists work.

4.   Discussion

Speech training systems are basically designed for two different user groups:

1. Methods for speech handicapped persons especially for hearing impaired children:
    Visual feedback is particularly effective for hearing impaired persons, for whom the auditory feedback does not work properly, so they have troubles with the speech learning process.
2. Methods for Computer-Assisted Language Learning:
    With the increase of international communication in foreign language, oral communication is especially important. Today a demand has arisen for a self-learning paradigm for speaking foreign languages. In the self-language learning process the reference speaker is not present; thus the acoustic and visual information of speaking are missing.

Both methods can use the same technical environment and speech processing possibilities, but the didactical material must be different. These didactical structures of speech training systems are very important. The effectiveness of a speech training system depends upon the teaching treatment in a big extent. On the other hand, these systems are technically based on speech technology. As speech technology develops, the effectiveness of such systems will improve and their usefulness will increase.

Acknowledgements

This research has been supported by the European Union in the framework of the Inco-Copernicus Program (Contract no. 977126) and by the Hungarian Scientific Research Foundation.

The author is grateful to Anne-Marie Öster (KTH-Kungl. Tekniska Högskolan), Zdravko Kacic (Universityí of Maribor), Peter Roach (University of Reading), Peter Barczikay (Robot Control Software Ltd.) for their friendly and useful cooperation.

References

[1] Abberton, E. and Fourcin, A. "Visual feedback and the acquisition of intonation in Lenneberg." *Foundations of Language Development*, Vol.2. pp. 157-165, 1975.

[2] Anderson-Hsieh, J. "Interpreting visual feedback in computer-assisted instruction on suprasegmentals." *CALICO Journal*, 11(4): 5-22, 1994.

[3] Alvarez, A., Martínez R., Gómez P., Domínguez J.L. "A signal processing technique for speech visualization." *ESCA-STILL98,* pp. 33-36, 1998.

[4] Bernstein, L. and Benoît, C. "For speech perceptions by human or machines, three senses are better than one." *Proc. Int. Conf. Spoken Lag. Proc.*, pp. 1477-1480, 1996.

[5] Beskow, J., Dahlquist, M., Granström, B., Lundeberg, M., Spens, K-E. and Öhman, T. "The Teleface project - isability, feasibility and intelligibility." *Proc. Fonetik97,* 1997.

[6] de Bot, K. "Visual feedback of intonation: Effectiveness and induced practice behavior." *Lang. Speech* 26(4): 331-350, 1983.

[7] Campbell, R., *et al*. "Hearing by eye 2 II." *Psychology Press*, 1998.

[8] Cole, R., Carmell, T., Connors, P., Macon, M., Wouters, J., de Villiers, J., Tarachow, A., Massaro, D., Cohen, M., Beskow, J., Yang, J., Meier, U., Waibel, A., Stone, P., Fortier, G., Davis, A., Soland, C. "Intelligent animated agents for interactive language training." *ESCA-STILL98,* pp. 163-166, 1998.

[9] Cole, R., Massaro, D. W., de Villiers, J., Rundle, B., Shobaki, K., Wouters, J., Cohen, M., Beskow, J., Stone, P., Connors, P., Tarachow, A., Solcher, D.."New tools for interactive speech and language training: Using animated conversational agents in the classrooms of profoundly deaf children." *Proc. ESCA/Socrates Workshop on Method and Tool Innovations for Speech Science Education (MATISSE)*,1999.

[10] Crystal, D. *Clinical Linguistics*. New York: Harper, 1981.

[11] Delmonte, R., Petrea, M., Bacalu, C. "Slim prosodic module for learning activities in a foreign language." Proc. *Eurospeech,* pp. 669-672, 1997.

[12] Gibbon, F.E. and Hardcastle, W. J. "Deviant articulation in a cleft plate child following late repair of the hard palate: A description and remediation procedure using electropalatography." *Clinical Ling. Phonetics* 3: 93-110, 1989.

[13] W. J. Hardcastle, F. E. Gibbon and W. Jones. "Visual display of tongue-palate contact: Electropalatography in the assessment and remediation of speech disorders." *Br. J. Dis. Comm.* 26: 41-74, 1991.

[14] Hiller, S., Rooney, E., Lefevre, J.P. and Jack, M. "SPELL: An automated system for computer-aided pronunciation teaching." *Proc. Eurospeech,* 1993.

[15] ISLE *"Interactive Spoken Language Education."* Annual Report. http://www.ec-isle.org, 1999.

[16] ISTRA *"Indiana Speech Training Aid Features."* Bloomington, IN: Communication Disorders Technology, Inc. http://www.comdistec.com/istra_faq.shtm, 2003.

[17] Itakura, F. "Minimum prediction residual principle applied to speech recognition." *IEEE Trans. Acoust. Speech Sig. Proc.* 23: 67-72, 1975.

[18] James, E. "The acquisition of prosodic features of speech using a speech visualizer." *IRAL*, 14(3): 227-243, 1976.

[19] Kawai, G. and Hirose, K.A. "CALL system using speech recognition to train the pronunciation of Japanese long vowels, the mora nasal and mora obstruents." *Proc. Eurospeech*, 1997.

[20] Kent, R.D. and Read, C. *The Acoustic Analysis of Speech.* San Diego: Singular, pp. 158-164, 1992.

[21] Luettin, J. and Thacker, N.A. "Speechreading using probabilistic models." *Computer Vision and Image Understanding* 65:163-178, 1997

[22] Markham, D. and Nagano-Madesen, Y. *Proc. Int. Conf. Spoken Lang. Proc.*, pp. 1473-1476, 1996.

[23] Massaro, D.W. *Perceiving Talking Faces: From Speech Perception to a Behavioural Principle.* Cambridge, MA: MIT Press, 1998. [Information about the facial animation software developed at the University of California, Santa Cruz, is available at http://mambo. ucsc.edu/psl/pslfan.html]

[24] Narusa, J. "Computer-aided spoken language training with enhanced visual and auditory feedback." *Proc. Eurospeech,* pp. 183-186, 1999.

[25] Rabiner, L.R. and Levinson, S.E. "Isolated and connected word recognition - theory and selected application." *IEEE Trans. Comm.* 29(5): 621-659, 1981.

[26] Sakoe, H. and Chiba, S. "Dynamic programming algorithm optimization for spoken word recognition." *IEEE Trans. Acoust. Speech Sig. Proc.* 26: 43-49, 1978.

[27] Spaai, G.W. and Hermes, D.J. "A visual display for the teaching of intonation." *CALICO Journal* 10(3):19-30, 1993.

[28] Stibbard, R.M. "Teaching English intonation with a visual display of fundamental frequency." *The Internet TESL Journal*, II(8), August 1996.

[29] Vicsi, K. "The most relevant acoustical microsegment and its duration necessary for the recognition of unvoiced stops." *Acoustica* 48: 53-58, 1981.

[30] Vicsi, K., Matilla, M. and Berényi, P. "Continuous speech segmentation using different methods." *Acoustica* 71: 152-156, 1990.

[31] Vicsi, K. "A product oriented teaching and training system for speech handicapped children." *Proc. Speech and Language Technology for Disabled Persons Workshop*, pp. 177, 1993.

[32] Vicsi, K. *et al.* "LIAS: Language-independent automatic segmentation technique using SAMPA labeling of phonemes." *1st Int. Conf. Lang. Res. Educ.*, pp. 1-317, 1998.

[33] Vicsi, K., Csatári, F., Bakcsi, Z. and Tantos, A. "Distance score evaluation of the visualised speech spectra at audio-visual articulation training." *Proc. Europseech*, pp. 1911-1914, 1999.

[34] Vicsi, K., Roach, P., Öster, A., Kacic, Z, Barczikay, P., Tantos, A., Catári, F., Bakcsi, Z. and Sfakianaki, A. "A multimedia, multilingual teaching and training system for children with speech disorders." *Int. J. Speech Tech.* 3: 289-300, 2000.

[35] Vicsi, K. *et al.* "A multilingual multimodal Speech Training System, SPECO." *Proc. Eurospeech,* pp. 2807-2810, 2001.

[36] Wallace, J. L., Russell, M., Brown, C., Skilling, A. "Applications of speech recognition in the primary school classroom." *ESCA – Still 98 Workshop Proc.,* pp. 21-24, 1998.

[37] Zwicker, E. *Psychoakustik.* Berlin: Springer Verlag, 1982.

[38] Zwicker, E. and Terhardt, E. "Analytical expressions for band rate and critical bandwidth as a function of frequency." *J. Acoust. Soc. Am.* 68: 1523, 1980.

Dynamics of the Singing Voice

Dynamics of Speech Production and Perception
P. Divenyi et al. (Eds.)
IOS Press, 2006

Dynamics of the Singing Voice

David WESSEL[1], Pierre DIVENYI[2,3], and Adam LAMMERT[2,3]
[1]*Center for New Music and Audio Technology, University of California, Berkeley, USA*
[2]*Veterans Affairs Medical Center, Martinez, California USA*
[3]*East Bay Institute for Research and Education, Martinez, California, USA*

According to Leonard Meyer, one of the most prominent figures of the philosophy of music, music is a dynamic process in which both the emotional and the informational components are continuous functions of time [1]. The consequences of this statement are many, the most important among them being that considering music as a sequence of notes as its elements is as laden with the same problems as is considering speech as a sequence of phonemes. The note, not even a note-complex such as a chord or a tone cluster, is meaningless in itself; it has to be embedded in a longer context – a phrase or some other structure – before it is able to convey emotion or information, i.e., meaning. This being said, it is clear that the analogy between speech and music rapidly breaks down when one starts comparing the two dynamic processes crucial for the human condition. What is common to both is the desire to express something in time, that this desire engenders a temporal program – cognitive with an emotional collateral (or emotional with a cognitive collateral) – and that this program will drive the talker or the performer to realizing an acoustic output created by muscular activity based on the program. However, the message in the outputs differs: speech does have a semantic component that music lacks. Conversely, the temporal flow of music, even in cases when its beats are uneven, rests on a slow (i.e., low-frequency) fluctuation to which the listener's temporal expectations are synchronized; while some temporal expectations are present in the person listening to speech, these expectations are much more lenient.

Perhaps because speech and music are more complementary than synonymous activities, their intersection – songs – have been with us probably from the earliest manifestations of both in the history of mankind. What is interesting in sung lyrics as well as in the human voice made into a musical instrument is, arguably, the necessity of each one accommodating the demands of the other. Both chapters in this section explore the intersection of speech dynamics and the singing voice. One chapter shows how dynamics can convey musical information in unexpected ways, while the other shows how speech dynamics and musical meter can compromise to reach a common goal.

Hiroshi Riquimaroux's chapter examines how changes in the amplitude envelope of a human voice might be enough to carry intonation when pitch and spectral detail are removed from the sung examples. His previous research [2][3] has suggested that intonation might still be conveyed in a signal, despite deliberate removal of information regarding the fundamental frequency. Although this information seems essential, the amplitude envelope alone may be enough for listeners to extract the intonation of a speaker's voice. Taking this finding further, experimental results in the chapter appear to show that subjects are remarkably capable of identifying the tunes that are sung. How can this be so? Indeed, tempo-specific rhythmic patterning plays a powerful role in melody recognition – just consider how the opening rhythm alone of Beethoven's 5'th Symphony evokes its melodic pattern. Riquimaroux's amplitude envelopes and crude spectral contours generated by using a noise vocoder provide additional cues. On the one hand, his subjects appear to hear melodic pitches in the absence of fundamental frequencies, but only further experiments would tell the extent to which they could identify the tonalities (keys) of the tunes as well.

The chapter by Jaan Ross and Ilse Lehiste concerns sung Estonian folk songs. In the chapter, the emphasis is on the relationships among the durations of phonetic elements, consonants and vowels, in spoken and sung examples of the same texts. The authors compare spoken and sung data from the same performer making the study of special interest. The structure of the ratios of the phonetic element durations differ in the spoken and sung versions. On the whole, temporal ratio invariance was not observed. As the authors point out, the metrical structure of the music and its alignment or misalignment with duration relationships required for lexical and/or grammatical differences play a role in the transforming the quantities in the sung versions of the texts. There remains an interesting question for further research: Is the lack of duration ratio invariance between spoken and sung text due to just the addition of musical constraints or does tempo also play a role? For the most part, song is slower than speech. Vowels are elongated and the temporal proportions change. In general, temporal proportions do not scale with tempo. One very telling example is the ratio of successive long and short durations in jazz swing. This long/short ratio is typically large at slow tempi, e.g. 0.75, and much closer to 0.5 at very rapid tempi [4]. It would indeed be interesting to know how the temporal quantity oppositions behave in Estonian when it is spoken at either a rapid or slow rate.

Thus, the chapter presents an intricate interplay of metrical structure in the songs with the prosody of the Estonian language. Estonian is a language which uses phoneme duration to differentiate between lexical and grammatical structures. However, putting words to music requires that durations, especially those of vowels, be adjusted to some extent to fit the rhythm. Obviously, linguistic information carried by prosody must compete with strict metrical structures of folksongs when the speech takes on the role of lyrics. The chapter shows how, rather than either prosody or rhythm winning out completely, the songs present us with an intricate compromise between music and meaning.

References

[1] Meyer, L.B. Emotion and Meaning in Music, Chicago: Univ. Chicago Press, 1956.
[2] Obata, Y. and Riquimaroux, H. "Speech perception based on temporal amplitude change with spectrally degraded synthetic sound." Trans. Tech. Comm. Psychol. Physiol. Acoust. Soc. Jpn. H-99-6, 1999.
[3] Obata, Y. and Riquimaroux, H. "Intelligibility of synthesized Japanese speech sound made of band noise - preliminary study for a speech recognition processor utilizing central auditory function." Trans. Tech. Comm. Psychol. Physiol. Acoust. Soc. Jpn. J-2000-3, 2000.
[4] Friberg, A and Sundstrom, A. "Swing ratios and ensemble timing in jazz performance: Evidence for a common rhythmic pattern." Music Perception 19: 333-349, 2002.

Dynamics of Speech Production and Perception
P. Divenyi et al. (Eds.)
IOS Press, 2006

309

The Extent to Which Changes in Amplitude Envelope Can Carry Information for Perception of Vocal Sound Without the Fundamental Frequency or Formant Peaks

Hiroshi RIQUIMAROUX
Department of Knowledge Engineering and Computer Sciences
Doshisha University
Kyotanabe, Kyoto, Japan

Abstract. Perception of Japanese songs with lyrics consisting of noise-vocoded speech sounds are described here. After training, normal-hearing subjects were able to recognize Japanese sentences (12-16 morae) composed of four-band noise-vocoded speech sounds. These sentences contained no information about the fundamental frequency or formant peaks but only slow temporal changes in the amplitude envelope. Further, the subjects could also perceive melody of songs with lyrics, where the acoustic signals were replaced by four noise bands without the fundamental frequency present. The results indicate that internal pitch streams might be created by lyrics, which are extracted from the temporal amplitude envelopes of noise-vocoded speech sounds. The findings suggest that lyrics could create melodies in the central nervous system without fundamental frequency information. The results also indicate that some melodies could be created even from scats without lyrics.

Keywords. Vocoder, envelope modulation, pitch, Japanese

Introduction

It has been believed that frequency information is essential for speech perception, e.g., formants and the fundamental frequency. However, recent studies adopting processed speech made of noise bands have revealed that amplitude envelope information also plays an important role in speech perception [3][1]. Not only sentence recognition, but also intonation can be identified with the processed noise speech. Japanese sentences can be recognized by means of the processed noise speech without the fundamental frequency or precise formant information. Intonation can also be identified without the fundamental frequency. In Japanese a difference in intonation makes a total difference in the meaning of a word. So, these findings have suggested that the amplitude envelope carries important information for supra-segmental speech perception ([2], Figure 1).

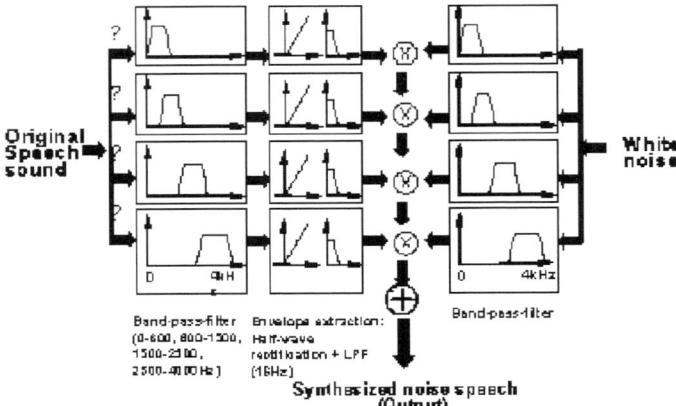

Band-pass-filter   Envelope extraction: Band-pass-filter
(0-600, 800-1500,   Half-wave
1500-2500,   rectification + LPF
2500-4000 Hz)   (16Hz)

**Synthesized noise speech
(Output)**

Figure 1. Four-band speech processor. This figure schematically shows how to produce synthesized 4-band noise speech.

Then, we plan to bring our previous findings to a new field, melody of song perception/ recognition. In other words, we examine if melodies of songs synthesized by the processed noise bands can be recognized.

Ordinarily, melody of a song is carried by a sequential change in the voice pitch, which would be decided by the fundamental frequency. Our synthesized songs have been composed of four noise bands, 0-600, 600-1500, 1500-2500 and 2500-4000 Hz. Therefore, being buried in a noise band, the fundamental frequency cannot be identified as a frequency but a noise band. Unless the fundamental frequency goes across the boarder of noise bands, no frequency would change. So, the pitch would not change if the change in the fundamental frequency stays within the same band. In these situations, melody is difficult to recognize or identify if it is decided only by the change in the fundamental frequency. Here, we selected parts of songs with the same rhythm pattern in order to test if processed noise bands could convey sequential change in the pitch of a song, i.e. the melody. We compared regular songs with lyrics to those without lyrics, i.e., scats.

1. Experiment 1: Songs With Lyrics

1.1 Methods

1.1.1 Original songs

"Sakura" (Cherry blossoms), *"Tulips"*, *"Chouchou"* (Butterflies), and *"Akatombo"* (Red dragonflies) were used as original songs. Melodies of these four songs are well known. *"Sakura"*, *"Tulips"* and *"Chouchou"* are made of an identical rhythm pattern and a similar melodic contour, while *"Akatombo"* contains a totally different rhythm pattern and melodic contour. *"Chouchou"* is not the one that is best known. The lyrics of the first half are identical to the best known, "Chouchou Chouchou". However, the lyrics of the second half are different. The lyrics used in the present experiment are less well known than the other one. Two male (M1 and M2) and two female singers (F1 and F2)

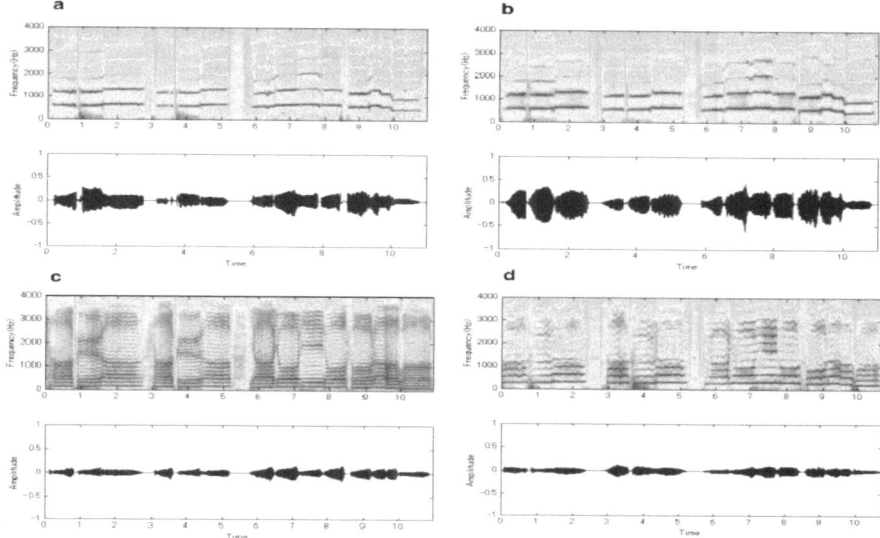

Figure 2. Sound spectrograms and temporal amplitude patterns of "Sakura" sung by four different singers (a, b: females, c, d: males). Upper panels: sound spectrograms, Lower panels: temporal amplitude patterns.

sang these four songs to the pre-recorded accompaniment of piano through headphones (Figure 2). These songs were digitally recorded with sampling rate of 8 kHz and 16-bit resolution. To increase similarity in rhythm patterns of the former three songs, tempo of accompaniment was synchronized.

1.1.2 Synthesizing processed noise speech

In the present study four-band processed speech sound was synthesized for stimuli which were previously reported ([2], Figure 1). The original speech sounds were divided into four bands (0-600, 600-1500, 1500-2500 and 2500-4000 Hz) by passing it through four band-pass filters (IIR infinite impulse response). Then, the amplitude envelope was extracted from each band by half-wave rectification and low-pass filtering (< 16 Hz, [3]). Each amplitude envelope was multiplied with the noise with the same bandwidth. Passing white noise through the same four band-pass filters explained above made the bands of noise. Normally distributed random numbers generated the white noise. Then, output waveforms from each band were added to create a degraded noise speech ([2], Figure 1).

1.1.3 Subjects

Five subjects with normal hearing (hearing loss less than 15 dB) were employed after pure tone screening test. They were native Japanese males aging between 22 and 23 years old. They were trained to listen to 20 Japanese sentences, each of which was made of 12 to 16 morae. The training could improve their ability to recognize sentences with processed noise bands dramatically. We started the experiment after confirming that their

Song title and singer	Subj. 1	Subj. 2	Subj. 3	Subj. 4	Subj. 5
Chouchou F1	x	x	x	x	x
Chouchou F2	x	x	x	x	x
Chouchou M1	o	o	x	x	x
Chouchou M2	o	x	x	x	x
Tulips F1	o	o	o	o	o
Tulips F2	o	o	o	o	o
Tulips M1	o	o	o	o	o
Tulips M2	o	o	o	o	o
Sakura F1	o	o	o	o	o
Sakura F2	o	o	o	o	o
Sakura M1	o	o	o	o	o
Sakura M2	o	o	o	o	o
Akatombo F1	o	o	o	o	o
Akatombo F2	o	o	o	o	o
Akatombo M1	o	o	o	o	o
Akatombo M2	o	o	o	o	o

Table 1. Identification of melodies of degraded songs made of 4-band noise. O: Subject could identify the melody. x: Subject could not identify the melody. F: female singer. M: male singer. Chouchou: Butterflies in Japanese. Sakura: Cherry blossoms in Japanese. Akatombo: Red dragonflies.

acuity was more than 80% even when they listened to a novel sentence [1].

1.1.4 Procedure

Experiments were carried out in a sound attenuated chamber. A computer itself was put outside the chamber to prevent noise, while its monitor was put within the chamber. Subjects listened to melodies through a pair of headphones (STAX Lambda Signature) following the instruction on the monitor. They were asked to identify the songs that they heard. Answers were written down on paper. No information about the songs was given to the subjects. The correct answers were not given to them even after the experiments. Each subject judged sixteen songs, four singers times four songs. Sixteen songs were divided into two sessions. A ten-minute rest was provided between the two sessions. Songs were presented with random order. Same songs were not consecutively presented. Duration of each part was kept almost identical in order to prevent subjects from utilizing duration to identify the melodies.

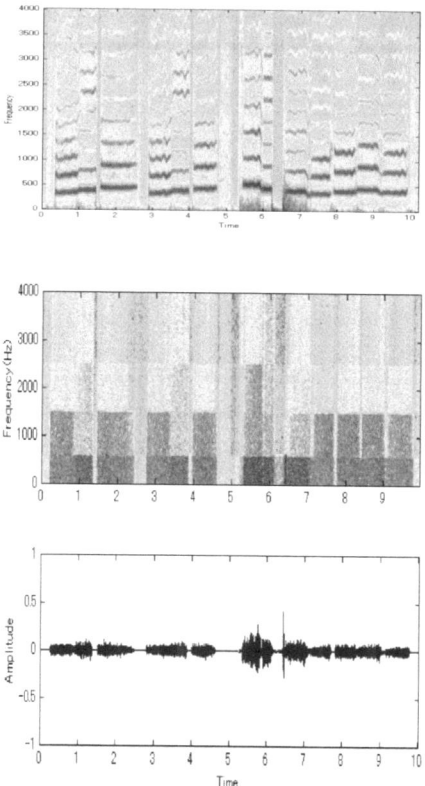

Figure 3. Sound spectrograms of song of "Tulips" before and after passing through 4-band noise speech processor. Top: original sound. Middle: song replaced by 4-band noise. Bottom: temporal amplitude change in the processed song.

1.2 Results

Results are shown in Table 1. Circles (o) indicate correct answers, while crosses (x) represent wrong or no answers. Singers are identified as F1, F2, M1 and M2. Correct answers were 71 out of 80 trials (4 songs x 4 singers x 5 subjects). *"Akatombo"*, *"Sakura"* and *"Tulips"* got a perfect score (20/20). On the contrary, correct answers were only 3 out of 20 for *"Chouchou"*.

1.3 Discussion

Percent correct in total was 88.8% (71/80). Taking look at individual songs *"Akatombo"*, *"Sakura"* and *"Tulips"* got a perfect score, 100% correct (20/20). On the contrary, only 15% (3/20) was correct for *"Chouchou"*. The present results indicate a melody could be recognized only by the amplitude envelope information without the fundamental frequency if both the melody and the lyric are known. The lyric of the second half of *"Chouchou"* is not well known. This might be the reason that its melody

Song title and singer	Subj. 1	Subj. 2	Subj. 3	Subj. 4	Subj. 5
Chouchou F1	x	Δ	x	x	x
Chouchou F2	Δ	Δ	x	Δ	Δ
Tulips F1	Δ	Δ	x	x	x
Tulips F2	x	o	x	x	x
Sakura F1	o	o	o	x	o
Sakura F2	o	x	o	o	x
Akatombo F1	o	o	o	o	o
Akatombo F2	o	o	o	o	o

Table 2. Identification of melodies of degraded scat songs. O: Correct. Δ : Confused with other song. x: Could not answer at all. See caption for Table 1.

was not correctly recognized.

In the present experiment, the fundamental frequency of female voices crossed the boundary between the first and the second noise bands when they sang *"Sakura"*. However, the fundamental frequencies of male voices stayed within the first noise band all the time. Nevertheless, subjects correctly identified the melody of *"Sakura"* despite the fact that for some singers the fundamental frequency moved between the first and the second bands but for other singers it did not. We might translate that subjects judged the melody by utilizing amplitude envelope information even when an uncertainty in frequency information existed.

Subjects could correctly judge melodies although *"Sakura"* and *"Tulips"* are made of the same rhythmic pattern and have a similar melodic contour. This finding suggests that subjects listened to the songs and identified the melody by transferring amplitude envelope information into pitch information.

2. Experiment 2: Songs with Scat

Findings of Experiment 1 revealed that, when the lyrics were known, melodies could be identified even when the songs were composed of processed noise bands. So, we decided to examine effects of phonemic information on melody perception. Here, we used songs identical to those in Experiment 1 but we replaced the lyrics by scat.

2.1 Methods

We used the same songs, *"Akatombo"*, *"Sakura"*, *"Tulips"*, and *"Chouchou"*, which were employed in Experiment 1. Two female singers (F1 and F2) who participated in Experiment 1 sang these songs with the scat "rarara". These original songs were processed in the same way as in Experiment 1 (Figures 1 and 4). Five subjects who partici-

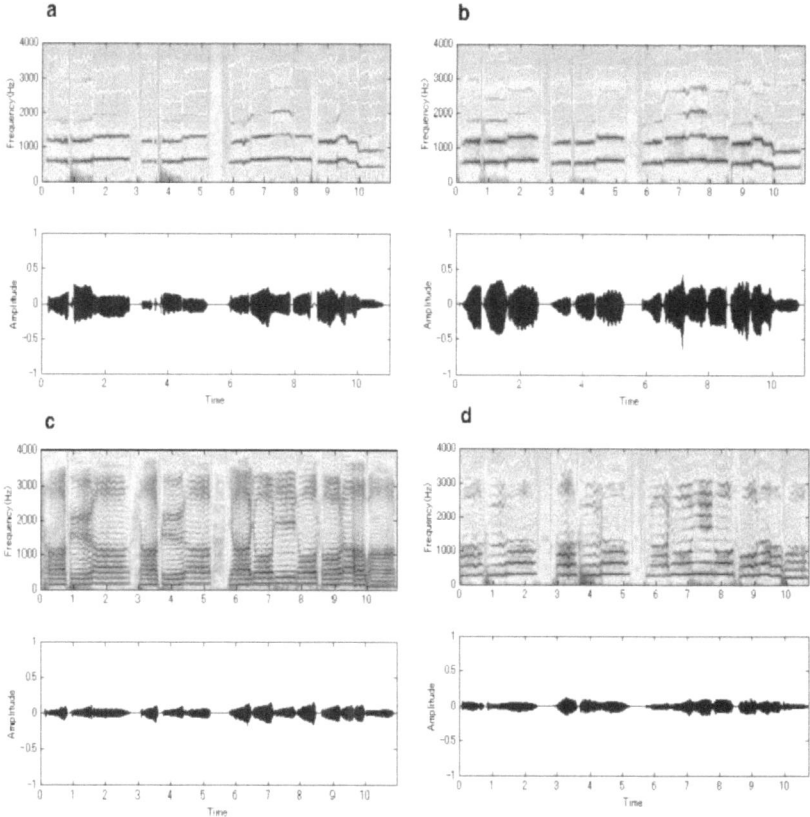

Figure 4. Sound spectrograms and temporal amplitude patterns of scat song "Tulips" before and after passing
through 4-band noise speech processor. Upper two panels: original scat song. Lower two panels:
song replaced by 4-band noise. Compare to Figure 3.

pated in Experiment 1 also joined Experiment 2. The experimental procedure used was
also the same as the one used in Experiment 1.

2.2 Results

Results are summarized in Table 2. Circles (o) indicate correct answers, triangles (Δ)
represent incorrect answers, and crosses (x) show no answers. Singers are identified as
F1 and F2. In total, there were 18 correct answers out of 40 trials (8 songs times 5 subjects). In other words, the percent correct was 45%. For the song *"Akatombo"*, the correct ratio was 10 our of 10, or 100%, for*"Sakura"*, it was 7 out of 10, or 70%, but for
"Chouchou" it was 0 out of 10, i.e., 0%.

Song title and singer	Subj. 1	Subj. 2	Subj. 3	Subj. 4	Subj. 5
Chouchou F1	x	Kagome	x	x	x
Chouchou F2	Sakura	Kagome	x	Kagome	Sakura
Tulips F1	Sakura	Chouchou	x	x	x
Tulips F2	x	o	x	x	x
Sakura F1	o	o	o	x	o
Sakura F2	o	x	o	o	x
Akatombo F1	o	o	o	o	o
Akatombo F2	o	o	o	o	o

Table 3. Confusion matrix for degraded scat songs. Triangular symbols in Table 2 are replaced by confused song titles. For details see caption of Table 1.

2.3 Discussion

"*Akatombo*" was correctly identified 100%. However, the recognition of other songs were worse than that found in Experiment 1, showing difficulty in recognizing melodies carried by scat without fundamental frequency or phonemic information. In order to discuss the reason for incorrect answers, the confusion matrix is shown in Table 3.

"*Chouchou*" was often confused with "*Sakura*" and "*Kagome*". "*Tulips*" was also confused with "*Sakura*" and "*Chouchou*". The common factors for these confusions appear to be the rhythm pattern. All of these songs possess similar rhythm patterns. Identification of melodies of songs without the fundamental frequencies appears to be difficult when the rhythmic patterns are identical and melodic contours are similar. However, one has to note that "*Akatombo*" was correctly identified 100% of the time. So, even scat melody made of degraded noise bands can be identified when the rhythmic pattern is unique. It is likely that we utilize amplitude envelope, which is translated into pitch by the central auditory system.

Therefore, hearing-impaired people might perceive melodies by pathways, which are not normally used, activated by training by means of processed speech with noise bands. This is how we utilize plasticity of the brain for melody perception.

Amplitude envelope of the scat, Ra-Ra-Ra, looks less clear than that of the ordinary lyric singing. Absence the fundamental frequency and lacking clear change in amplitude envelope would make perception of melody carried by degraded noise band scat very difficult.

3. Conclusion

After listening to about twenty Japanese sentences (12-16 morae each) composed of speech processed by four noise-bands, subjects with normal hearing were able to recognize these sentences. They could also perceive the melody of songs with lyrics, where the acoustic signal was replaced by four noise bands. Furthermore, these subjects could identify a melody of songs without lyric (scat) processed in the same way. The results indicate that subjects can perceive melodies by extracting pitch from amplitude envelope information when fundamental frequency information is not available. The findings suggest that lyrics alone may create melodies in the central nervous system without any fundamental frequency information present.

Acknowledgements

The author wishes to express his great appreciation to those students who cooperated in the experiments. The present research was partially supported by a Grant-in-Aid for Scientific Research in Priority Area (B) "Prosody and Speech Processing", Special Research Grants for the Development of Characteristic Education from the Promotion and Mutual Aid Corporation for Private Schools in Japan, and a grant to RCAST at Doshisha University from the Ministry of Education, Culture, Sports, Science and Technology of Japan.

References

[1] Obata, Y. and Riquimaroux, H. "Speech perception based on temporal amplitude change with spectrally degraded synthetic sound." *Trans. Tech. Comm. Psychol. Physiol. Acoust. Soc. Acoust. Soc. Jpn.* H-99-6, 1999.
[2] Obata, Y. and Riquimaroux, H. "Intelligibility of synthesized Japanese speech sound made of band noise – preliminary study for a speech recognition processor utilizing central auditory function." *Trans. Tech. Comm. Psychol. Physiol. Acoust. Soc. Acoust. Soc. Jpn.* H-2000-3, 2000.
[3] Shannon, R.V., Zeng, F.G., Kamath, V., Wygonski and Ekelid, M. "Speech recognition with primarily temporal cues." *Science* 270: 303-305, 1995.

Dynamics of Speech Production and Perception
P. Divenyi et al. (Eds.)
IOS Press, 2006

Quantity Oppositions in Spoken Estonian and Their Transformation in Folksongs

Jaan ROSS[1] and Ilse LEHISTE[2]

[1]*Department of Arts, University of Tartu, Estonia*
[2]*Department of Linguistics, Ohio State University, Columbus, Ohio, USA*

Abstract. Estonian is a language in which duration is used contrastively within the prosodic system to signal lexical and/or grammatical differences. The quantity system is ternary, distinguishing between short, long, and overlong degrees. It is also hierarchical, making use of contrastive durations at the level of segments, syllables, and prosodic feet. The metrical structure of old Estonian folksongs employs the so-called Kalevala line, a system likewise based on quantity, but using just two categories, short and long. The Kalevala line can be described as consisting of four trochaic (long-short) metric feet, or of eight syllables arranged in a sequence where odd-numbered positions are metrically strong (carry metrical stress or ictus) and even-numbered syllables are metrically weak (off-ictus). Words are stressed on the first syllable in Estonian, and long and overlong first syllables must occur in metrically strong positions (i.e. as first syllables of the trochaic feet). A conflict between the metre and word-level stress arises in the case of words with a short stressed initial syllable: the quantity rules require that such syllables be placed in off-ictus positions, even though they carry lexical stress. As a result, the metric foot in which the short-quantity word begins contains a word boundary. Such metric feet are referred to as 'broken feet', and the lines in which such feet occur are called 'broken lines'. The paper describes an acoustic analysis of broken lines found in sung old folksongs. While contrastive vowel durations are neutralized in singing, musical rhythm superimposed on the lines is manifested by slightly greater duration of notes representing odd-numbered positions in the line. However, broken lines deviate from this pattern in a way that represents a compromise between lexical stress and musical rhythm.

Keywords. Estonian, metrical structure, duration, word stress, folksongs

Introduction

The topic of our research is the relationship between use of duration in the prosodic structure of the language, the metrical structure of the folksongs, and the realization of the quantity patterns in singing. We use the methodology of acoustic phonetics, namely spectrographic analysis of recorded samples of speech and song. We restrict the analysis to samples from a specific historical singing tradition characteristic of the majority of the so-called Baltic-Finnic cultures, including Estonian and Finnish. Peoples representing these cultures inhabit the eastern shores of the Baltic Sea in the north-eastern part of

Europe. Their singing tradition is usually referred to as the Kalevala or runic singing tradition; sometimes these songs are also referred to as old folksongs, to distinguish them from newer folksongs that exhibit a different structure. A comprehensive ethnomusicological overview of the tradition is provided by Rüütel [8].

From a typological perspective, Estonian and Finnish (as well as other Baltic-Finnic minority languages) are remarkable due to their unusually complex prosodic systems [1]. Both languages make lexical as well as grammatical use of contrastive duration – the feature of quantity. In Finnish, vowels can be contrastively short or long in any syllable, and consonants can be contrastively short or long (i.e. single versus geminate) anywhere except in word-initial and word-final position. The Estonian quantity system is even more complicated. In the first place, the system is hierarchical: duration is contrastive at the level of segments, syllables, and higher-level units, displaying a hierarchy of many-to-one mappings (different segmental combinations mapping into a smaller number of contrastive syllable durations, and contrastive syllable combinations mapping into higher-level units like prosodic feet). The second peculiarity of the Estonian system is the fact that it is ternary: there are three-way oppositions at every level – segments, syllables, and metric feet. The distinctive quantities are called short, long, and overlong, and are conventionally referred to as Q1, Q2, and Q3. Vowel duration is contrastive in the first syllable of a word. Consonants can be in the contrastive three quantities within a prosodic foot, and in a two-way opposition between prosodic feet and in final position; there is no durational contrast in consonants in word-initial position.

It is evident that in singing, the durational or quantity constraints inherent in the language have to compete with constraints from other domains than speech. These additional temporal constraints are, firstly, metrical, i.e. related to regular repetition of strong and weak timing units, and, secondly, rhythmical, i.e. related to more fine-grained and individual timing patterns characteristic to music (of which singing is a part). In principle it is possible to unite metrical and rhythmical features of music and to view them as two sides of a single coin (and thus be able to speak about metro-rhythmical properties of music). In the present study, however, we prefer to consider the metre and the rhythm as separate entities, for reasons which, as we hope, will become evident in due course. Thus the topic of our study is the temporal structure of Estonian folksongs looked at from three aspects: the prosodic structure of the language, the metric structure of the verse, and the rhythmic and melodic structure of the songs. In particular, we are investigating the ways in which these three aspects interact: the way in which the language is adapted to the requirements of the metre (and, conversely, the way in which the metre reflects the prosodic structure of the language), and the way in which the metre interacts with the musical structure of the folksongs.

Next we will very briefly outline the way the three above components – speech prosody, metre, and musical rhythm – are expected to operate by themselves. As to Estonian prosody, it has been a matter of debate at which level (phoneme, syllable, or prosodic foot or disyllabic sequence) the ternary quantity oppositions primarily operate. According to Lehiste [3], the optimal level for the description of quantity oppositions is the prosodic foot. Among other characteristics, the foot as an entity has a tendency toward isochrony, which is achieved through complementarity in the duration of the two syllables of which it consists: short, long, and overlong first syllables are followed by successively shorter second syllables. The three contrastive quantity degrees are characterized by specific ratios between the two syllables (the S1/S2 ratio). For words in the short quantity (Q1), this ratio is approximately 2/3, for words in the long quantity (Q2), it is 3/2, and for words in the overlong quantity (Q3), the S1/S2 ratio is approximately 2/1. When the consonants are in short quantity, the S1/S2 ratio can be represented by the ratio between the vowels (the V1/V2 ratio). Note that in words of Q1, i.e. words with a short initial syllable, the unstressed second syllable is phonetically longer than the stressed first syllable. Unstressed second syllables can be open or closed; closed second syllables are considered to be long.

A comprehensive survey of metre in the Kalevala song repertoire has been presented by Leino [4]. The basic structural unit in the Kalevala songs is the line; no regular higher-order structures (e.g. stanzas) normally emerge. There are two complementary ways to define the structure of the line. Traditionally the line is described as a trochaic tetrametre: all lines consist of four feet, and each foot consists of two positions, of which the first is long and carries metrical stress (ictus), while the second is short and lacks metrical stress (non-ictus). The use of the term 'trochaic' is somewhat ambiguous, since in contemporary usage the term is also used to refer to a metric foot whose first syllable is stressed and second syllable is unstressed. According to this description, the folksong lines would be trochaic regardless of whether quantity rules are followed or not. The other way to define the line is to describe it as a sequence of eight positions, of which the odd-numbered positions are strong (and carry metrical stress) and the even-numbered positions are weak. The metrically strong positions correspond to the first syllables of trochaic feet. As such they are expected to be long, and to carry metrical stress.

Normally a position is filled with a single syllable (and a single tone in the melody), but, due to different reasons, numerous exceptions may apply. According to Lippus [5], about 70 percent of the Estonian folksong repertoire consists of regular trochaic tetrametric lines.

The metrical structure of the folksongs places certain constraints on the way in which lexical items can be used to fill the eight positions in the line. The so-called quantity rules regulate the placement of stressed word-initial syllables into the line: the first syllables of words in long and overlong quantity *must* be placed in metrically strong positions, and the first syllables of words in short quantity *must be excluded* from metrically strong positions. Unstressed syllables are not subject to quantity rules; thus in the case of a trisyllabic Q2 or Q3 word, its unstressed third syllable may occupy a metrically strong position, regardless of whether it is short (open) or long (closed). The application of the quantity rules is not always very rigid; our own data, for example, show that they are followed more consistently with regard to trisyllabic Q1 words than Q2 and Q3 words, or with regard to disyllabic and quadrisyllabic words [7]. Since the ictus position in the Kalevala songs is contrasted to off-ictus positions both on the basis of stress and duration, it is reasonable to expect that syllables filling metrically strong positions are, on the average, acoustically longer than those filling metrically weak positions. This expectation has indeed been confirmed [6].

There is relatively little rhythmic variation to be found in the old Estonian folksongs. A trochaic tetrametric line is usually coupled with an isochronous string of tones of more or less equal duration, a syllable in the text corresponding to a tone in the melody (which brings about a neutralization of durational oppositions in vowels). An early notation [2] of an old Estonian folksong line is given in Figure 1. The first two bars correspond to the eight-syllable verse line; the following four bars represent the refrain. In

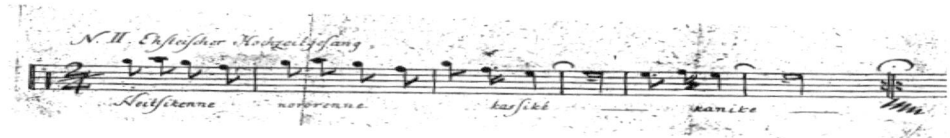

Figure 1. An early notation of a wedding song by Hupel [2]. The notation consists of an isochronic eight-tone melody, followed by a refrain of meaningless fillerwords *kasike, kanike.*[1]

traditional singing, the rhythm and melody remain the same for the whole duration of the song, creating a rather monotonous effect. In general, there is no fixed association between texts and melodies; the texts and melodies are combined freely with each other in actual performance. One might assume that it is the monotonous regularity of the melody that makes such a relationship possible.

1. Broken Lines

The term 'broken line' is applied to lines in which short stressed word-initial syllables occur in off-ictus position. All words are stressed on the initial syllable; according to the quantity rules, long and overlong initial syllables occur in positions where word stress and metrical stress coincide, but short initial syllables occur in positions where word stress is in conflict with metrical stress. One can only speculate about how and why the quantity rules came into being; in the recorded folksong corpus, they are used for stylistic purposes to considerable effect. Frequently one finds a series of parallel lines (a stylistic device of the folksongs) with regular trochaic rhythm, wrapped up with a broken final line.

The question we are concerned with in this paper is the way in which the basic conflict between word stress and metrical stress is solved in sung and spoken versions of Estonian folksongs. Duration is involved in this in more ways than one.

In traditional descriptions of the metre of the folksongs, the duration of unstressed syllables is frequently overlooked. The reason for this is probably the fact that in establishing word-level quantity, the duration of the stressed first syllable determines the duration of the following unstressed syllable. But the second syllable can be phonetically fairly long for two reasons: it can contain a half-long vowel (if the word is in Q1), or the second syllable can be long by virtue of being closed by a final consonant. An example of a broken line illustrates the situation.

Table 1 presents the schematic structure of a broken line, *karguti kanad kesalta* ('made the hens run from the fallow field'). Its eight positions are filled with three words, two of them trisyllabic (*karguti* and *kesalta*), one disyllabic (*kanad*). The words *kanad* and *kesalta* are in the short quantity. In a spoken version of this line, stress would fall on the first syllable of each word, which would correspond to positions 1, 4, and 6. Positions 4 and 6 are metrically weak, but they contain the stressed short initial syllables of the two short-quantity words. The metrically strong position 5 is filled with the second syllable of *kanad*, which contains a half-long vowel; the metrically strong position 7 is filled with a closed syllable, which counts as long.

	kar-	gu(t)-	ti	ka-	nad	ke-	sal(t)-	ta
Position number	1	2	3	4	5	6	7	8
Metrical strength	+		+		+		+	
Word stress	+			+		+		
Syllable length	+	+			+		+	

Table 1. Schematic structure of a broken folksong line, *karguti kanad kesalta.* The rows represent the eight positions of the line and indicate the metrically strong positions, the syllables carrying word stress, and the phonetic length of the syllables.

The broken foot consisting of positions 3 and 4 is filled with the short third syllable of *karguti*, followed by the stressed short initial syllable of *kanad*. The second broken foot in the line, consisting of positions 5 and 6, is filled with the second syllable of *kanad* and the stressed initial syllable of *kesalta*. But *–nad* is phonetically long, both by virtue of containing the half-long vowel that occurs in the second syllable of short-quantity words, and by virtue of being closed. The same applies to the second syllable of *kesalta.* Thus the only metric foot that does not in fact consist of a long syllable followed by a short syllable is the second foot.

2.   Materials and Method

The material analyzed in the present study consists of recordings of singing and speech (including recitation) by a single performer, K.K., from southern Estonia (Karksi). The materials were recorded on tape in the years 1960-61 and 1971-73 under fieldwork conditions. Currently the recordings are kept in the Estonian Folklore Archives in Tartu, Estonia. The materials sung by K.K. consist of four separate songs, one of them performed twice. The total number of recorded verse lines in these songs amounts to 160. Details concerning the four songs, including their archival references, melody notations, original texts and their English translations can be found in [7] (pp. 151-160, i.e. items 8 to 11 in the Appendix). More than a hundred of the total of about 160 verse lines come from a single longer song (item 10); the other three (items 8, 9, and 11) are much shorter.

The recorded interviews during which the three shorter songs were taped also contain recited verse lines and free conversation. The recited lines are mostly repetitions of the sung lines; thus we have parallel sung and spoken realizations of these three songs.

The acoustic analysis of the recordings was carried out by the second author at the Linguistics Laboratory of the Ohio State University, using a Kay Elemetrics Computerized Speech Laboratory (model 4300). Durations of all segmental sounds were measured from broad-band spectrograms, using established measurement procedures.

3.   Results

3.1 The longer song

The song consists of more than 100 lines, of which 28 are broken. This equals nearly 25 per cent, which is more than the average of 18 per cent typical for the singer's region

	N	V1		V2	
		Duration (msec)	**St. Deviation**	**Duration (msec)**	**St. Deviation**
Broken feet	21	296	41.0	311	52.6
Trochaic feet	10	338	37.2	303	36.1

Table 2. Average durations of V1 and V2 in broken and trochaic CVCV feet in the longer song by K.K. Broken feet contain a word boundary between V1 and V2. The duration difference between the vowels occurring in broken and trochaic feet is statistically significant for V1 but not for V2.

[9]. In these broken lines, there were 21 occurrences of metric feet consisting of two short syllables and containing a word boundary: the first syllable was an unstressed short syllable, and the second syllable constituted the initial, stressed syllable of a Q1 word.

These metric feet represent the classic manifestation of the conflict between word stress and metrical structure – the short, stressed word-initial syllable occurring in a metrically unstressed position. We will refer to such metric feet as 'broken feet'. The song also contained ten instances in which words with the same CVCV structure constituted metric feet, word stress and verse ictus both occurring on the first syllable. Since the first syllable was short, these words actually represent a violation of the classical metric structure of a folksong line.

Table 2 presents average durations of V1 and V2 in broken and trochaic CVCV feet in the longer song by K.K. Initial and final metric feet were excluded from the calculations because of possible boundary effects. The contrastive sounds in CVCV words are vowels, and thus the durations of the two vowels can be used to represent the prosodic shape of the word. Analysis of variance showed that the duration of the first vowel (V1) is significantly different depending on whether or not the foot contains a word boundary (p=.012). For the second vowel (V2), however, the difference between the two conditions was not statistically significant.

As we have reported earlier [7], the quantity oppositions in vowels are neutralized in the sung versions of folksongs. The rhythmic structure of the songs is manifested by slightly longer durations of the first notes of the two-note sequences that correspond to metric feet. Given the neutralization of oppositions, the somewhat greater duration of the first syllable (tone) reflects metrical and musical stress. The broken feet differ from this general pattern by having a shorter first vowel and a longer second vowel. What this means is that metrical and musical stress are not signaled by longer duration, as is the case with regular trochaic metric feet.

The trochaic metric feet with which the broken feet are compared in Table II actually constitute instances of violation of the quantity rules, since these metric feet consist of CVCV words with a short stressed initial syllable falling in a metrically strong position. If these words were produced in speech, they would have a half-long vowel in the second syllable, with a ratio between syllables of approximately 2/3. In the performance of this song by K.K., the first syllable is in fact 35 msec longer than the second syllable, and the S1/S2 ratio in these words is 1.12. In one of our earlier studies [6] we found that in productions by another singer, the ratio between the two syllables of metric feet in trochaic lines was 1.18, which is rather close to the value obtained in the present study for metric feet with a CVCV structure.

A comparison of vowel durations in Table II yields some insights regarding the role

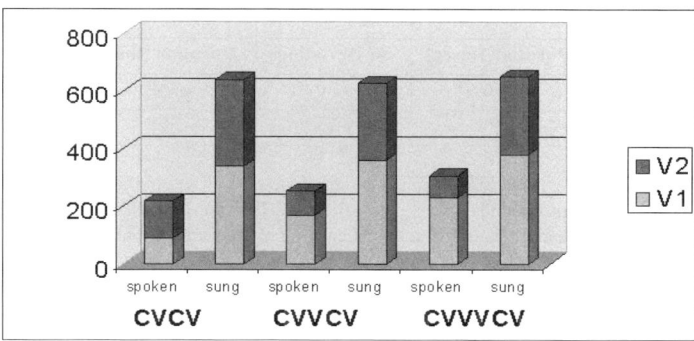

Figure 2. Comparison of average V1 and V2 durations (msec) in spoken and sung performances. The spoken words were extracted from narrative portions interspersed between recordings of the songs. The values for the sung version of the word in short quantity are repeated from Table 2; the other values were calculated from measurements made of these types of words in the full version of the longer song. CVCV = short quantity (Q1), CVVCV = long quantity (Q2), CVVVCV = overlong quantity (Q3).

of metrical and word-level stress. The difference between V1 durations in trochaic versus broken feet is 42 msec. This statistically significant difference could be attributed to the presence versus absence of word-level stress on the first vowel, since in both cases, the first syllable carries metrical and musical stress. The duration of V2 is longer by 8 msec in broken feet compared to trochaic feet. This might be attributed to the presence of word-level stress on the second syllable of broken feet, but this difference is statistically not significant, and probably below the perceptual threshold.

It might be appropriate to say at this point that the singer does indeed use the regular three-way prosodic oppositions when she speaks the language. The average durations of vowels in three word types are given in Figure 2 for both speech and singing. The spoken words were extracted from narrative portions interspersed between recordings of the songs by K.K. The three word types are symbolized as CVCV (Q1), CVVCV (Q2), and CVVVCV (Q3). The values for the sung version of the word in short quantity are repeated from Table I; the other values were calculated from measurements made of these types of words in the full version of the longer song.

Figure 2 shows that the singer uses the standard three-way quantity patterns in her speech; the CVCV word has a half-long second syllable, and the duration of V1 increases while the duration of V2 decreases with successively higher quantity degrees. Figure 2 shows also that this singer, too, neutralized vowel durations in singing (like the singers whose productions we have analyzed earlier). And Figure 2 illustrates also the considerable difference in tempo between speech and song.

3.2 Shorter songs

The recordings of shorter songs provide an opportunity for direct comparison of spoken and sung texts. The shorter songs contained a larger number of violations of the quantity rules – words with a stressed short initial syllable occurring as regular metric feet, with metrical and musical stress on the short first syllable. Figure 3 shows the average durations of vowels in CVCV words, occurring in spoken and sung versions of the three

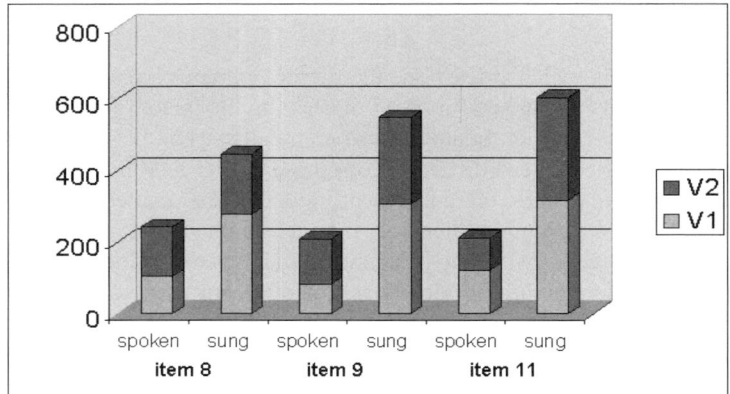

Figure 3. Average V1 and V2 durations (msec) of Q1 words in recited and sung versions of the three shorter
songs ([7], items 8, 9, and 11).

short songs. In these short-quantity words, too, the spoken versions correspond basically
to the standard prosodic model. The first syllable is shorter, the second syllable contains
the half-long vowel, and the ratio between the durations of the syllables is 0.86 (the generalized 2/3 ratio would correspond to 0.67). The sung versions resemble the patterns
observed in the longer song, with a longer first syllable; the ratio between the vowel
durations is 1.30 (in the longer song this ratio was equal to 1.12).

In some instances, it was possible to compare identical words in the recited and
sung versions. Three examples of Q1 words are given on Figure 4. These examples were
taken from one of the shorter songs (item 9 in [7]). All words occurred as regular metric
feet, that is, they carried word-level, metrical and musical stress on the first syllable.
Here the half-long vowel of the second syllable is particularly clearly manifested in the
spoken versions; the average ratio is 0.65, almost exactly corresponding to the 2/3 ratio
for words in short quantity. The sung versions were produced with differences in tempo,
but the neutralization of the durational differences is clear in all instances; the overall
vowel duration ratio for the sung version was 1.47.

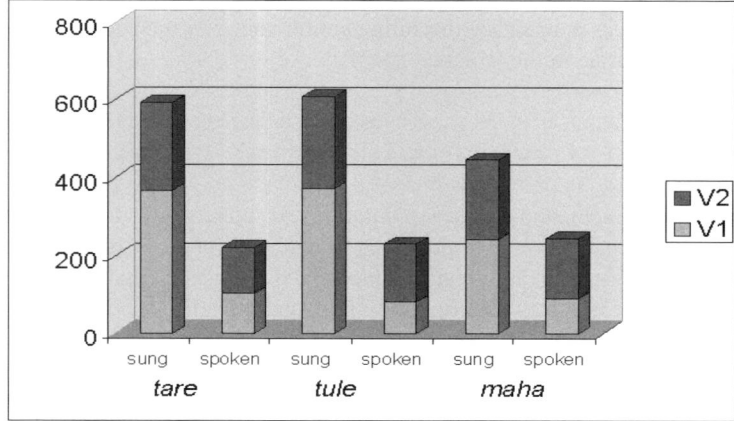

Figure 4. Average V1 and V2 durations (msec) for the three Q1 words *tare, tule*, and *maha* occurring in
recited and sung versions of one of the three shorter songs ([7], item 9).

4. Discussion

Broken lines are lines in which at least one metric foot contains a word boundary. Such metric feet – 'broken feet' – arise as a result of obeying the quantity rules that exclude initial syllables of words in short quantity from metrically strong positions. Our studies show that broken feet are indeed different from those metric feet that do not contain a word boundary. In regular lines, there is a clearly documented tendency to produce the initial syllable of a foot with greater length. Although in musical transcription notes of equal duration are traditionally used to designate both notes of the foot, the extra length of the first syllable/note may be confidently assumed to contribute to the establishment and perception of musical rhythm.

But in broken metric feet, the second syllable has equal or even greater duration than the first, even though the first syllable carries musical and metrical stress. And since the singer knows the language, she knows also that these second syllables are first syllables of words. All other words that occur in the line are assigned positions where their stressed first syllables also carry musical and metrical stress.

One possible reason for lengthening the first syllable of CVCV words is analogy – generalization from the long and overlong words to the short-quantity words. This would explain the process from internal reasons, without external influence. It would also imply that for some reason, words have become more important than metric feet – word structure dominates metrical structure.

Another possible reason – even more speculative than the first one – is connected with the fact that the recordings were made close to the end of continuous transmission of traditional folksong performance. There is no doubt that the singers must have been exposed to and familiar with singing styles where word stress and musical beat were regularly associated. Here the source of influence would be stress-timing in songs available as models in the cultural environment.

However, there was no stress-timing in the narrative portions of the recordings – the speakers continued to use the traditional quantity patterns in their speech. And in instances where the broken lines were produced as sequences containing trisyllabic feet with stressed first syllables, there was no compression of unstressed syllables to equalize the durations of trisyllabic and disyllabic feet. Whatever the reasons, the ultimate outcome of the process is bringing the sung version closer to the spoken version, without initiating any change in the language itself.

5. Conclusions

A comparative acoustical study of vowel durations in spoken and sung versions of folksongs by the same performer demonstrates that (1) differences between contrastive duration patterns of Estonian are greatly reduced in singing as compared to speech; (2) a more detailed study of vowel durations in short-quantity (Q1) CVCV words showed consistency in the production of durational patterns by the same performer for different song productions and for different words within the same production; (3) CVCV-type metric feet demonstrate different patterns of vowel duration, depending on whether the two syllables belong to the same word or are separated by a word boundary.

Acknowledgment

Parts of this chapter have been presented during METHODS XI: Eleventh International Conference on Methods in Dialectology, 5-9 August 2002, University of Joensuu, Finland.

Endnote

1. According to contemporary Estonian ortography, the line should be spelled as *neitsikene, noorukene, kaasike, kaanike.*

References

[1] Engstrand, O. and Krull, D. "Durational correlates of quantity in Swedish, Finnish and Estonian: Cross-language evidence for a theory of adaptive dispersion." *J. Phonetics* 51: 80-91, 1994.

[2] Hupel, A.W. *Topographische Nachrichten von Lief- und Ehstland II*. Riga: Hartknoch, 1777.

[3] Lehiste, I. "Search for phonetic correlates in Estonian prosody." In *Estonian Prosody: Papers from a Symposium*, I. Lehiste and J. Ross (eds.), Tallinn: Institute of Estonian Language, pp. 11-35, 1997.

[4] Leino, P. *Language and Metre. Metrics and the Metrical System of Finnish*. Helsinki: Suomalaisen Kirjallisuuden Seura, 1986.

[5] Lippus, U. *Linear Musical Thinking. A Theory of Musical Thinking and the Runic Song Tradition of Baltic-Finnish Peoples*. Helsinki: University of Helsinki, 1995.

[6] Ross, J. and Lehiste, I. "Timing in Estonian folk songs as interaction between speech prosody, meter, and musical rhythm." *Music Perception* 15: 319-333, 1998.

[7] Ross, J. and Lehiste, I. *The Temporal Structure of Estonian Runic Songs*. Berlin: Mouton de Gruyter, 2001.

[8] Rüütel, I. "Estonia, traditional music." In *The New Grove Dictionary of Music and Musicians* (2nd ed.), S. Sadie (ed.), pp. 342-347, 2001.

[9] Särg, T. "Karksi regilaulude värsiehitusest esituse põhjal (The versification of Karksi runo songs based on their performance)." In *Regilaul – keel, muusika, poeetika*, T. Jaago and M. Sarv (eds.), Tartu: Estonian Literary Museum and University of Tartu, pp. 195-238, 2001.

Speech Processing and the Auditory Cortex

Dynamics of Speech Production and Perception
P. Divenyi et al. (Eds.)
IOS Press, 2006

Speech Processing and the Auditory Cortex

Christoph E. SCHREINER
Coleman Memorial Laboratory
University of California
San Francisco, California USA

The neural representation of speech sounds in human auditory cortex is one of the main unresolved issues in auditory neuroscience. Comprehension of its rules and implementations is critical since it constitutes the dominant interface to the most human of all brain functions: language. Further, remediation of receptive communication disorders, both of peripheral or central origins, would benefit tremendously from detailed knowledge of the nature of communication sound representation. Yet, progress toward this goal is slow. One of the reasons is that direct access to human central physiology at a high level of resolution, i.e., involving single neurons and neuronal networks, is very limited. Non-invasive imaging methods have added immensely to our knowledge of speech and language processing albeit at a spatial and temporal resolution that has not reached neuronal levels. Animal models of communication sound encoding, for example in birds, bats and monkeys, are being increasingly studied (e.g., [2]). Even the representation of speech sounds in the auditory cortex of animals has been considered, although that approach has limitations since "The biological relevance of stimuli is the most important prerequisite for sensory physiology" [1]. Animal models of communication sound encoding are highly pertinent, because they maintain biological stimulus and task relevance while allowing a high resolution exploration of the underlying coding and representation principles at the neuronal level. At the same time psychophysical considerations of basic principles of speech perception need to be taken into account to derive the most plausible scenarios and conditions for realistic speech representation in humans. This has to be combined with an increased effort to delineate the layout of the human auditory system.

The following contributions cover three critical facets of contemporary approaches to the study of the central nervous basis of speech sound representation and perception. Reductionist approaches to coding of simple and complex sounds in the peripheral and early central auditory system have shown neuronal selectivities to various elemental stimulus properties, including frequency, intensity, amplitude modulation frequency, and direction and speed of frequency sweeps. By contrast, no clear neurophysiological evidence has been obtained that is indicative of a category-based of call-specific encoding of communication sounds, at least between the cochlea and the earliest stages of cortical sound representation. However, sensitivity of neural responses to specific combinations of echolocation sounds has been obtained even at subcortical levels [3], and a similar features sensitivity may be envisioned for speech coding.

Shamma *et al.* describe in their review a two-stage, bottom-up model of speech representation that combines decomposition of the incoming speech or speech-like sounds as performed in the peripheral auditory system with an early cortical transformation of the representation into more complex combinations of spectral and temporal features. The first, peripheral stage provides representation of acoustic stimuli in a spectrogram-like fashion based on relatively simple band-pass filters for different stimulus aspects. The second stage, reflecting properties identified for primary auditory cortex, provides a more complex recombination and refinement of representation that emphasizes combined spectro-temporal properties that may be of special relevance for the identification of communication sounds. The latter stage results in selective filters that are specific to particular ranges of spectral and temporal modulation, constituting effectively a multi-resolution spectro-temporal representation. In this scheme, linear and non-linear spectro-temporal combinations activate a specific set of filters across primary auditory cortex, corresponding to a vector or distributed coding of important elements of auditory events. The author hypothesizes that distance measures in the multi-dimensional representation space may relate to 'perceptual distance'. Combined, this approach provides a state-of-the-art quantitative estimate of the cortical representation of stimulus properties, decomposed along several dimensions derived from physical attributes.

A crucial issue is, however, whether such a stimulus-based point of view captures all aspects, or even the essence, of the early cortical representation of speech sounds. To what extent and in which form do neural representations relate to the perception of sounds and to processing tasks that are reflected in speech perception. Indeed, beginning already at the level of the inferior colliculus, principles of processing appear to be increasingly object-, task-, and perhaps action-related. Examples of identifiable task-specific central processing streams are reflected in the Doppler-shift and echo-delay maps in bats [3], and the proposed 'what' and 'where' pathways in primates [4]. Other necessary central processing tasks include perceptual robustness in background noise and, of special relevance for communication sounds but not limited to them, object equivalencies across sound source variability that may augment processes of signal categorization. Further support for some representational dissociation of stimulus and perception comes from context-dependence of a perceived sound. These phenomena suggest that global, top-down processes play a role in the transformation of an acoustics-based peripheral representation into a object- or task-based central representation. In the chapter by Nelken and Ahissar, an intriguing conceptual framework is outlined that postulates a central representation of sounds that is more object-based and amenable to top-down influences and higher-order processing that appear necessary to account for many context-dependent influences in speech perception but are also evident in more basic perceptual aspects such as pitch and sound localization. The 'Reverse Hierarchy Theory' combines many facets that have been found to operate in the perceptually expressed interpretation of the physical structure of sounds.

The delineation of sound- and, especially, speech-sound-related areas in human auditory cortex is at the core of efforts to unravel the parallel and hierarchical structural base of speech processing. The chapter by Gaschler-Markefski and colleagues sketches an up-to-date picture of human cortical field parcellation using fMRI technology. Of special significance is that several areas become more distinct when applying task- or object-based stimulation schemes, as opposed to pure stimulus-based approaches.

Combined, the chapters indicate that auditory cortical research is entering an exciting phase. Multiple and sophisticated analytical approaches to studies of speech and communication sounds in animal and human models seem to provide a fulcrum for major advances in this field.

References

[1] Hauser, M.D. and Konishi, M. *The Design of Animal Communication*. Cambridge, MA: MIT Press, 1999.

[2] Kanwal, J.S. "Processing species-specific calls by combination-sensitive neurons in an echolocating bat." In T*he Design of Animal Communication*, M.D. Hauser and M. Konishi (eds.). Cambridge, MA: MIT Press, pp. 133-158, 1999.

[3] O'Neill, W.E. "The bat auditory cortex." In *Hearing by Bats*, A.N. Popper and R.R. Fay (eds.), New York: Springer Verlag, pp. 416-480, 1995.

[4] Romanski, L.M., Tian, B., Fritz, J., Mishkin, M., Goldman-Rakic, P.S. and Rauschecker, J.P. "Dual streams of auditory afferents target multiple domains in the primate prefrontal cortex." *Nat. Neurosci.* 2: 1131-1136, 1999.

Dynamics of Speech Production and Perception
P. Divenyi et al. (Eds.)
IOS Press, 2006

Analysis of Speech Dynamics in the Auditory System

Shihab SHAMMA

Center for Auditory and Acoustic Research
Institute for Systems Research
Electrical and Computer Engineering Department
University of Maryland
College Park, Maryland, USA

Abstract. Speech understanding involves the integration and identification of acoustic cues that are distributed over multiple time scales ranging from the sub-millisecond intervals associated with spectral estimates, to the few-millisecond periods of the fundamental frequency (f_0), to the tens of milliseconds spanning phonemic and syllabic segments, and the longer time scales involved in perceiving words and sentences. In this short article we review experimental findings from auditory cortical areas that concern the encoding of such temporal dynamics in various stages of auditory processing, emphasizing the implications of these findings to the perception of speech timbre.

Keywords. Auditory cortex, speech dynamics, auditory transformations

Introduction

The speech signal in its journey in the auditory system from the eardrum to the cortex undergoes a profound transformation from a simple one-dimensional temporal pressure waveform to an elaborate multidimensional representation of a wide variety of dynamic and spectral features that have been deemed valuable for speech processing and intelligibility. Examples of such features include the selectivity to speed and direction of frequency modulated (FM) tones which resemble formant transitions in speech [19], and sensitivity to different rates of amplitude modulated (AM) tones [17], to sound onsets [13], to complex spectro-temporal modulation features [18], and to elaborate combinations found in species-specific vocalizations. The existence and functional relevance of these spectrotemporal feature detectors has often been associated with extensive physiological response maps in numerous auditory structures [6][18].

To understand and utilize this representation, we must recognize that a key ingredient in the analysis of speech is the detection and integration of acoustic cues that are distributed over multiple time-scales. These range from the sub-millisecond intervals associated with spectral estimates, to the few-millisecond periods of the fundamental frequency, to the tens-of-milliseconds spanning phonemic and syllabic segments, and the longer time scales involved in perceiving words and sentences. Features on all these time scales need to be extracted and processed sequentially, and often simultaneously, so as to be combined and identified. The brief review below is limited in its scope in two fundamental ways: It concerns concepts of auditory processes operating at the faster time scales (less than a second) found in the early and cortical auditory pathways where animal experimentation is possible. Furthermore, they are based on extrapolations from experiments that employ simpler stimuli than speech (such as tones, ripples, and noise with various amplitude and frequency modulations), and hence the models discussed are not specific to speech perception.

Much of what is known about the auditory representation of these cues comes from experimental studies in various animal species. Especially well studied are the early stages of the cochlea and cochlear nucleus, and the later cortical stages [21][24][25][6][2][22][16][8]. By contrast, the physiological underpinnings of the linguistic processes remain highly elusive despite extensive investigations employing a host of new human fast-imaging technologies and computational models over the last decade [20][14]. These techniques do not yet have the resolution to give a clear insight into single units and the neural circuits and their responses and representations.

1.   Overall View of Auditory Transformations

The acoustic spectrum is extracted early in the auditory pathway at the cochlear nucleus, the first stage beyond the auditory nerve. It is then projected to the auditory cortex via a tonotopically organized pathway through the midbrain and thalamus. The representation of the spectral profile in the early stages of cochlear filtering, the auditory nerve, and some subdivisions of the cochlear nucleus and the binaural Superior Olivary Complex is relatively well understood. Beyond that, however, the response properties and functional organization of the Inferior Colliculus, Medial Geniculate Body, and the cortex are more vague. As with other cortical sensory areas, the auditory cortex is subdivided, with a primary auditory field (AI) at its center, surrounded by a belt of secondary areas that are distinguishable both anatomically and physiologically [6].

The neural correlates of the acoustic spectrum undergo substantial transformations between the auditory-nerve and the cortex. Perhaps the most obvious change is the apparent progressive loss of temporal dynamics, from rapid phase-locking to individual spectral components (< 4 kHz), down to moderate rates of synchrony in the midbrain (< 1 kHz), to the much lower rates of modulations seen in the cortex (< 30 Hz) [17][16]. These latter time-scales are commensurate with the dynamics of the vocal tract in speech, with the rate of change of pitch in musical melody, with the transient dynamics that differentiate a struck from a bowed string (e.g., a piano versus a violin), and with the rhythms of percussion instruments. Another important change in the nature of the neural responses is the emergence of more complex selectivity to combined spectral and temporal features. For instance, compared to the relatively simple tuning curves and dynamics of auditory-nerve fiber responses, cortical cells typically exhibit elaborate spectral and temporal selectivity as noted earlier.

A model of auditory processing is described briefly below that reflects these major transformations in a two stage process (Figure 1). The first is called the *early* stage; it captures cochlear and midbrain processing by transforming the acoustic stimulus to an auditory time-frequency spectrogram-like representation that combines relatively sim-

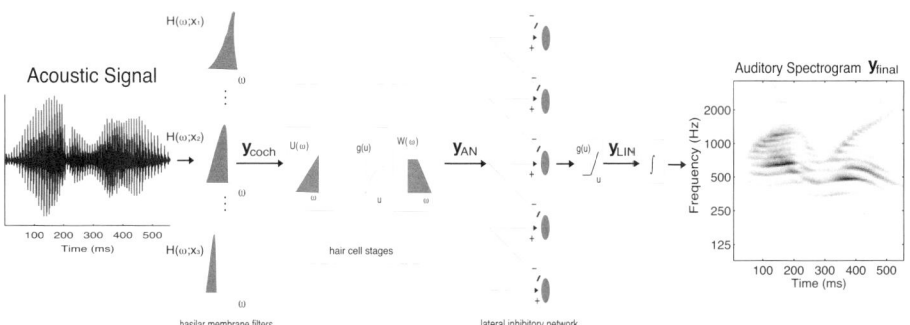

Figure 1. A schematic model of the early stages in auditory processing. Cochlear analysis is followed by auditory-nerve responses due a speech phrase /right away/. Lateral Inhibitory Network detects and enhances the presence of discontinuities such as edges, peaks, and other fast changing spatial features in its input pattern, thus extracting the auditory spectrogram.

ple bandpass spectral selectivity with moderate temporal dynamics. The second is called *cortical* stage because it reflects the more complex spectrotemporal analysis presumed to take place in mammalian AI.

2. Early Auditory Transformations

In the first stage, the acoustic signal is transformed into an auditory spectrogram - a representation resembling the well-known "spectrogram" of speech. It is the end-result of three steps (Figure 1): frequency analysis in the cochlea, combined with detection and temporal smoothing in the hair cells, and a final edge-enhancement and temporal integration in the cochlear nucleus. A simplified view of the auditory spectrogram is to think of it as the output of a bank of constant-Q bandpass filters with center frequencies (CF) that are uniformly spaced along a *logarithmic* (tonotopic) frequency axis. A detailed mathematical description of this model is available in [28][27].

A unique aspect of cochlear filters is that they encode not simply the instantaneous power of each frequency band, but rather preserve or explicitly encode the rapidly modulated waveforms of the frequency components falling within the band. This is strictly true in the lower CF bands (< 2000 Hz). At higher CF (> 4000 Hz), the hair cell stage following each filter smooths out the output waveform replacing it with the instantaneous power output as in the usual spectrogram. Aside from these fast modulations, cochlear outputs at all CFs may become modulated due to formant transitions or other dynamic features of speech, or they may also beat at the fundamental frequency (of the voice) because of interactions among signal components that pass within their bandwidths. These latter modulations are identical to the so-called f_0 modulations (striations) typically seen in traditional broadband spectrograms of speech.

These three types of temporal modulations are depicted in more detail in auditory spectrogram (Figure 2(a)) where the output waveform from an auditory channel at CF=750 Hz (Figure 2(b)) is shown in response to the speech signal "*We've done our part*". The response encodes the three temporal scales simultaneously. At the top of Figure 2(b) are the slowest gross modulations (approximately 4 bursts per second) that

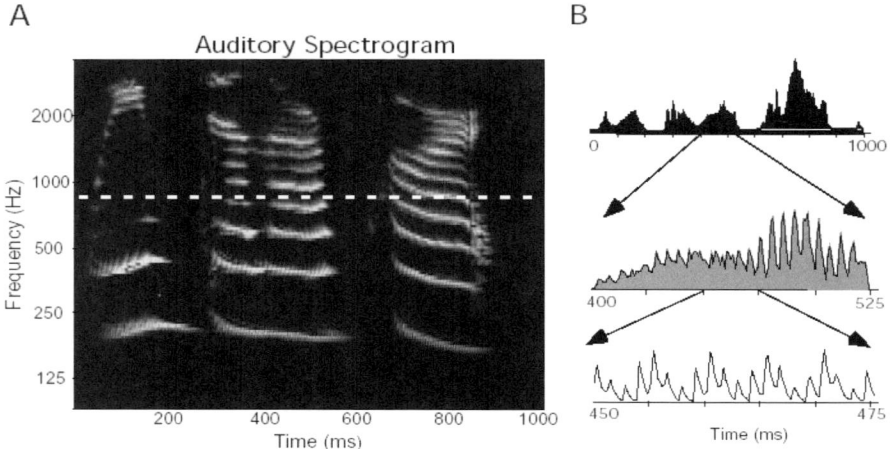

Figure 2. Temporal modulations in an auditory spectrogram of a speech sentence /We've done our part/ with a pitch of approximately 200 Hz. The dashed line marks the auditory channel at 750 Hz whose temporal modulations are depicted to the right at different time scales. At the coarsest scale (top panel), the slow modulations (few Hz) roughly correlate with the different syllabic segments of the utterance. At an intermediate scale (middle panel), modulations due to inter-harmonic interactions occur at a rate that reflects the fundamental (approximately 200 Hz) of the signal. At the finest scale (bottom panel), the fast temporal modulations are due to the frequency component driving this channel best (around 750 Hz).

reflect the rise and fall of energy in this frequency band during the speech utterance. These slow modulations reflect the succession of syllables, and hence are affected by the dynamics of the vocal tract, movement of the formants, and onsets and offsets of consonants that are directly responsible for the intelligibility of the speech signal. The middle plot illustrates the intermediate-rate modulations (about 200 Hz) that are due to interactions among partially resolved harmonics that fall within the bandwidth of the cochlear filter in this band. The depth and shape of these modulations are sensitive to the relative phase of the interacting components and, therefore, reflects the timbre of the sound being voiced, harsh, or whispered. Furthermore, these modulations decrease as the interacting harmonics within a filter bandwidth become more resolved, and hence they largely disappear in responses dominated by low order (well resolved) harmonics as in the CF< 300 Hz region in Figure 1 (and CF < 700 in Figure 2). Finally, the bottom plot of Figure 2(b) depicts the responses at the finest (fastest) temporal scale that reflect the acoustic frequency components (around 800 Hz) that carry the energy of the stimulus in this band. As mentioned earlier, these fast modulations disappear in high CF channels (> 4 kHz) leaving only the f0 modulations as "carriers" of the all-important slow modulations of speech in these bands. In general, this overall picture of the modulations remains the same up the auditory pathway, with the one major exception being that there is a progressive decrease in the maximum fast rates possible to under a few hundred Hertz at the collicular and thalamic stages [6][17].

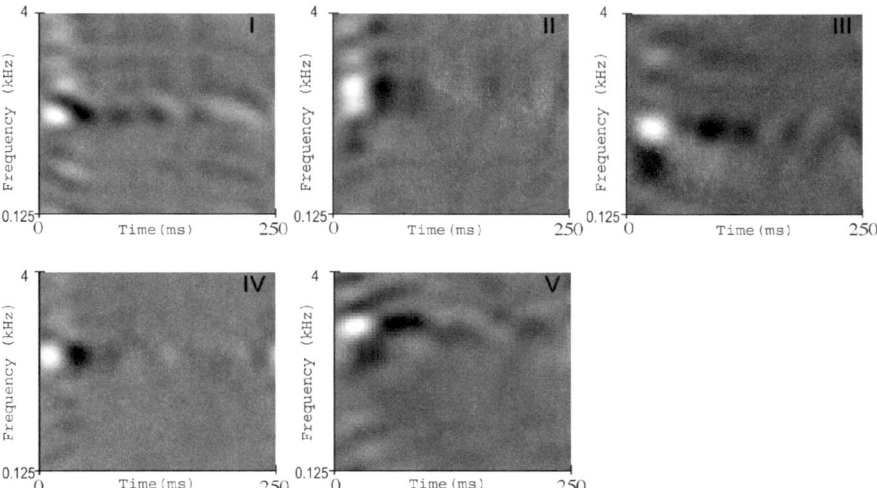

Figure 3. Example Spectrotemporal Response Fields (STRFs) from the AI of ferret primary auditory cortex.

3. Auditory Cortical Physiology

The *cortical* stage of the model is strongly inspired by extensive data and ideas gained from physiological and psychoacoustical experiments over the last decade. Specifically, much insight has been gained from measurements of the Spectro-Temporal Response Fields (STRF) of AI cells. Examples of the wide variety of STRFs are shown in Figure 3, with different spectral bandwidths (also called *scales*), asymmetries, dynamics (*rates*), and directional preferences (peaks sweeping *up* or *down* in frequency) [9]. Some units are broadly tuned (i, ii) and hence are most responsive to low density ripples; Others are narrowly tuned (iv) and respond well to fine features of the profile and to high density ripples. STRFs also exhibit a variety of asymmetric inhibitory surrounds, e.g., contrast the symmetrically inhibited STRF in unit (iv) with the asymmetric STRF in (iii). Finally, STRFs may be slow (iii, v) or fast (iv), or selective to upward (iii) and downward-moving (v) ripples. From a functional and psychoacoustical perspective, such rich variety implies that each STRF acts as a *selective filter* specific to a particular range of spectral resolutions (or *scales*) and tuned to a limited range of temporal modulations *rates*. The collection of all such STRFs then would constitute a filter bank spanning the broad range of psychoacoustically observed scale and rate sensitivity in humans and animals [4][11]. Consequently, each spectrotemporal feature in the spectrogram will activate a unique pattern of filters. A map of responses across the entire filterbank, therefore, provides a unique characterization of the spectrogram, one that is sensitive to the short-time spectral shape and temporal dynamics of the stimulus.

Evidence of the importance of spectrotemporal modulations in the perception of complex sounds has come from experiments in which systematic degradations of the speech signal were correlated with the gradual loss of intelligibility [10][23]. All such experiments have consistently pointed to the importance of the slow temporal (< 30 Hz) and broad spectral modulations in conveying a robust level of intelligibility [10][7][12]. In fact, the relationship between the temporal modulations and speech intelligibility has long been codified in the formulation of the widely used Speech Transmission Index (STI) [15]. In an extension of such ideas, and inspired by the neurophysiological data briefly reviewed here, we formulated and tested a Spectro-Temporal Modulation Index (STMI) [4][11] which assesses the integrity of *both* the spectral and temporal modulations in a signal as a measure of intelligibility. The STMI proved reliable in capturing the deleterious effects of noise and reverberations, as well as of previously difficult to characterize distortions such as nonlinear compression, phase jitter, and phase shifts [11].

In summary, there is physiological and psychoacoustical evidence that the auditory system, particularly at the level of AI, analyzes the dynamic acoustic spectrum of the stimulus extracted at its earlier stages. It does so by explicitly representing its spectro-temporal modulations by employing arrays of spectrally and temporally selective STRFs. A mathematical formulation of these computations is available in [5] together with details of methods to invert the representations back to the acoustic stimulus in order to hear the effects of arbitrary manipulations.

4. Applications of Multiresolution Auditory Processing

The perception of speech is critically dependent on the faithful representation of spectral and temporal modulations in the auditory spectrogram. Therefore, an intelligibility index which reflects the integrity of these modulations can be effective regardless of the source of the degradation. Such a *spectro-temporal modulation index* (STMI) was derived using the representation of speech modulations in the above multiresolution auditory model. It was validated by comparing its predictions of intelligibility to those of the classical *Speech Transmission Index (STI)* and to error rates reported by human subjects listening to speech contaminated with combined noise and reverberation. The STMI in principle can handle difficult and nonlinear distortions such as phase-jitter and shifts, to which the STI is not sensitive [11].

In another example of the effectiveness of the auditory model, it was used to account for the detection of phase of complex sounds such as phase differences between the envelopes of sounds occupying remote frequency regions, and between the fine structures of partials that interact within a single auditory filter [3]. The approach was simply to interpret the discrimination between two stimuli as being proportional to the distance (or difference) measured between their cortical representation in the model. Discriminations successfully modeled in this way included phase differences between pairs of bandpass filtered harmonic complexes, and between pairs of sinusoidally amplitude modulated tones, discrimination between amplitude and frequency modulation, and discrimination of transient signals differing only in their phase spectra ("Huffman sequences").

We believe that this approach can be successfully extended beyond these two applications to explain the complex phenomena associated with "auditory scene analysis" and "informational masking". For example, it is well known that two sounds (A,B) are more readily streamed when they differ in timber, pitch, or other perceptual qualities [1]. We hypothesize that this "perceptual distance" can be directly measured from the cortical multiresolution spectrotemporal representation of these sounds. And, therefore, it is possible to predict or test the effects of manipulating this distance on the perception of streaming in a variety of sequences.

Acknowledgements

This work has been supported in part by a grant from the Office of Naval Research under the ODDR and MURI97 Program to the Center for Auditory and Acoustic Research.

References

[1] Bregman, A.S. *Auditory Scene Analysis: The Perceptual Organization of Sound*. Cambridge, MA: MIT Press, 1991.

[2] Calhoun, B. and Schreiner, C. "Spectral envelope coding in cat primary auditory cortex." *J. Aud. Neurosci.* 1: 39-61, 1995.

[3] Carlyon, R. and Shamma, S. "An account of monaural phase sensitivity." *J. Acoust. Soc. Am.* 114: 333-348, 2003.

[4] Chi, T., Gao, Y., Guyton, M.C., Ru, P. and Shamma, S.A. "Spectro-temporal modulation transfer functions and speech intelligibility." *J. Acoust. Soc. Am.* 106: 2719-2732. 1999.

[5] Chi, T., Ru, Y. and Shamma, S.A. "A muliscale model of auditory processing." *Speech Communication, 2004..*

[6] Clarey J., Barone, P., and Imig, T. "Physiology of thalamus and cortex." In *The Mammalian Auditory Pathway: Neurophysiology*, D. Webster, A.N. Popper and R.R. Fay (eds.), New York: Springer Verlag, pp. 232-334, 1992.

[7] Dau, T., Puschel, D. and Kohlrausch, A. "A quantitative model of the 'elective' signal processing in the auditory system. II. Simulation and measurements." *J. Acoust. Soc. Am.* 99: 3623-3631, 1996.

[8] deCharms, R.C., Blake, D.T. and Merzenich, M.M. "Optimizing sound features for cortical neurons." *Science* 280: 1439-43, 1998.

[9] Depireux, D., Simon, J., Klein, D. and Shamma, S. "Spectro-temporal response field characterization with dynamic ripples in ferret primary auditory cortex." *J. Neurophysiol.*, 85: 1220-1234, 2001.

[10] Drullman, J., Festen, J. and Plomp, R. "Effect of envelope smearing on speech perception." *J. Acoust. Soc. Am.* 95: 1053-1064, 1994.

[11] ElHilali, M., Chi, T. and Shamma, S. "A spectro-temporal modulation index (STMI) for assessment of speech intelligibility." *Speech Communication, 2002.*

[12] Greenberg S., Arai, T. and Silipo, R. "Speech intelligibility derived from exceedingly sparse spectral information." *Proc. Int. Conf. Spoken Lang. Proc.*, 1998.

[13] Heil, P. "Representation of sound onsets in the auditory system." *Audiol. Neurootol.* 6: 167-172, 2001.

[14] Horwitz, B., Friston, K. and Taylor, J. "Neural modelling and functional brain imaging: An overview." *Neural Networks* 13: 829-846, 2000.

[15] Houtgast, T., Steeneken, H.J.M. and Plomp, R. "Predicting speech intelligibility in rooms from the modulation transfer function. I. General room acoustics." *Acoustica* 46: 60, 1980.

[16] Kowalski, N, Depireux, D. and Shamma, S. "Analysis of dynamic spectra in ferret primary auditory cortex: I. Characteristics of single unit responses to moving ripple spectra." *J. Neurophysiol.* 76: 3503-3523, 1996.

[17] Langner, G. "Periodicity coding in the auditory system." *Hear. Res.* 6. 115-142, 1992.

[18] Lyon, R. and Shamma, S. "Auditory representation of timbre and pitch." In *Auditory Computation*, H. Hawkins, M. McMullen, A.N. Popper,and RR.. Fay (eds.), New York: Springer Verlag, pp. 221-270, 1996.

[19] Nelken, I. and Versnel, H. "Responses to linear and logarithmic frequency-modulated sweeps in ferret primary auditory cortex." *Eur. J. Neurosci.* 12: 549-62, 2000.

[20] Poeppel, D. *Brain and Speech: special issue Cog. Science*, 21(5), 2001.

[21] Sachs, M.B. and Young, E.D. "Encoding of steady state vowels in the auditory-nerve: Representation in terms of discharge rate," *J. Acoust. Soc. Am.* 66: 470-479, 1979.

[22] Shamma, S., Versnel, H. and Kowalski, N. "Ripple analysis in ferret primary auditory cortex: I. Response characteristics of single units to sinusoidally rippled spectra." *Aud. Neurosc.* 1: 233-254, 1995.

[23] Shannon, R., Zeng, F.-G., Wygonski, J., Kamath, V. and Ekelid, M. "Speech recognition with primarily temporal cues." *Science* 270: 303-304, 1995.

[24] Young, E.D. and Sachs, M.B. "Representation of steady-state vowels in the temporal aspects of the discharge patterns of populations of auditory-nerve fibers." *J. Acoust. Soc. Am.* 66: 1381-1403, 1979.

[25] Young, E. "The cochlear nucleus." In *Synaptic Organization of the Brain*, G.M. Shepherd (ed.), New York: Oxford University Press, pp. 131-157, 1997.

[26] Winslow, R. and Sachs, M. "Effect of electrical stimulation of olive-cochlear bundle on auditory nerve responses to tones in noise." *J. Neurophysiol.* 57(4): 1002-1021, 1987.

[27] Wang, K. and Shamma, S.A. "Self-normalization and noise-robustness in early auditory representations." *IEEE Trans. Speech Audio Proc.* 2(3): 421- 435, 1994.

[28] Yang, X., Wang, K. and Shamma, S.A. "Auditory representations of acoustic signals." *IEEE Trans. Inform. Theory*, 38(2): 824, 1992.

Dynamics of Speech Production and Perception
P. Divenyi et al. (Eds.)
IOS Press, 2006

343

High-level and Low-level Processing in the Auditory System: The Role of Primary Auditory Cortex

Israel NELKEN[1] and Merav AHISSAR[2]
[1]*Dept. of Neurobiology, The Silberman Institute of Life Sciences*
Hebrew University, Jerusalem, Israel
[2]*Department of Pyschology*
Hebrew University, Jerusalem, Israel
[1,2]*The Interdisciplinary Center for Neural Computations*
The Hebrew University, Jerusalem, Israel

Abstract. In spite of a large number of studies at different levels of the auditory system, there is still no satisfactory physiological account for the perception of speech. We argue here that many of the problems in creating such an account are common to other processing tasks of the auditory system, such as the extraction of pitch and sound localization. These difficulties are related to the global aspects of these percepts, which depend on integrating information over large bandwidth and on temporal context. We describe a possible framework for a solution - the Reverse Hierarchy Theory, recently formulated to account for difficulties of similar character in the relationships between visual psychophysics and the physiology of the visual system. We show that the concepts of Reverse Hierarchy Theory can be easily mapped into the auditory system, and that it generates natural explanations to some perplexing features of auditory perception of global structures such as pitch, space and speech. We argue that in the context of Reverse Hierarchy Theory, primary auditory cortex seems to occupy a pivotal role in that it generates auditory objects over which higher-order processing tasks can be performed.

Keywords. Auditory cortex, speech, sound localization, pitch, processing levels, reverse hierarchy theory

Introduction

In spite of a large number of studies at different levels of the auditory system, there is still no satisfactory physiological account for the perception of speech. We argue here that many of the problems in creating such an account are common to other processing tasks of the auditory system, such as the extraction of pitch and sound localization. These difficulties are related to the global aspects of these percepts, which depend on integrating information over large bandwidth and on temporal context. We describe a possible framework for a solution – the Reverse Hierarchy Theory, recently formulated to account for difficulties of similar character in the relationships between visual psychophysics and the physiology of the visual system. We show that the concepts of Reverse Hierarchy Theory can be easily mapped into the auditory system, and that it generates natural explanations to some perplexing features of auditory perception of global structures such as pitch, space and speech. We argue that in the context of Reverse Hierarchy Theory, primary auditory cortex seems to occupy a pivotal role in that it generates auditory objects over which higher-order processing tasks can be performed.

1.   Speech Perception from the Point of View of an Auditory Physiologist

The study of coding of speech signals in neural activity has a long and distinguished past (reviewed in [13]). However, although these studies shed light on how specific acoustic features, relevant to speech perception, could be coded in the auditory system, some of the hardest and most interesting questions about speech perception are still unanswered.

For an auditory physiologist, one possible context for studying the coding of speech sounds is as follows. We assume here that the speech signal is the only relevant sensory input. In order to avoid the influence of semantic context, we assume that the speech sound is e.g. a consonant-vowel-consonant non-sense syllable. Under these circumstances, we assume that in order to correctly identify the syllable, it is necessary to correctly identify each of the three phonemes [2]. We are therefore looking for a brain signal that will be as unambiguously as possible related to each of the phonemes.

Under these circumstances, speech perception should be easy – there is a finite number of vowels and consonants (a few tens, maybe 100-200 [34]). Furthermore, these sounds are different from each other on a large number of features that have (or should have) clear acoustic correlates. We could for example look for a brain region in which neurons act as 'phoneme detectors': they are active if, and only if, the specific phoneme they respond to was perceived. This is of course a naïve, caricatural view of speech perception given the complexity in the structure of speech sounds. This setup also doesn't explicitly take into account questions such as the large redundancy that exists in speech sounds, the reliability of the detection of speech in background noise, coarticulation effects and so on. Nevertheless, most electrophysiological studies of speech coding are performed under these assumptions. Such studies identified features that could be used by a (admittedly, half mythical) 'next layer' that should be activated according to the phonemic identity of the speech sound [55][8][43].

Why then is understanding speech perception so hard? We would like to invoke four reasons here: (1) the wideband character of speech sounds; (2) the generalizing nature of the phonemic space; (3) the discrete character of the phonemic space; and (4) the effect of context.

Consider first a simple, continuous, isolated vowel sound. A basic difficulty, from the point of view of an auditory physiologist, is the fact that the identity of such a sound depends on information in a wide frequency band, consisting of many octaves. For example, telephone lines transmit sound energy between about 500 Hz and 4000 Hz – at least 3 octaves. In contrast, the basic auditory processing is all narrowband. The basic auditory perceptual channel, the critical band, has a width of about 1/6 octave in humans. Critical bands are often considered to be related to the bandwidth of auditory neurons in the auditory nerve [39] or in the inferior colliculus [14]. If speech is processed through the same channels, single neurons in the core pathway of the auditory system cannot be used for speech perception (without detracting from their ability to extract important features that are relevant for speech perception!). The perceptual correlate of this statement is the fact that decomposing a speech sound into its critical band components results in many signals, none of which sounds like speech. Thus, in some sense, speech is a non-linear construct of multiple non-speech components. Somewhere on the way between a critical-band component and the full broad-band speech, the non-speech becomes speech.

The next difficulty is the generalizing nature of the speech perceptual space: different physical sounds can be perceived as the same phoneme. Thus, whatever is the nature of the phoneme detectors, they should generalize across many physical realizations of the same speech sound. For example, a given vowel can be performed by an adult or a child; by an adult male or female; voiced or whispered; or it can be synthesized by a low-quality LPC vocoder. These realizations of the same phoneme 'sound' differently – we are certainly able to tell them apart, but they share the same phonemic label. The difficulty for the electrophysiologist is that most neurons in the auditory system that have been studied thus far will be influenced by the nuisance parameters, probably more strongly than by the phonemic label. Thus, we have in fact a pretty good theory of why different realizations of the same phoneme sound differently, but no theory for what gives them the same label. In other words, most of what we know about the auditory system is related to a high-fidelity description of the physics of the sounds, and not about extracting invariants.

The previous problem is compounded by the fact that the phonemic space is in fact discrete. Most studies of acoustic features in the auditory system, from the auditory nerve to the auditory cortex, are consistent with a continuous representation of acoustic features, rather than with discrete representations. For example, although different neurons have different best frequencies, it is usually accepted that firing rate depends continuously on stimulus frequency. Similarly, the linear representation of stimulus features that is inherent in the spectro-temporal receptive fields [53][11][44][33] is inherently continuous: although STRFs have preferred frequency, bandwidth, temporal frequency and so on, the responses they predict vary continuously with the similarity between a stimulus and the receptive field, due to the linearity of the similarity calculation. There are only a few studies [49][12][50] in which an electrophysiological correlate of categorical perception has been proposed.

However, the most cited reason for the hard nature of speech perception is co-articulation [20]. Co-articulation refers to the fact that speech sounds differ according to their temporal context. The result is that the same physical sound can receive two different phonemic labels, according to the context in which it is presented. Thus, the phonemic identity of a sound depends not only on the immediate acoustic input, but also on a temporal context that may last as long as a few hundreds of milliseconds. For the electrophysiologist, this means that the mythical phoneme detectors should be influenced not only by the current sound input, but also by past and possibly also future context. Although we (the electrophysiologists) all know that context is important, we tend to describe our neurons in terms of relatively short past – 10 ms or so in the auditory nerve, maybe 100 ms or so in cortex. Very few studies explicitly manipulated context. These studies demonstrated a strong influence of temporal context in auditory cortex, and under the appropriate conditions, even as low as the inferior colliculus [46][28][29][54].

Many of the theories proposed for speech perception are attempts to circumvent these difficulties. For example, the lack of simple acoustic invariants for phonemes led to the motor theory of speech perception and to direct perception theories, which suggest that speech is perceived in terms of vocal tract gestures [16]. However, these theories do not by themselves solve the problem of the auditory physiologist, since we assumed that the acoustic input is the only input to the system. Thus, the hypothesized motor or gestural invariants are functions of the acoustic waveform, and should be extracted by purely auditory processing.

The most radical attempt to solve this problem is the modular theory of Liberman and his coworkers, which assumes that the human auditory system contains a special 'module' for speech perception [25]. This module is activated by speech sounds and preempts other auditory processes. Liberman and Mattingly argued that this process should occur very early in the auditory system, leading to a 'speech mode' of sound perception, in which speech sound identity is directly perceived, and the perception of other acoustic features is suppressed.

This theory is unsatisfactory to the electrophysiologist: Since speech is a human activity not shared by other animals, the existence of a speech module would make it impossible to relate our understanding of electrophysiology (mostly studied in animals) to speech processing. However, we know that many aspects of speech perception, including some rather fine effects, can be mimicked by other mammals [24] and even birds, the japanese quails [27]. In fact, there is no reason to assume that early processing in the human auditory system is different qualitatively from that of other mammals. Both the anatomical substrates, and all the psychophysical information currently available both in humans and in animals, suggest great similarities, rather than differences.

2. Is Speech Special?

However, the most powerful argument against a special module for speech is possibly the fact that the difficult aspects of speech perception are also shared by other auditory computational tasks. In fact, the difficulties mentioned above for an electrophysiological theory of speech perception, namely the wideband character, the generalization across disparate physical structures, and the temporal contextual effects, are shared by both pitch perception and space perception. Some aspects of pitch perception are even thought to be categorical [5]. Thus, although pitch and space have a continuous perceptual space, they share with speech many hard aspects, some of which have been used to argue that speech is special.

Consider pitch first. A multi-component harmonic complex with a missing fundamental can be decomposed into multiple components, none of which evokes the pitch of the whole complex. If the complex contains only resolvable harmonics, any single critical band cannot be used by itself to signal pitch. It can be argued that high-frequency, non-resolvable components can be used to extract the inherent periodicity that is present in stimuli evoking pitch. However, sounds that contain only resolved harmonics generate very strong pitch sensation, even stronger than that evoked by high-frequency sounds with no resolved harmonics. Thus, the pitch system must be able to cope with the problem of extracting period information by integrating information across multiple peripheral channels. More complex situations can exist as well: for example, dichotic pitch requires integration of information from the two ears, and neither of the monaural signals has a pitch by itself. Thus, pitch is a non-linear construct of its components.

The same pitch can also be evoked by many different physical sounds: for example, a harmonic complex, a segment of iterated-ripple noise, an AABBCC sound (consisting of a random noise segment of pitch period followed by a copy of itself, followed by another random noise segment of the same duration which is followed by itself, and so on), or a sinusoidally amplitude-modulated high-frequency sine wave, would all create the same pitch. All four can be used for playing melodies. Thus, there must be a mechanism that generalizes across the very different physical structure of these sounds, and assigns to all of them the same pitch value.

Finally, this mechanism is also context-dependent. This can be seen, for example, from the possibility of changing the pitch of a harmonic complex by catching one of its components into a different auditory stream [9][10]. When one of the components of a harmonic complex is slightly mistuned, the pitch of the complex is shifted. However, when the mistuned component is given a different context, e.g. by starting it before the whole complex or by embedding it in a fast stream of repeated pure tones of the same frequency, the pitch shift is reduced or eliminated.

Spatial perception and lateralization have similar properties. The spatial percepts created by a binaural wideband sound, and by its narrowband components, can be dramatically different [51]. In these experiments, a delay of 1.5 ms was imposed on noise bands centered at 500 Hz. Since the period of a 500 Hz tone is 2 ms, an interaural delay of 1.5 ms imposed on a 500 Hz tone is interpreted as a delay of –0.5 ms (that is, the sound is lateralized to the lagging side). The same is true for narrow noise bands centered at 500 Hz, but wider frequency bands are lateralized to the leading ('correct') side. Similarly, in free-field, there are consistent errors of localization (mostly in elevation) for narrow noise bands, but not for wide noise bands [32][31]. Spatial perception also generalizes across physical characteristics: the same lateralization or localization can be created by sounds with widely different acoustic structure. Finally, spatial perception also shows contextual effects. For example, when presenting a pair of noise bursts with a very short time interval between them, each from a different location, the perception of the second one is suppressed. This effect is called the law of the first waveform [4] or the precedence effect [58][18][57][26]. When the second burst is loud enough, it is nevertheless heard, and the minimal level above which the second click is perceived is called the echo threshold. This threshold is not fixed, and can be manipulated: a long series of burst pairs, in which the 2nd burst would come from the left, would increase the echo threshold, whereas if the position of the 2nd burst is suddenly shifted, it will be perceived at lower levels [17].

Is then understanding speech perception harder than understanding pitch and space perception? In some sense yes, because the low-level correlates of pitch and space are much better understood. For example, pitch is intimately related to periodicity (although the relationships are not one-to-one), whereas space is related to binaural disparities and monaural spectral structure. However, the harder questions related to pitch and space are as poorly understood as those related to speech. For example, there is still no accepted model of pitch psychophysics, with two families of models, one based mostly on temporal processing and the other based mostly on spectral processing, neither of which can explain all experimental results satisfactorily [35]. Furthermore, although there are a number of elegant studies of the extraction of low-level correlates of pitch [6][7], there is no accepted location in the brain where pitch is represented (as opposed e.g. to the spectral structure of the sound). It has been proposed that pitch is already represented in the inferior colliculus, and that periodicity maps are present in auditory cortex [45]. Some of these studies, however, lacked important control. For example, we [37] recently showed that periodotopic maps exist in the ferret auditory cortex, but these maps are different for sinusoidally amplitude-modulated sines, band-passed click trains, and iterated ripple noise. Such maps, that do not generalize across different realizations of the same pitch, cannot be considered as pitch maps.

The situation regarding spatial processing is somewhat better, in that we know about the presence of a space map in the superior colliculus of mammals (and in its homologue, the optic tectum, of birds). Furthermore, we know that this space map is generated from subcortical inputs, certainly in birds [23] but probably also in mammals [22]. However, auditory cortex is known to participate in spatial processing, and although there are no known space maps in auditory cortex, many cortical fields contain neurons that are sensitive to the location of sounds in space. Some of these fields project to the superior colliculus, but the role of these projections in the generation of the space map is unknown [30]. Furthermore, most studies of spatial processing have been performed in 'dry' space, using a single sound source. Spatial processing is much more than that. For example, humans (and presumably other animals too) are capable of assigning direction to multiple concurrent sound sources. Such questions are only now starting to be tackled in electrophysiological research [52][48].

Thus, although pitch and space have a continuous perceptual space, whereas speech is much more discrete, we conclude that most of the 'hard' aspects of pitch and space processing in the auditory system are similar, and as unsolved, as those of speech processing. There is a global aspect to the processing of speech, pitch and space that is hard to capture with our current models of auditory processing, because these models are local, both in time and in frequency – neurons in the core pathway are narrowband, and most current studies of neural responses ignore the effects of context, both spectral and temporal, on neuronal responses.

3.   Parallels with Visual Psychophysics: The Reverse Hierarchy Theory

The same conflict between local and global aspects of stimuli and of perception can be also found in the visual system. The immediate perception of global features, such as faces or illusory contours, is well known. Such phenomena led to the gestalt models of perception [41][56] in which it is assumed that "… the properties of the parts are determined by the laws of structure of the whole …" [56] and to Gibson's direct perception theory [15], both of which also influenced models of speech perception.

The known physiology of the visual system, however, hardly supports perception of global structures before the analysis of their parts. Instead, we know that simple feature detectors of spots of light (in the retina and the LGN) somehow create line detectors and more complex feature detectors in primary visual cortex. This information further flows along the visual pathway, and finally generates rather complex feature detectors, culminating e.g. in the well known 'face detectors' in monkeys [38][42]. Studies in humans also suggest the presence of high visual areas that are sensitive to global structures, such as faces [21]. Thus, coding of complex features, such as faces, seems to occur late in the visual system, rather than early.

Recently, the Reverse Hierarchy Theory has been proposed as a way around these types of difficulties. The main aspect of the Reverse Hierarchy Theory is the separation between the bottom-up processing hierarchy on the one hand, and conscious perception, which follows along the reverse direction, on the other hand [1][19]. Bottom-up processing is the initial fast processing sequence, which is typically probed by single unit receptive field properties. This processing progresses from simple feature detection to increasingly more complex and abstract representations, which are aimed at getting closer to the distal stimulus (in contrast with its proximal representation on the retina). For example, in the visual system, single neurons show a gradual increase in invariance to the position and illumination, which are important features of the proximal stimulus. Conscious perception does not follow this processing scheme. On the contrary – initial conscious perception reflects higher-level representations. Thus, our initial visual percept follows the "real" size of objects rather than their retinal size. Bottom-up fast processing subserves our ability to get the "gist" of scenes quite fast, in about a tenth of a second, which is where our conscious perception begins.

Initial conscious perception is thus global and holistic, unlike the basic local characteristics of low-level representations, and yet it is crude. If more details are important, scrutiny (i.e. further processing time) is required. Under these conditions we search for further details at lower-level representations, which are better suited for finding fine details. Thus later conscious perception reflects lower-level representations, and hence the Reverse Hierarchy terminology. It follows that when we need crude categorical identification, we can do it fast, based on high-level global representations. However, when a specific item needs be identified, after our first initial glimpse yields a crude category, we search backwards to lower level representations in order to acquire more detailed information.

The same type of reasoning can be applied to the auditory system. For example, in the case of pitch processing, a limited form of periodicity, for example periodicity within the narrow band peripheral filters, could be extracted early. But this periodicity is only one feature of the conscious percept of pitch, as discussed above. The Reverse Hierarchy Theory suggests that, because of its global temporal and spectral aspects, pitch is a high-level construct, resulting in its being perceived globally and holistically, late in the bottom-up processing hierarchy. Space is similar – although features that underlie spatial perception, such as interaural time and level differences, are computed early, the initial global spatial percept is based on cruder high-level representations.

The same argument can be applied for speech perception. Neurons all over the early auditory system are sensitive to important acoustic features of speech, but the perception of speech is global, and therefore high. This hypothesis provides a natural explanation for the intuitive notion of the 'speech mode' of auditory perception, which is insensitive to possible large changes in the physical qualities of sounds. The speech mode is hypothesized here to be the conscious correlate of the activity in a high-level, global representation of the spectro-temporal structure, which has crude resolution in terms of the basic acoustic features of the speech sounds (e.g. Pols and van Son, this volume). It preempts the perception of low-level acoustic correlates, when we are not asked to attend to them. In order to be able to make fine distinctions about the physical details of the sound, it is necessary to follow the reverse hierarchy of the bottom-up processing stream, requiring scrutiny and further processing time.

4. Implications: The Role of Primary Auditory Cortex in Auditory Perception

Neurons that code for pitch, space or speech should have properties that mirror the properties of the resulting percepts. The activity of such neurons should be affected by sound energy in a sufficiently wide frequency band; these neurons should be sensitive to context; and they should be insensitive to some, possibly large, changes in the physical structure of sounds, while being extremely sensitive to other, possibly small, changes, provided that these changes have to do with the global aspects of sound encoded by these neurons. The Reverse Hierarchy Theory makes the additional prediction that these neurons would be found relatively high in the ascending auditory system.

Our results in the primary auditory cortex of cats seem to partially fit this description. For example, neurons in AI show strong temporal context dependence [54]. In this study, pairs of pure tones were presented in an oddball paradigm. One of the two tones was presented with high probability ('standard') and the other one at a low probability ('deviant'). The responses to a frequency, when deviant, were larger than the responses to the same frequency, when standard. This difference was inversely related to the probability of the deviant and to the frequency separation between the two tones, but was still significant overall for a frequency separation of 4% when the deviant appeared 10% of the time and the standard 90% of the time. Similar effects were shown also for amplitude deviants. The stimulus-specific adaptation occurred even for interstimulus intervals of 2 seconds, but were not significant for intervals of 4 seconds. Contextual effects related to large changes in stimulus parameters can be demonstrated as early as the IC [47], but fine-level contextual effects seem to be absent in the MGB, and are first expressed only in auditory cortex [54].

Neurons in primary auditory cortex show other useful properties for high-level representation of sounds. They show also simultaneous context dependence [36][3] in the sense that responses can be affected by frequency components outside the neuronal tuning curve, even when these components are weaker than stimulus energy within the tuning curve. They are also 'promiscuous' – they respond to many different sounds in ways that are not always clearly related to the low-level features of these sounds [3]. The simultaneous contextual effects are already apparent, at least to some extent, in the auditory thalamus, but not in the IC [59][60].

The common denominator of all of these results is that neurons in auditory cortex seem to be exquisitely sensitive to weak and rare acoustic components – they can respond to mixtures of strong and weak acoustic components as if they heard only the weak components, both when the strong component is tonal and the weak component is noise [3], and when the strong component is noise and the weak component is tone [36]. Furthermore, neurons in auditory cortex respond differentially to rare acoustic components [54].

Going back to the Reverse Hierarchy Theory, the global aspects of sounds that are encoded by neurons in auditory cortex should be related to the invariance properties of the responses of the same neurons. The sensitivity to weak and rare acoustic components suggest that neurons in primary auditory cortex are dealing with the extraction of acoustic components from mixtures – in other words, in auditory scene analysis.

Our results suggest therefore that pitch, space and speech are not encoded as such in the activity of neurons in primary auditory cortex. Rather, primary auditory cortex builds auditory objects, to which later processing can assign pitch, spatial location, or phonemic identity. The primary auditory cortex is therefore at an intermediate stage in the processing hierarchy – whereas it is already sensitive to spectro-temporal context, this sensitivity is related to the creation of auditory objects rather than to the computations of their properties. In this respect, we hypothesize that pitch, space and speech perception are related to higher processing stages. In fact, it has been suggested that at least in primates [40] there are separate space and object processing streams in the auditory system, similar to the dorsal and ventral processing streams of the visual system. Although the evidence for these streams is weak, it is tempting to hypothesize that if they exist, they may operate on the auditory objects created in primary auditory cortex.

The role of primary auditory cortex is therefore pivotal in the auditory system. Whereas lower processing stages (at least up to the IC) seem to encode with high fidelity the physical properties of sounds, activity in primary auditory cortex seem to be related already to the interpretation of the physical structure of sounds, rather than with the physical structure itself. We therefore hypothesize that primary auditory cortex supplies the object representation on which all further auditory processing operates. The extensive anatomical projections from primary auditory cortex to both higher auditory areas and lower processing stations, such as the auditory thalamus and the IC, seem to support its central position both within the bottom-up processing hierarchy, and within the reverse, top-down interpretation hierarchy.

So where should we look for speech coding in the auditory system? The account of the auditory system given here suggest that we should see some speech-related activity in primary auditory cortex, but only in the sense that regularities in the speech signals can be used to bind together information in different frequency bands and create the appropriate temporal contexts for interpreting the speech sounds. Somewhere beyond primary auditory cortex there may be phoneme detectors. These could well lie beyond the core auditory system.

One intriguing possibility is that these speech coding neurons would be found in areas that have motor functions. Finding phoneme detectors in motor areas should not be more surprising than finding the auditory space map in a nucleus that subserves important motor functions, namely the superior colliculus. Such a finding would vindicate in part the intuition of Liberman and Mattingly [25], but with an important twist. Speech perception is so immediate and effortless not because it is early in the sensory stream, but because it is late in the sensory stream and therefore 'closer' to consciousness. The realization that speech perception can be both immediate and effortless, but also crude in terms of the physical structure of speech sounds, is the contribution of the Reverse Hierarchy Theory.

References

[1]   Ahissar, M. and Hochstein, S. "Task difficulty and the specificity of perceptual learning." *Nature* 387: 401-406, 1997.
[2]   Allen, J.B. "Harvey Fletcher's role in the creation of communication acoustics." *J. Acoust. Soc. Am.* 99: 1825-1839, 1996.
[3]   Bar-Yosef, O., Rotman, Y. and Nelken, I. "Responses of neurons in cat primary auditory cortex to bird chirps: effects of temporal and spectral context." *J. Neurosci.* 22: 8619-8632, 2002.
[4]   Blauert, J. *Spatial Hearing.* Cambridge, MA: MIT Press, 1997.
[5]   Burns, E.M. and Campbell, S.L. "Frequency and frequency-ratio resolution by possessors of absolute and relative pitch: Examples of categorical perception." *J. Acoust. Soc. Am.* 96: 2704-2719, 1994.

[6] Cariani, P.A. and Delgutte, B. "Neural correlates of the pitch of complex tones. II. Pitch shift, pitch ambiguity, phase invariance, pitch circularity, rate pitch, and the dominance region for pitch." *J. Neurophysiol.* 76: 1717-1734, 1996.

[7] Cariani, P.A. and Delgutte, B. "Neural correlates of the pitch of complex tones. I. Pitch and pitch salience." *J. Neurophysiol.* 76: 1698-1716, 1996.

[8] Chi, T., Gao, Y., Guyton, M.C., Ru, P. and Shamma, S. "Spectro-temporal modulation transfer functions and speech intelligibility." *J. Acoust. Soc. Am.* 106: 2719-2732, 1999.

[9] Ciocca, V. and Darwin, C.J. "Effects of onset asynchrony on pitch perception: Adaptation or grouping?" *J. Acoust. Soc. Am.* 93: 2870-2878, 1993.

[10] Darwin, C.J., Hukin, R.W. and al-Khatib, B.Y. "Grouping in pitch perception: evidence for sequential constraints." *J. Acoust. Soc. Am.* 98: 880-885, 1995.

[11] Depireux, D.A., Simon, J.Z., Klein, D.J. and Shamma, S.A. "Spectro-temporal response field characterization with dynamic ripples in ferret primary auditory cortex." *J. Neurophysiol.* 85: 1220-1234, 2001.

[12] Eggermont, J.J. "Representation of a voice onset time continuum in primary auditory cortex of the cat." *J. Acoust. Soc. Am.* 98: 911-920, 1995.

[13] Eggermont, J.J. "Between sound and perception: Reviewing the search for a neural code." *Hear. Res.* 157: 1-42, 2001.

[14] Ehret, G. and Merzenich, M.M. "Complex sound analysis (frequency resolution, filtering and spectral integration) by single units of the inferior colliculus of the cat." *Brain Res.* 472: 139-163, 1988.

[15] Fodor, J.A. and Pylyshyn, Z.W. "How direct is visual perception?: Some reflections on Gibson's 'Ecological Approach'." *Cognition* 9: 139-196, 1981.

[16] Fowler, C.A. "Listeners do hear sounds, not tongues." *J. Acous. Soc. Am.* 99: 1730-1741, 1996.

[17] Freyman, R.L., Clifton, R.K. and Litovsky, R.Y. "Dynamic processes in the precedence effect." *J. Acoust. Soc. Am.* 90: 874-884, 1991.

[18] Gaskell, H. "The precedence effect." *Hear. Res.* 12: 277-303, 1983.

[19] Hochstein, S. and Ahissar, M. "View from the top: Hierarchies and reverse hierarchies in the visual system." *Neuron* 36: 791-804, 2002.

[20] Holt, L.L. and Kluender, K.R. "General auditory processes contribute to perceptual accommodation of coarticulation." *Phonetica* 57: 170-180, 2000.

[21] Kanwisher, N., McDermott, J. and Chun, M.M. "The fusiform face area: A module in human extrastriate cortex specialized for face perception." *J. Neurosci.* 17: 4302-4311, 1997.

[22] King, A.J., Jiang, Z.D., and Moore, D.R. "Auditory brainstem projections to the ferret superior colliculus: Anatomical contribution to the neural coding of sound azimuth." *J. Comp. Neurol.* 390: 342-365, 1998.

[23] Konishi, M., Takahashi, T.T., Wagner, H., Sullivan, W.E. and Carr, C.E. "Neurophysiological and anatomical substrates of sound localization in the owl." In: *Auditory Function*, G.M. Edelman, W.E. Gall and W.M. Cowan (eds.),New York: Wiley, pp 721-745, 1988.

[24] Kuhl, P.K. "Theoretical contributions of tests on animals to the special-mechanisms debate in speech." *Exp. Biol.* 45: 233-265, 1986.

[25] Liberman, A.M. and Mattingly, I.G. "A specialization for speech perception." *Science* 243: 489-494, 1989.

[26] Litovsky, R.Y., Colburn, H.S., Yost, W.A. and Guzman, S.J. "The precedence effect." *J. Acoust. Soc. Am.* 106: 1633-1654, 1999.

[27] Lotto, A.J., Kluender, K.R. and Holt, L.L. "Perceptual compensation for coarticulation by Japanese quail (Coturnix coturnix japonica)." *J. Acoust. Soc. Am.* 102: 1134-1140, 1997.

[28] Malone, B.J. and Semple, M.N. "Effects of auditory stimulus context on the representation of frequency in the gerbil inferior colliculus." *J. Neurophysiol.* 86: 1113-1130, 2001.

[29] Malone, B.J., Scott, B.H. and Semple, M.N. "Context-dependent adaptive coding of interaural phase disparity in the auditory cortex of awake macaques." *J. Neurosci.* 22: 4625-4638, 2002.

[30] Meredith, M.A. and Clemo, H.R. "Auditory cortical projection from the anterior ectosylvian sulcus (Field AES) to the superior colliculus in the cat: an anatomical and electrophysiological study." *J. Comp. Neurol.* 289: 687-707, 1989.

[31] Middlebrooks, J.C. "Narrow-band sound localization related to external ear acoustics." *J. Acoust. Soc. Am.* 92: 2607-2624, 1992.

[32] Middlebrooks, J.C. and Green, D.M. "Sound localization by human listeners." *Ann. Rev. Psychol.* 42: 135-159, 1991.

[33] Miller, L.M., Escabi, M.A., Read, H.L. and Schreiner, C.E. "Spectrotemporal receptive fields in the lemniscal auditory thalamus and cortex." *J. Neurophysiol.* 87: 516-527, 2002.

[34] Moore, B.C.J. *An Introduction to the Psychology of Hearing* (2nd ed.). London: Academic Press, 1982.

[35] Moore, B.C.J. "Frequency analysis and pitch perception." I: *Human Psychophysics*, W.A. Yost, A.N. Popper and R.R. Fay (eds.), New York: Springer Verlag, pp. 56-115, 1993.

[36] Nelken, I., Rotman, Y. and Bar-Yosef, O. "Responses of auditory-cortex neurons to structural features of natural sounds." *Nature* 397: 154-157, 1999.

[37] Nelken, I., Bizley, J.K., Nodal, F.R., Ahmed, B., Schnupp, J.W. and King, A.J. "Large-scale organization of ferret auditory cortex revealed using continuous acquisition of intrinsic optical signals." *J. Neurophysiol.*, 2004.

[38] Perrett, D.I., Hietanen, J.K., Oram, M.W., Benson, P.J. "Organization and functions of cells responsive to faces in the temporal cortex." *Phil. Trans. Royal Soc. Lond. B Biol. Sci.* 335: 23-30, 1992.

[39] Pickles, J.O. "Normal critical bands in the cat." *Acta Otolaryngol* 80: 245-254, 1975.

[40] Rauschecker, J.P. and Tian, B. "Mechanisms and streams for processing of 'what' and 'where' in auditory cortex." *Proc. Natl. Acad. Sci.* (USA) 97: 11800-11806, 2000.

[41] Rock, I. and Palmer, S. "The legacy of Gestalt psychology." *Sci. Am.* 263: 84-90, 1990.

[42] Rolls, E.T. "Neurophysiological mechanisms underlying face processing within and beyond the temporal cortical visual areas." *Phil. Trans. Royal Soc. Lond. B Biol. Sci.* 335: 11-20, 1992.

[43] Ru, P., Chi, T., and Shamma, S. "The synergy between speech production and perception." *J. Acoust. Soc. Am.* 113: 498-515, 2003.

[44] Schnupp, J.W., Mrsic-Flogel, T.D. and King, A.J. "Linear processing of spatial cues in primary auditory cortex." *Nature* 414: 200-204, 2001.

[45] Schulze, H., Hess, A., Ohl, F.W. and Scheich, H. "Superposition of horseshoe-like periodicity and linear tonotopic maps in auditory cortex of the Mongolian gerbil." *Eur. J. Neurosci.* 15: 1077-1084, 2002.

[46] Spitzer, M.W. and Semple, M.N. "Responses of inferior colliculus neurons to time-varying interaural phase disparity: Effects of shifting the locus of virtual motion." *J. Neurophysiol.* 69: 1245-1263, 1993.

[47] Spitzer, M.W. and Semple, M.N. "Transformation of binaural response properties in the ascending auditory pathway: influence of time-varying interaural phase disparity." *J. Neurophysiol.* 80: 3062-3076, 1998.

[48] Spitzer, M.W., Bala, A.D. and Takahashi, T.T. "Auditory spatial discrimination by barn owls in simulated echoic conditions." *J. Acoust. Soc. Am.* 113: 1631-1645, 2003.

[49] Steinschneider, M., Schroeder, C.E., Arezzo, J.C. and Vaughan, H.G., Jr. "Speech-evoked activity in primary auditory cortex: Effects of voice onset time." *Electroencephalogr. Clin. Neurophysiol.* 92: 30-43, 1994.

[50] Steinschneider, M., Volkov, I.O., Noh, M.D., Garell, P.C. and Howard, M.A. "Temporal encoding of the voice onset time phonetic parameter by field potentials recorded directly from human auditory cortex." *J. Neurophysiol.* 82: 2346-2357, 1999.

[51] Stern, R.M., Zeiberg, A.S. and Trahiotis, C. "Lateralization of complex binaural stimuli: A weighted-image model." *J. Acoust. Soc. Am.* 84: 156-165, 1988. [published erratum appears in *J. Acoust. Soc. Am.* 90: 2202, 1991].

[52] Takahashi, T.T. and Keller, C.H. "Representation of multiple sound sources in the owl's auditory space map." *J. Neurosci.* 14: 4780-4793, 1994.

[53] Theunissen, F.E., Sen, K. and Doupe, A.J. "Spectral-temporal receptive fields of nonlinear auditory neurons obtained using natural sounds." *J. Neurosci.* 20: 2315-2331, 2000.

[54] Ulanovsky, N., Las, L. and Nelken, I. "Processing of low-probability sounds by cortical neurons." *Nat. Neurosci.* 6: 391-398, 2003.

[55] Versnel, H. and Shamma, S.A. "Spectral-ripple representation of steady-state vowels in primary auditory cortex." *J. Acoust. Soc. Am.* 103 :2502-2514, 1998.

[56] Westheimer, G. "Gestalt theory reconfigured: Max Wertheimer's anticipation of recent developments in visual neuroscience." *Perception* 28: 5-15, 1999.

[57] Yost, W.A. and Soderquist, D.R. "The precedence effect: revisited." *J. Acoust. Soc. Am.* 76: 1377-1383, 1984.

[58] Zurek, P.M. "The precedence effect and its possible role in the avoidance of interaural ambiguities." *J. Acoust. Soc. Am.* 67: 953-964, 1980.

[59] Checkik, G., Anderson, M.J., Bar-Yosef, O., Young, E.D., Tishby, N and Nelken, I. "Transformations of stimulus representations in the ascending auditory pathway." *Neuron*, in press.

[60] Las, L., Stern, e.A. and Nelken, I. "Representation of tone in fluctuating maskers in the ascending auditory system." *J. Neurosci.* 25: 1503-1513, 2005.

Dynamics of Speech Production and Perception
P. Divenyi et al. (Eds.)
IOS Press, 2006

Definition of Human Auditory Cortex Territories Based on Anatomical Landmarks and fMRI Activation

Birgit GASCHLER-MARKEFSKI, André BRECHMANN, Gregor Rafael SZYCIK,
Thomas KAULISCH, Frank BAUMGART and Henning SCHEICH
Leibniz-Institute for Neurobiology
Magdeburg, Germany

Abstract. The parcellation of human auditory cortex into functional fields is unclear when using anatomical criteria exclusively. On the basis of comparative anatomical studies of non-human primates, the dorsal plane of the temporal lobe, as well as the lateral aspect of the superior temporal gyrus, should contain a large number of anatomically (and functionally) distinct fields in the human auditory cortex. Functional magnetic resonance imaging (fMRI) can be used to elucidate this issue by delineating the loci of activation in response to various acoustic signals. Because of the large anatomical variability of folds of the human temporal lobe and their variable topographic relation to the rest of the brain, it is difficult to establish the specific identity of such activation foci across individuals. Using a special form of fMRI, in which the acoustic background noise is kept to a minumum, we sought to differentially activate auditory territories on the superior temporal plane using a variety of simple and complex acoustic stimuli presented in the context of controlled auditory tasks. Four distinct areas in human auditory cortex could be distinguished using a combination of structural landmark delineation and differential functional activation.

Keywords. Human auditory cortex, low noise fMRI, anatomical landmarks, functional parcellation

Introduction

The parcellation of the human auditory cortex into functional fields is essentially unclear. Based on comparative evidence from non-human primate auditory cortices a large number of fields are expected on the dorsal plane of the temporal lobe and on the lateral aspect of the superior temporal gyrus. At present the only potential correlates of different auditory cortex fields in fMRI studies are multiple foci of activation which can be observed with various stimulus regimes. But in view of the large gross-anatomical variability of folds of the human temporal lobe and of their variable topographic relation to the rest of the brain it is a major problem to establish the identities of such activation foci across individuals. Using low acoustic noise functional magnetic resonance imaging and several classes of simple and complex acoustic stimuli in combination with controlled auditory tasks we attempted to differentially activate auditory territories on the superior temporal plane. So far, four areas have been distinguished by a structural landmark delineation and differential functional activation.

1. Low-noise MRI Measurement and Acoustical Stimulation

In recent years functional magnetic resonance imaging (fMRI) has become the method of choice to analyze human brain activity. This technique is based on the blood oxygen-level dependent (BOLD) change of signal intensity, the underlying mechanisms of which are still under discussion [44][12][30][15][41]. A series of suitably configured MR-images reveals the amount and concentration of the intrinsic blood contrast-agent deoxyhemoglobin in specific areas of the brain. The analysis of such a time series only yields statistical power if a minimum number of (temporal) sample points are provided. Thus rapid scanning procedures (Echo Planar Imaging, EPI) are used very often in fMRI-experiments. The acoustic noise of MRI-scanners causes severe problems for clinical routine [11][57] and especially for auditory experiments as described in this chapter. Though very efficient in terms of temporal resolution EPI causes severe problems due to its inherent high acoustic noise emission. Even with effective ear protection, scanner noise interference with the acoustic stimuli can not be ruled out. Several strategies have been proposed to minimize the direct interaction of noise and acoustical stimulation [18][28][60]. However, the problem of noise generation still remains and may have several effects in addition to the stressful experience which influences the subjects' attention and autonomous nervous system functions. A different approach to this problem is to directly avoid high noise levels by using different imaging protocols (FLASH) at the expense of slower imaging [22]. The EPI-sequence reaches a noise level of up to 125 dB while FLASH type sequences produces acoustic noise levels of "only" 105 dB on our scanner (Bruker BioSpec 3T/60cm with an asymmetric gradient system (30 mT/m)). In a multi-step procedure we further reduced the background noise by 50 dB to nearly inaudible levels at the expense of slower imaging. The use of a FLASH sequence offers the possibility of slowing down the gradient switching without affecting the image quality. Together with an optimized excitation pulse and modified spoiler gradients this reduced the noise level by >30 dB below 500 Hz. The headphone system and a foam cushion (see below) gave >20 dB suppression of background noise for frequencies above 0.5 kHz and more than 30 dB suppression at 2 kHz. Furthermore, the scanner room is lined with an acoustic wall lining to suppress reverberation. All these measures add up to a "low noise" imaging protocol with a noise peak level of 54 dB SPL at the subject's ear.

Capsules from commercially available headphones were modified by removing their magnets and integrating them into ear muffs [2]. The ear muffs were attached to a foam cushion that is routinely used for immobilizing the subjects head. The pressure holding the muffs against the skin is stronger than with a typical headband, but it is still tolerable to subjects. Close fit, enhanced by the liquid-filled rims of the ear muffs, produces efficient MRI gradient noise suppression for frequencies above 0.5 kHz.

The operating principle is distinct from normal operation but still yields efficient sound radiation with sound pressure levels of up to 115 dB over a wide range of frequencies (0.2kHz-30kHz). The headphone's coils are magnetic dipoles that in normal patient position are oriented perpendicular to the homogenous magnetic field of the scanner and therefore exert a torque, which in turn leads to a partial tilt of the speaker's diaphragm. A stiff diaphragm together with a soft suspension and an asymmetrical current entry to the voice coil ensures a satisfying low frequency response without audible distortions. This set can in principle be connected to the headphone sockets of any commercial audio amplifier without modifications. However, to prevent destructive interactions between the radio-frequency system of the scanner and the audio system some design features like shielded and terminated cables, galvanic separation and a proper grounding to earth are necessary. In extensive tests [2] the phones and their leads have proven compatibility with the MRI-system, i.e. neither interference with the gradient and high-frequency fields nor a disturbance of the static field homogeneity in the volume of interest could be detected.

2. Auditory Cortex Territories Based on Anatomical Landmarks

In animals the functional parcellation of the auditory cortex into multiple distinct fields is largely based on functional gradients (e.g. tonotopic organization) or neuronal response properties (for reviews see [42][58][54][56][45][20][34][50][35]). This type of distinction between fields is not available for the human auditory cortex.

At present, the only potential correlates of different auditory cortex fields in fMRI studies are multiple foci of activation which have been observed with various stimulus regimes. But in view of the large gross-anatomical variability of folds of the human temporal lobe [49][46][39] establishing the identities of such activation foci across individuals is a major problem. It seems possible to achieve this if landmarks can be found which across individuals relate to subdivisions of human auditory cortex and can be identified by anatomical MR imaging.

For an indirect approach to this problem a number of histological schemes of parcellation of the human temporal lobe are available[21][9][47][63][3][4][62][32][7][23][49][52]. In spite of differences in detail among those studies they contain important landmarks concomitant with histological areas. In order to optimally relate such landmarks to fMRI activation patterns it is useful to keep the plane of imaging parallel to the dorsal surface of the temporal lobe on both hemispheres. Then fMRI activations appear as multiple stripes which resemble the stripe-like histological schemes.

The primary area defined by the most stringent definitions of thalamic projections and of koniocortex is always found on first Heschl's gyrus. It covers the anteromedial slope of the gyrus and reaches to a variable degree posteriorly up to or somewhat over the convexity of first Heschl's gyrus. This restriction was noticed by Flechsig [21] and Pfeifer [47] in their studies of the ontogenetic myeloarchitecture at certain stages of development which revealed that the thalamic projection was unaffected by the later developing association systems. A similar topographic definition of the primary area based on cytoarchitectonic features was given by Brodmann [9] who termed it Area 41, by von Economo and Horn [62] who termed it TC1 and by Galaburda and Sanides [23] who termed it KAm. In our fMRI studies we always see a stripe-like, spatially coherent activation which is topographically in accordance with the primary area defined in the above cited studies (for further details see Section 4). Consequently a territory T1 was defined which covers this area (see Fig. 1).

A stripe-like area of less pronounced koniocortex parallel to Heschl's gyrus lies posteriorly adjacent to the extreme manifestation of koniocortex. The anterior border of this cytoarchitectonic area (BA 41/42 border [9], area TC1/TBC border [62], area KAm/ KAlt border [23][33]) was placed by these authors on the convexity or the posterior slope of Heschl's gyrus. This area reaches to a variable degree into the second trans-

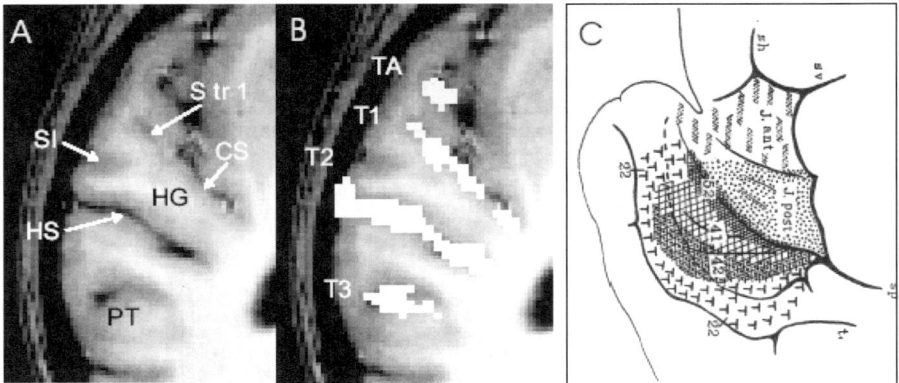

Figure 1. Relationship between activation and anatomical landmarks used for parcellation of auditory cortex. (A) Anatomy of the surface of the right temporal lobe of one subject. Labels indicate landmarks used to divide auditory cortex into different territories. CS Circular sulcus; HG Heschl's gyrus, HS Heschl's sulcus, PT Planum temporale, S tr 1 First transverse sulcus, SI Intermediate sulcus. (B) Patterns of fMRI-activation of the same subject obtained with pure tone stimuli. The stripe-like pattern of activation in T1 follows the rostromedial slope of HG and in T2 it is centered on Heschl's sulcus. These two stripes of activation remained separated from one another. (C) Scheme of auditory Brodmann's areas [9]. BA 41 and BA 42 is located roughly parallel to each other and parallel to Heschl's gyrus, resembling the stripe-like pattern of activation in T1 and T2. The territory TA on the anterior surface of the superior temporal lobe anterior of Heschl's gyrus and the territory T3 on the planum temporale may correspond to the anterior part and the posterior part of BA22, respectively.

verse sulcus (Heschl's sulcus) or reaches over this sulcus on the planum temporale. Using the second transverse sulcus as a center-landmark we defined a territory largely corresponding to the above described anatomical area and termed it T2 [55]. Like T1 it reliably contains stripe-like and largely coherent fMRI activation (see Figure 1) with many types of stimuli.

A functional dissociation of areas presumably corresponding to T1 and T2 has been found in a study of middle latency auditory evoked potentials through intracerebral recording in auditory cortex of humans [40]. The authors suggested that an area referred to as KAm by Galaburda and Sanides [23] is the chief generator of the N30 component and that an area corresponding to KAlt is the chief generator of the P50 component.

An additional area on the anterior surface of the superior temporal lobe anterior of Heschl's gyrus showed distinct fMRI activation with certain stimulus and task regimes [25][55]; (see Figure 1, as well as Sections 4.2 and 4.3) and has been termed TA. It may correspond to the cytoarchitectural area ProA of Galaburda and Sanides [23] and the anterior part of Brodmann area 22 (see Fig. 1).

The large remaining surface of the planum temporale posterior to T2 has been defined as territory T3. It includes the posterior wall of the Sylvian fissure which presumably exhibits the same cytoarchitecture as the most posterior part of the superior temporal lobe (area Tpt) [24][23] and the posterior part of Brodmann area 22 (see Figure 1).

Although we used a "region of interest" approach, thereby taking the interindividual anatomical variability into account, one has to keep in mind that the relationship between histological features and anatomical landmarks is not necessarily constant

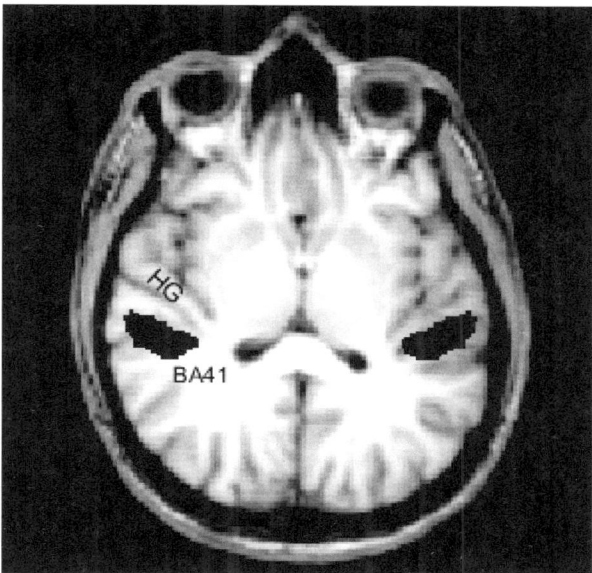

Figure 2. Location of Brodmann's area 41 (BA 41, black). Derived from [59] using the Talairach Deamon
[37] and superimposed on a Talairach transformed individual brain slice in parallel to the superior
temporal plane. Note the posterior displacement of BA 41 in relation to 1st Heschl's gyrus (HG).

across individuals. Presumably, all of the territories defined in these studies may still
contain several functional areas.

3.   Auditory Brodmann Areas in Talairach-Space

As stated in the previous paragraph interindividual variability of the brain-anatomy is a
serious problem for the parcellation of the human auditory cortex. One approach to this
problem which is often used in functional imaging studies is the Talairach transformation [59] in combination with the coordinates of Brodmann areas (BA).

    We tested the reliability of such an approach. The 3D-dataset of the brain of ten sub-
jects was Talairach transformed by using BrainVoyager 2000™. The template of BA 41
(primary auditory cortex) was derived from [59] using the Talairach Deamon [37]. Then
we determined the overlap between the template of BA 41 and the area of Heschl's
gyrus identified in each individual brain. On average 14.6% ± 11.2% of BA 41 was
located on Heschl's gyrus on the left hemisphere and 4.6% ± 4.9% on the right hemisphere. Overall, there was a strong tendency for posterior displacement of BA 41 (Figure 2). Comparing the location of BA 41 and 42 in Talairach space with the original
figure by Brodmann (see Fig. 1C, [9]) a significant mismatch becomes evident: In
Talairach space BA 41 occupies the medial two thirds of Heschl's gyrus and BA 42 the
lateralmost aspect. In Brodmann's figure BA 41 and BA 42 are located roughly parallel
to each other and parallel to Heschl's gyrus, resembling our definition of T1 and T2 (see
Fig. 1B and 1C).

    These results show that using the Talairach coordinates of the Brodmann areas to

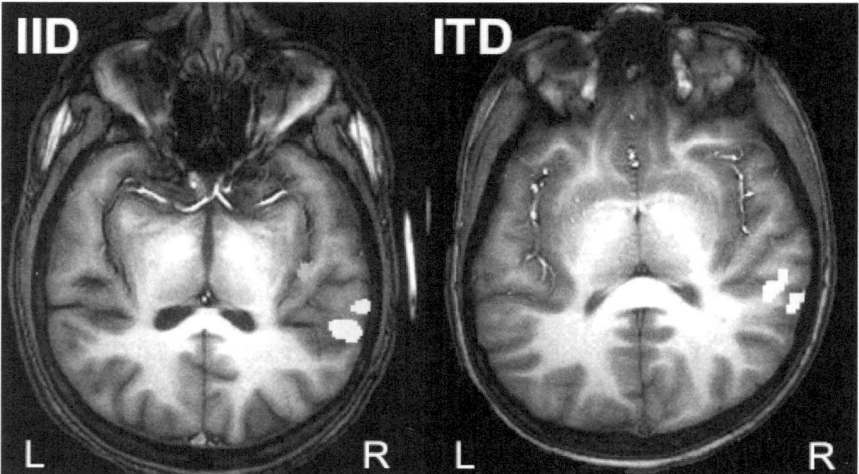

Figure 3. Parameter-independence of movement-sensitive fMRI activation in human auditory cortex. The activations in the white areas in the right planum temporale in two subjects were obtained during perceived motion of an auditory object generated by interaural phase shifts of envelopes of an amplitude-modulated sound (interaural intensity difference, IID, left panel), or by changing interaural onset delays of a pure tone (interaural time difference, ITD, right panel), respectively.

describe the location of fMRI activation in auditory cortex is misleading. In contrast, reliable landmarks (Heschl's gyrus and 1st Heschl's sulcus) allow to match the spatial fMRI patterns to individual anatomical variations, which we described in the previous paragraph.

4.   Auditory Cortex Areas Based on Acoustical fMRI Experiments

In the following paragraph four recent findings of differential fMRI activation in the human auditory cortex are described. The direct interaction of noise and acoustical stimulation was minimized by the low noise MRI measurement (see Section 1). Using several classes of simple and complex acoustic stimuli in combination with controlled auditory tasks, we attempted to differentially activate auditory territories on the superior temporal plane.

4.1 A motion-sensitive map in auditory cortex

A small area on the lateral planum temporale, dominantly or sometimes exclusively activated on the right side, was identified in recent fMRI studies using motion percepts generated by time-variant interaural cues through headphones [1]. One motion cue is a changing interaural level relationship of stimuli (interaural intensity difference, IID). In this case a slow amplitude modulation of a carrier sound was generated which in the case of the control stimulus had the same phase of the modulation cycle at both ears. This sound was not perceived as having any specific location in space. Conversely, if amplitude-phase cycles of the identical stimuli were slowly shifted interaurally the percept was that of a sound source slowly moving back and forth in azimuth.

With fMRI these two stimuli generated very strong and spatially similar activations in primary and non-primary areas of auditory cortex. The subtraction of the two activation patterns, however, yielded a reliable signal intensity increase with the motion stimulus laterally on the right planum temporale (Fig. 3, left panel). Interestingly, a very similar activation increase was obtained with a different interaural cue and a different type of carrier stimulus (Fig. 3, right panel). These were short tone bursts of constant frequency presented with simultaneous onset at the two ears (control) or with successively changing onset between the two ears (motion). The latter contains interaural time differences (ITD) as a motion cue. While the control condition did not generate any location percept of the sound source the ITD cue led to the percept of small azimuthal jumps of source location.

The similarity of the spatial location of signal increase for IID and ITD cues in the right planum temporale is relevant for assumed hemispheric specializations for extracorporeal space analysis by the right hemisphere. Obviously not only visual space cue analysis and multimodal space cue processing is lateralized to the right hemisphere [6][5] but also auditory space cue analysis. Whether this relates in any way to a proposed "dorsal stream" of auditory space analysis in the auditory cortex [53] remains to be determined.

The immediate relevance to the present subject is that the motion-selective area in right auditory cortex is neither stimulus specific nor motion-cue-specific, and thus does not fulfill the criteria of an area specialized for specific acoustic features in a bottom-up concept. Rather, the generation of explicit motion percepts seems to be the common denominator. This is further underlined by fMRI experiments using a third motion cue, namely head-related transfer functions using a moving sound source (obtained by a twin microphone array in an artificial human head), which generates a vivid space percept of movement all around the head. In this case the motion area on the planum temporal is even more strongly activated, but on both sides, and with a dominant activation on the right side (unpublished).

4.2 Foreground-background decomposition

In further low-noise fMRI studies on the human auditory cortex [55] a mechanism which may relate to the "Cocktail-Party-Effect" [13] was analyzed. While Cherry [13] assumed the effect to be a sound localization problem, it is now clear that several other acoustic cues can be used to solve such a problem [65][64]. Some lines of experiments have led to the concept that an anterior area on the superior surface of the temporal lobe, anterior to Heschl's gyrus, may be an area of central importance in foreground-background decomposition. Several mechanisms relevant in this context may converge in this area, previously named territory TA [55] (see also Sections 2 and 3).

The experiment addressed the question of how, in a series of complex tones (notes of different musical instruments), matching pairs (instrument and note identical) are identified in the presence of a continuous background. This background consisted of a loud saw tooth frequency modulation of a tone which masked the fundamental and lower harmonic frequencies of the instrument notes. This constellation is a simplified version of the task that a conductor has while monitoring different instruments in an orchestra.

In version I of the experiment the total effect of instrument notes, background and discrimination task was determined in auditory cortex as referred to interval periods without any stimulation. This revealed strong bilateral activation in all previously known primary and non-primary subdivisions of auditory cortex (territories TA, T1, T2, T3, see also Sections 2 and 3).

Version II of the experiment served to isolate the effect of the foreground-dependent task. The described situation was the same as version I but the background alone continued though the reference periods. The FM background was calibrated to maximally activate primary-like areas in auditory cortex. Consequently, by referring foreground plus background to the background alone it was expected that much of the primary-like activation in auditory cortex would cancel out. This was indeed the case. Of the original activation determined in version I merely the activity in the anterior area TA was maintained in version II and was not significantly different. This suggests that in contrast to the other areas the background alone had very little direct influence on TA and did not appreciably influence the effect of the foreground task in this area.

4.3 Retrieval of encoded instrument or melody

Not distinguished in the experiment described above was the possibility that TA contained additional specializations for auditory tonal matching-to-sample tasks or more generally speaking for tasks involving tone sequence - (melody) perception [17][66].

The issue of tone sequence processing in the auditory cortex has been tackled in the awake monkey auditory cortex with single unit recordings [31][61][26][27] and with bilateral ablation experiments [43]. Specific unit responses related to a delayed matching-to-sample task were preferentially found in belt areas around the primary auditory cortex. Conversely ablation impaired the performance in such tasks when belt areas were included. A recent study in the monkey cortex has more specifically searched for mechanisms which permit the temporal integration of sequences of different tones [10]. Forward and backward interactions between the responses to consecutive tones were found which were different from masking effects seen over short intervals.

A recent fMRI study [25] addresses this issue with respect to learning using a melody retrieval task. Arbitrary four note sequences (melodies) played by different instruments were encoded keeping either the melody or the instrument constant. In the consecutive retrieval period various melody-instrument-combinations were presented and the task was either to retrieve the encoded instrument (control-task) or the encoded melody (melody-task).

As a result the right territory TA (definition see also Section 2) showed significantly larger activation during the (tone-) sequence retrieval condition than during the target instrument detection task with the same acoustic material.

The retrieval experiment used a short term memory task (retrieval over seconds) and the melody retrieval requires recognition of a "temporal Gestalt". Therefore it may be assumed that memory-guided processing in TA is of a more general type related to sequential analysis applying to both. In this context it should be noted that true sequential analysis per definition requires at least a short term memory process.

It could be argued that TA activation could be explained mainly by differential involvement of filters specialized for stimulus properties. Melody retrieval as well as instrument retrieval used melodies as common stimulus aspect. Thus the difference of TA activation between the two tasks may not be due to the stimulus material but rather to the selectively memory guided type of processing that is performed in TA on the given stimulus material. This is a "top down" characteristic that has also been attributed to the late auditory evoked potentials (AEP) such as the N400 wave which are sometimes called endogenous responses [36]. Late AEP are typically found to extend from the region of primary AC anteriorly or posteriorly over the cortex.

The retrieval experiment extends the previous characterization of a secondary human auditory cortex field as being involved in auditory foreground-background decomposition [55] (see paragraph FOREGROUND-BACKGROUND DECOMPOSITION). The specificity of TA activity was demonstrated with respect to the decomposition, i.e. the separation of the two simultaneous sound patterns. The analysis of the retrieval experiments also attributes specificity to TA with respect to the sequential listening aspect which is characteristic of the Cocktail Party effect. Thus it is not unlikely that TA contains mechanisms which relate to various components of selective listening capabilities under jamming conditions which are biologically of fundamental importance.

4.4 Sound level dependency of auditory territories

The relationship between acoustic stimulus level and blood-oxygen-level-dependent (BOLD) response in the auditory cortex is of considerable interest for at least two reasons. First, different auditory fields could potentially differ in BOLD response to varying sound levels of acoustic stimuli. Generally, an increase in sound pressure level (SPL) of pure tones above threshold leads to monotonically increasing response rates and to a larger recruitment of primary and secondary auditory cortex neurons as described in animals. Second, ambient scanner noise is a confounding factor in fMRI investigations of the auditory cortex because it leads to a constant, considerable increase in baseline activity.

Sound level dependent activation of the four human auditory territories was studied using a very low noise functional MR imaging sequence (48dB SPL peak) and frequency modulated tones of 5 stimulus levels (36dB to 102dB) in combination with a pure tone detection task [8]. By using a simple pure tone detection paradigm and introducing the very low sound level of 36 dB (12 dB below the scanner noise) this task implies a simplified cocktail-party problem. With this we addressed the question of how the pattern of activation in the auditory cortex changes with intelligibility of presented stimuli.

Activation of territory T1 showed the most robust level-dependence both in terms of activated volume and BOLD signal intensity. T2 also showed a good correlation of level with activated volume, but in contrast to T1, not with BOLD signal intensity. These findings are compatible with level coding mechanisms observed in animal AC [48][51] and demonstrate that, based on level-dependent activation, T1 and T2 can be distinguished.

A systematic increase of activation with level was not observed for TA and T3 on planum temporale. Thus these areas might not be specifically involved in processing the overall intensity of frequency modulated tones.

The territory TA showed little activation and no level dependence for intermediate and high levels of stimuli. But TA of the left hemisphere exhibited its highest activation when the FM sound-level fell 12 dB below scanner noise. This supports the previously suggested special involvement of this territory in foreground-background decomposition tasks.

5. Conclusion

The above described studies demonstrate the suitability of using low noise fMRI in combination with the differentiation of auditory areas on the basis of functional knowledge. This chapter summarizes experimental evidence from the human auditory cortex that at least four auditory territories (TA, T1, T2, and T3) can be distinguished. These findings are based on a structural landmark delineation and differential functional activation on the superior plane of the temporal lobe in individual brains. This parcellation can be further differentiated by lateralization of functions even with non-speech sounds. Patterns of fMRI activation comparable to our functional parcellation of the auditory cortex have also been shown in studies of other laboratories examining cortical responses to speech sounds [14][29], to pulsed 1000 Hz sine tones [16] or dynamic ripples [38].

6. The Future

The number of auditory cortex fields in humans is not known but studies on monkeys suggest at least 15 functional fields [35]. Thus, the present parcellation of human auditory cortex described above has to be refined. As there are no further reliable anatomical landmarks the clusters of fMRI activation seen in each individual brain have to be characterized functionally. This is a major problem because, as recently stated by Eggermont [19], the similarities of neuronal response properties of auditory cortex fields outweigh the differences. Thus, the differences between fMRI activation of such functional fields will be rather small. Therefore, it is necessary to develop new paradigms with which distinct clusters of activation can be distinguished in each individual brain to establish identity of such areas across subjects.

References

[1] Baumgart, F., Gaschler-Markefski, B., Woldorff, M.G., Heinze, H.-J. and Scheich, H. "A movement-sensitive area in auditory cortex." *Nature* 400: 724-726, 1999.
[2] Baumgart, F., Kaulisch, T., Tempelmann, C., Gaschler-Markefski, B., Tegeler, C., Schindler, F., Stiller, D., and Scheich, H. "Electrodynamic headphones and woofers for application in magnetic resonance imaging scanners." *Med Phys* 25: 2068-2070, 1998.
[3] Beck, E. "Die myeloarchitektonische Felderung des in der sylvischen Furche gelegenen Teils des menschlichen Schläfenlappens," *J. Psychol. Neurol. Leipzig* 36: 1-21, 1928.
[4] Beck, E. "Die Myeloarchitektonik der dorsalen Schläfenlappenrinde beim Menschen." *J. Psychol. Neurol. Leipzig* 41: 129-262, 1930.
[5] Bisiach, E. and Berti, A. "Consciousness and dyschiria." In *The Cognitive Neurosciences*, M.S. Gazzaniga(ed.), Cambridge, MA: MIT Press, 1997.
[6] Bisiach, E. and Vallar, G. "Hemineglect in humans." In *Handbook of Neurophysiology*, Vol. 1, F. Boller and J. Grafman (eds.) Amsterdam: Elesevier, 1988.
[7] Braak, H. "The pigment architecture of the human temporal lobe." *Anat. Embryol.* 154: 213-240, 1978.
[8] Brechmann, A., Baumgart, F. and Scheich, H. "Sound-level-dependent representation of frequency modulations in human auditory cortex: a low-noise fMRI study." *J. Neurophysiol.* 87: 423-433, 2002.

[9] Brodmann, K. *Vergleichende Lokalisationslehre der Großhirnrinde.* Leipzig: Johann Ambrosius Barth, 1909.

[10] Brosch, M., Schulz, A., and Scheich, H. "Neuronal mechanisms of auditory backward recognition masking in macaque auditory cortex," *Neuroreport* 9: 2551-2555, 1998.

[11] Brummett, R.E., Talbot, J.M., and Charuhas, P. "Potential hearing loss resulting from MR imaging," *Radiology* 169: 539-540, 1988.

[12] Buxton, R.B., Wong, E.C., and Frank, L.R. "Dynamics of blood flow and oxygenation changes during brain activation: the balloon model," *Magn Reson Med* 39: 855-864, 1998.

[13] Cherry, E.C. "Some experiments on the recognition of speech, with one and with two ears," *J. Acous. Soc. Am.* 25: 975-979, 1953.

[14] Dhankhar, A., Wexler, B.E., Fulbright, R.K., Halwes, T., Blamire, A.M., and Shulman, R.G. "Functional magnetic resonance imaging assessment of the human brain auditory cortex response to increasing word presentation rates," *J Neurophysiol* 77: 476-483, 1997.

[15] Di Salle, F., Formisano, E., Linden, D.E., Goebel, R., Bonavita, S., Pepino, A., Smaltino, F., and Tedeschi, G. "Exploring brain function with magnetic resonance imaging," *Eur J Radiol* 30: 84-94, 1999.

[16] Di Salle, F., Formisano, E., Seifritz, E., Linden, D.E., Scheffler, K., Saulino, C., Tedeschi, G., Zanella, F. E., Pepino, A., Goebel, R., and Marciano, E. "Functional fields in human auditory cortex revealed by time-resolved fMRI without interference of EPI noise," *Neuroimage* 13: 328-338, 2001.

[17] Dowling, W.J. and Harwood, D.L. *Music Cognition* (Academic Press, Orlando), 1986.

[18] Edmister, W.B., Talavage, T.M., Ledden, P.J. and Weisskoff, R.M. "Improved auditory cortex imaging using clustered volume acquisitions." *Hum. Brain Mapping* 7: 89-97, 1999.

[19] Eggermont, J.J. "Representation of spectral and temporal sound features in three cortical fields of the cat. Similarities outweigh differences." *J. Neurophysiol.* 80: 2743-2764, 1989.

[20] Ehret, G. "The auditory cortex." *J. Comp. Physiol.* [A] 181: 547-557, 1998.

[21] Flechsig, P. "Bemerkungen über die Hörsphäre des menschlichen Gehirns," *Neurol. Zentralbl.* 27: 2-7, 50-57, 1908.

[22] Frahm, J., Merboldt, K.D., Hanicke, W., Kleinschmidt, A. and Boecker, H. "Brain or vein-oxygenation or flow? On signal physiology in functional MRI of human brain activation," *NMR Biomed.* 7: 45-53, 1994.

[23] Galaburda, A.M. and Sanides, F. "Cytoarchitectonic organization of the human auditory cortex," *J. Comp. Neurol.* 190: 597-610, 1980.

[24] Galaburda, A.M., Sanides, F. and Geschwind, N. "Human brain: Cytoarchitectonic left-right asymmetries in the temporal speech region," *Arch. Neurol.* 35: 812-817, 1978.

[25] Gaschler-Markefski, B., Baumgart, F., Tempelmann, C., Woldorff, M.G. and Scheich, H. "Activation of human auditory cortex in retrieval experiments: an fMRI study," *Neural Plast.* 6: 69-75, 1998.

[26] Gilat, E. and Perlman, I. "Single unit activity in the auditory cortex and the medial geniculate body of the rhesus monkey: Behavioral modulation." *Brain Res.* 324: 323-333, 1984.

[27] Gottlieb, Y., Vaadia, E. and Abeles, M. "Single unit activity in the auditory cortex of a monkey performing a short term memory task." *Exp. Brain Res.* 74: 139-148, 1989.

[28] Hall, D.A., Haggard, M.P., Akeroyd, M.A., Palmer, A.R., Summerfield, A.Q., Elliott, M.R., Gurney, E.M. and Bowtell, R.W. "'Sparse' temporal sampling in auditory fMRI," *Hum. Brain Mapping* 7: 213-223, 1999.

[29] Hashimoto, R., Homae, F., Nakajima, K., Miyashita, Y. and Sakai, K.L. "Functional differentiation in the human auditory and language areas revealed by a dichotic listening task." *Neuroimage* 12: 147-158, 2000.

[30] Hess, A., Lohmann, K., Gundelfinger, E.D. and Scheich, H. "A new method for reliable and efficient reconstruction of 3-dimensional images from autoradiographs of brain sections." *J. Neurosci. Methods* 84: 77-86, 1998.

[31] Hochermann, S., Benson, D.A., Goldstein, M.H.J., Heffner, H.E. and Hienz, R.D. "Evoked unit activity in auditory cortex of monkeys performing a selective attention task." *Brain Res.* 117: 51-68, 1976.

[32] Hopf, A. "Die Myeloarchitektonik des Isocortex temporalis beim Menschen." *J. Hirnforsch.* 1: 208-279, 1954.

[33] Hutsler, J.J. and Gazzaniga, M.S. "Acetylcholinesterase staining in human auditory and language cortices: regional variation of structural features." *Cereb Cortex* 6: 260-270, 1996.

[34] Kaas, J.H. and Hackett, T.A. "Subdivisions of auditory cortex and levels of processing in primates." *Audiol. Neurootol.* 3: 73-85, 1998.

[35] Kaas, J.H., Hackett, T.A. and Tramo, M.J. "Auditory processing in primate cerebral cortex." Curr. Opin. Neurobiol. 9: 164-170, 1999.
[36] Kraus, N. and McGee, T. "Electrophysiology of the human auditory system." In The Mammalian Auditory Pathway: Neurophysiology, A.N. Popper and R.R. Fay (eds.), New York: Springer Verlag, 1992.
[37] Lancaster, J.L., Woldorff, M.G., Parsons, L.M., Liotti, M., Freitas, C.S., Rainey, L., Kochunov, P.V., Nickerson, D., Mikiten, S.A. and Fox, P.T. "Automated Talairach atlas labels for functional brain mapping." Hum. Brain Mapping 10: 120-131, 2000.
[38] Langers, D.R., Backes, W.H. and van Dijk, P. "Spectrotemporal features of the auditory cortex: the activation in response to dynamic ripples." Neuroimage 20: 265-275, 2003.
[39] Leonard, C.M., Puranik, C., Kuldau, J.M. and Lombardino, L.J. "Normal variation in the frequency and location of human auditory cortex landmarks. Heschl's gyrus: Where is it?," Cereb. Cortex 8: 397-406, 1998.
[40] Liegeois-Chauvel, C., Musolino, A., Badier, J.M., Marquis, P. and Chauvel, P. "Evoked potentials recorded from the auditory cortex in man: Evaluation and topography of the middle latency components." Electroencephalogr. Clin. Neurophysiol. 92: 204-214, 1994.
[41] Matthews, P.M., Jezzard, P. and Evans, A.C. Methods for Neuroscience. Oxford: Oxford University Press, 2000.
[42] Merzenich, M.M., Roth, G.L., Andersen, R.A., Knight, P.L. and Colwell, S.A. "Some basic features of organization of the central auditory system." In Psychophysics and Physiology of Hearing, E.F. Evans and J.P. Wilson (eds.), London: Academic Press, 1977.
[43] Neff, W.D., Diamond, I.T. and Casseday, J.H. "Behavioral studies of auditory discrimination: central nervous system." In Handbook of Sensory Physiology, Vol. V/2, W.D. Keidel and W.D. Neff (eds.), Berlin: Springer Verlag, 1975.
[44] Ogawa, S., Tank, D.W., Menon, R., Ellermann, J.M., Kim, S.G., Merkle, H. and Ugurbil, K. "Intrinsic signal changes accompanying sensory stimulation: functional brain mapping with magnetic resonance imaging." Proc. Natl. Acad. Sci. (USA) 89: 5951-5955, 1992.
[45] Pandya, D.N. "Anatomy of the auditory cortex." Rev. Neurol. (Paris) 151: 486-494, 1995.
[46] Penhune, V.B., Zatorre, R.J., MacDonald, J.D. and Evans, A.C. "Interhemispheric anatomical differences in human primary auditory cortex: probabilistic mapping and volume measurement from magnetic resonance scans." Cereb. Cortex 6: 661-672, 1996.
[47] Pfeifer, R.A. "Myelogenetisch-anatomische Untersuchungen über das kortikale Ende der Hörleitung," Abh Math-Physik Kl sächs Akad Wiss Leipzig 37: 1-54, 1920.
[48] Phillips, D.P. and Orman, S.S. "Responses of single neurons in posterior field of cat auditory cortex to tonal stimuli," J Neurophysiol 51: 147-163, 1984.
[49] Rademacher, J., Caviness, V.S., Jr., Steinmetz, H., and Galaburda, A.M. "Topographical variation of the human primary cortices: implications for neuroimaging, brain mapping, and neurobiology," Cereb Cortex 3: 313-329, 1993.
[50] Rauschecker, J.P. "Cortical processing of complex sounds," Curr Opin Neurobiol 8: 516-521, 1998.
[51] Recanzone, G.H., Guard, D.C., and Phan, M.L. "Frequency and intensity response properties of single neurons in the auditory cortex of the behaving macaque monkey," J Neurophysiol 83: 2315-2331, 2000.
[52] Rivier, F. and Clarke, S. "Cytochrome oxidase, acetylcholinesterase, and NADPH-diaphorase staining in human supratemporal and insular cortex: Evidence for multiple auditory areas," Neuroimage 6: 288-304, 1997.
[53] Romanski, L.M., Tian, B., Fritz, J., Mishkin, M., Goldman-Rakic, P.S., and Rauschecker, J.P. "Dual streams of auditory afferents target multiple domains in the primate prefrontal cortex," Nat Neurosci 2: 1131-1136, 1999
[54] Scheich, H. "Auditory cortex: comparative aspects of maps and plasticity," Curr Opin Neurobiol 1: 236-247, 1991.
[55] Scheich, H., Baumgart, F., Gaschler-Markefski, B., Tegeler, C., Tempelmann, C., Heinze, H.J., Schindler, F., and Stiller, D. "Functional magnetic resonance imaging of a human auditory cortex area involved in foreground-background decomposition," Eur J Neurosci 10: 803-809, 1998.
[56] Schreiner, C.E. "Functional organization of the auditory cortex: maps and mechanisms," Curr Opin Neurobiol 2: 516-521, 1992.
[57] Sellers, M.B., Pavlidis, J.D., and Carlberger, T. "MRI acoustic noise," Int. J. Neuroradiol. 2: 549-560, 1996.

[58] Suga, N. "Cortical computational maps for auditory imaging," *Neural Networks* 3: 3-21, 1990.

[59] Talairach, J. and Tournoux, P. *Co-Planar Stereotaxic Atlas of the Human Brain* (Thieme, Stuttgart), 1988.

[60] Talavage, T.M., Edmister, W.B., Ledden, P.J. and Weisskoff, R.M. "Quantitative assessment of auditory cortex responses induced by imager acoustic noise," *Hum Brain Mapp* 7: 79-88, 1999.

[61] Vaadia, E., Gottlieb, Y., and Abeles, M. "Single-unit activity related to sensorimotor association in auditory cortex of a monkey," *J Neurophysiol* 48: 1201-1213, 1982.

[62] von Economo, C. and Horn, L. "Über Windungsrelief, Maße und Rindenarchitektonik der Supratemporalfläche, ihre individuellen und ihre Seitenunterschiede," *Z Neurol Psychiat* 130: 678-757, 1930.

[63] von Economo, C. and Koskinas, G.H. *Die Cytoarchitektonik der Hirnrinde des Erwachsenen Menschen* (Springer, Wien), 1925.

[64] Yost, W.A., Dye, R.H., Jr., and Sheft, S. "A simulated 'cocktail party' with up to three sound sources," *Percept Psychophys* 58: 1026-1036, 1996.

[65] Yost, W.A. and Sheft, S. "Auditory perception," in *Human Psychophysics*, edited by W.A. Yost, A.N. Popper and R.R. Fay (Springer, New York), 1993.

[66] Zatorre, R.J., Evans, A.C., and Meyer, E. "Neural mechanisms underlying melodic perception and memory for pitch,"*J Neurosci* 14: 1908-1919, 1994.

Dynamics of Speech Production and Perception
P. Divenyi et al. (Eds.)
IOS Press, 2006
© *2006 IOS Press. All rights reserved.*

Author Index